T0259079

Impact of Oral Health on Interprofessional Collaborative Practice

Editors

LINDA M. KASTE
LESLIE R. HALPERN

DENTAL CLINICS OF NORTH AMERICA

www.dental.theclinics.com

October 2016 • Volume 60 • Number 4

ELSEVIER

1600 John F. Kennedy Boulevard • Suite 1800 • Philadelphia, Pennsylvania, 19103-2899

http://www.dental.theclinics.com

DENTAL CLINICS OF NORTH AMERICA Volume 60, Number 4
October 2016 ISSN 0011-8532, ISBN: 978-0-323-46306-5

Editor: John Vassallo; j.vassallo@elsevier.com
Developmental Editor: Kristen Helm

Dental Clinics of North America (ISSN 0011-8532) is published quarterly by Elsevier Inc., 360 Park Avenue South, New York, NY 10010-1710. Months of issue are January, April, July, and October. Business and Editorial Offices: 1600 John F. Kennedy Boulevard, Suite 1800, Philadelphia, PA 19103-2899. Periodicals postage paid at New York, NY and additional mailing offices. Subscription prices are $280.00 per year (domestic individuals), $537.00 per year (domestic institutions), $100.00 per year (domestic students/residents), $340.00 per year (Canadian individuals), $695.00 per year (Canadian institutions), $410.00 per year (international individuals), $695.00 per year (international institutions), and $200.00 per year (international and Canadian students/residents). International air speed delivery is included in all *Clinics* subscription prices. All prices are subject to change without notice. **POSTMASTER:** Send address changes to *Dental Clinics of North America*, Elsevier Health Sciences Division, Subscription Customer Service, 3251 Riverport Lane, Maryland Heights, MO 63043. **Customer Service (orders, claims, online, change of address): Elsevier Health Sciences Division, Subscription Customer Service, 3251 Riverport Lane, Maryland Heights, MO 63043. Tel: 1-800-654-2452 (U.S. and Canada). Fax: 314-447-8029. E-mail: journalscustomer service-usa@elsevier.com (for print support); journalsonlinesupport-usa@elsevier.com (for online support)**.

Reprints. For copies of 100 or more, of articles in this publication, please contact the Commercial Reprints Department, Elsevier Inc., 360 Park Avenue South, New York, NY 10010-1710. Tel.: 212-633-3874; Fax: 212-633-3820; E-mail: reprints@elsevier.com.

The *Dental Clinics of North America* is covered in *MEDLINE/PubMed (Index Medicus), Current Contents/Clinical Medicine, ISI/BIOMED* and *Clinahl*.

Contributors

EDITORS

LINDA M. KASTE, DDS, MS, PhD
Diplomate, American Board of Dental Public Health; Professor, Department of Pediatric Dentistry, College of Dentistry, University of Illinois at Chicago, Chicago, Illinois

LESLIE R. HALPERN, MD, DDS, PhD, MPH
Associate Professor; Program Director, Department of Oral and Maxillofacial Surgery, Meharry Medical College, School of Dentistry, Nashville, Tennessee

AUTHORS

PAUL ARNSTEIN, RN, PhD, FNP-C, ACNS-BC
Adjunct Associate Professor, Nurse Practitioner Program, MGH Institute for Health Professionals; Clinical Nurse Specialist for Pain Relief, Massachusetts General Hospital, Boston, Massachusetts

ANTJE M. BARREVELD, MD
Assistant Professor, Department of Anesthesiology, Newton-Wellesley Hospital, Tufts University Medical School, Newton, Massachusetts; Department of Anesthesiology, Perioperative and Pain Medicine; Clinical Researcher, Brigham and Women's Hospital, Harvard Medical School, Boston, Massachusetts

HELENE BEDNARSH, BS, RDH, MPH
HASD/HIV Dental Program, Boston Public Health Commission, Boston, Massachusetts

BLASE P. BROWN, DDS, MS
Clinical Assistant Professor, Department of Oral Medicine and Diagnostic Services, College of Dentistry, University of Illinois at Chicago, Darien, Illinois

JOSEPH M. CALABRESE, DMD
Clinical Associate Professor; Assistant Dean of Students and Director of Geriatric Dental Medicine, Boston University Henry M. Goldman School of Dental Medicine; Director of Geriatric Dental Medicine, Boston Medical Center; Director of Dental Medicine, Hebrew Senior Life; Instructor, Harvard School of Dental Medicine, Boston, Massachusetts

MICHAEL D. COLVARD, DDS, PhD, MTS, MS
Director; Professor, Department of Oral Medicine and Diagnostic Sciences, Dental Medicine Responder Training Office, College of Dentistry, University of Illinois at Chicago, Chicago, Illinois

ROBERT BRUCE DONOFF, DMD, MD
Professor of Oral and Maxillofacial Surgery; Dean, Department of Oral and Maxillofacial Surgery, Harvard School of Dental Medicine, Boston, Massachusetts

CHERAE FARMER-DIXON, DDS, MSPH
Professor; Dean, Meharry Medical College, School of Dentistry, Nashville, Tennessee

CHRISTOPHER H. FOX, DMD, DMSc
Executive Director, International Association for Dental Research, Alexandria, Virginia

PAUL GLASSMAN, DDS, MA, MBA
Professor of Dental Practice; Director of the Pacific Center for Special Care, Arthur A. Dugoni School of Dentistry, University of the Pacific, San Francisco, California

SARA C. GORDON, DDS, MS, FRCD (Canada), FDSRCS (Edinburgh)
Professor of Oral Medicine; Associate Dean of Academic Affairs, Department of Oral Medicine, University of Washington, School of Dentistry, Seattle, Washington

LESLIE R. HALPERN, MD, DDS, PhD, MPH
Associate Professor; Program Director, Department of Oral and Maxillofacial Surgery, Meharry Medical College, School of Dentistry, Nashville, Tennessee

MAUREEN HARRINGTON, MPH
PhD Candidate; Director of Grant Operations and Community Education, Pacific Center for Special Care, Arthur A. Dugoni School of Dentistry, University of the Pacific, San Francisco, California

THOMAS C. HART, DDS, PhD
Volpe Research Center, Gaithersburg, Maryland

MICHELLE M. HENSHAW, DDS, MPH
Professor, Department of Health Policy and Health Services Research; Associate Dean of Global and Population Health, Boston University Henry M. Goldman School of Dental Medicine, Boston, Massachusetts

JEREMY L. HIRST, MS, MBA
Deputy Director, DuPage County, Office of Homeland Security and Emergency Management, Wheaton, Illinois

JAMES JAMES, MD, DrPH, MHA
Executive Director, Society for Disaster Medicine & Public Health, Rockville, Maryland

CAPT RENÉE W. JOSKOW, DDS, MPH, FAGD, FACD
US Public Health Service, Health Resources and Services Administration, Rockville, Maryland

LINDA M. KASTE, DDS, MS, PhD
Diplomate, American Board of Dental Public Health; Professor, Department of Pediatric Dentistry, College of Dentistry, University of Illinois at Chicago, Chicago, Illlinois

LAURA B. KAUFMAN, DMD
Clinical Assistant Professor, Department of General Dentistry, Boston University Henry M. Goldman School of Dental Medicine; Section of Geriatrics, Boston University School of Medicine, Boston, Massachusetts

RONALD J. KULICH, PhD, MS
Professor, Tufts University School of Dental Medicine; Lecturer, Department of Anesthesia, Critical Care and Pain Medicine, Massachusetts General Hospital, Harvard Medical School, Boston, Massachusetts

KATHY M. LITURI, RDH, MPH
Clinical Instructor and Oral Health Promotion Director, Boston University Henry M. Goldman School of Dental Medicine, Boston, Massachusetts

STEPHANIE McCLURE, MD, FACP
Professor; Vice Dean, Meharry Medical College, School of Medicine, Nashville, Tennessee

DANIEL M. MEYER, DDS
Chief Science Officer, American Dental Association, Chicago, Illinois

FREDERICK MORE, DDS, MS
Professor, Department of Epidemiology & Health Promotion, NYU College of Dentistry, New York, New York

CHARLES P. MOUTON, MD, MS
Professor, Department of Family and Community Medicine, Meharry Medical College, School of Medicine, Nashville, Tennessee

MAYSA NAMAKIAN, MPH
Program Manager, Pacific Center for Special Care, Arthur A. Dugoni School of Dentistry, University of the Pacific, San Francisco, California

DAVID E. PETERS, JD
Senior Director of Police Services; Commander of Support Services; UIC Police Department, University of Illinois at Chicago, Chicago, Illinois

POUL ERIK PETERSEN, DDS, Dr Odont, MSc (Sociology)
Professor, University of Copenhagen Faculty of Health Sciences, School of Dentistry, Copenhangen K, Denmark

DEBRA S. REGIER, MD, PhD
Genetics and Metabolism, Children's National Health System, Washington, DC

STEFANIE RUSSELL, DDS, MPH, PhD
Associate Clinical Professor, Department of Epidemiology & Health Promotion, NYU College of Dentistry, New York, New York

JEFFRY SHAEFER, DDS, MS, MPH
Assistant Professor, Department of Oral and Maxillofacial Surgery, Harvard School of Dental Medicine, Hingham, Massachusetts

JANET H. SOUTHERLAND, DDS, MPH, PhD
Professor, Department of Oral and Maxillofacial Surgery, Meharry Medical College, School of Dentistry, Nashville, Tennessee

PAUL SUBAR, DDS, EdD
Associate Professor of Dental Practice; Director, Special Care Clinic, Arthur A. Dugoni School of Dentistry, University of the Pacific, San Francisco, California

MACHELLE FLEMING THOMPSON, RDH, MSPH
Associate Professor; Assistant Dean, Clinical Affairs, Meharry Medical College, School of Dentistry, Nashville, Tennessee

SCOTT L. TOMAR, DMD, MPH, DrPH
Diplomate, American Board of Dental Public Health; Professor, University of Florida College of Dentistry, Gainesville, Florida

BENJAMIN J. VESPER, PhD, MBA
Research Assistant Professor, Department of Oral Medicine and Diagnostic Sciences, Dental Medicine Responder Training Office, College of Dentistry, University of Illinois at Chicago, Chicago, Illinois

RODRIGO VILLALOBOS, DDS, MSc, MS
Dean and Professor, Department of Restorative Dentistry, Dental School, Universidad Latina de Costa Rica (ULATINA), San Jose, Costa Rica

JENNIFER WEBSTER-CYRIAQUE, DDS, PhD
Professor, Department of Dental Ecology, University of North Carolina School of Dentistry, Chapel Hill, North Carolina

E. JOHN WIPFLER III, MD
Clinical Associate Professor of Surgery, Department of Emergency Medicine, University of Illinois College of Medicine; Attending Emergency Physician, Emergency Department, OSF Saint Francis Medical Center; Sheriff's Physician, Peoria County Sheriff's Office, Peoria, Illinois

DAPHNE YOUNG, DDS, MSPH
Professor; Program Director, General Practice Residency, Meharry Medical College, School of Dentistry, Nashville, Tennessee

Contents

> In 2009, the Interprofessional Education Collaborative (IPEC) was initiated. Its release of interprofessional collaborative practice (ICP) core competencies in 2011 was pivotal for the engagement of dentistry in patient-centered, collaborative efforts of interprofessional education (IPE) and ICP. Thereby, IPEC is helping to put into application, in North America, the 2010 World Health Organization (WHO) Framework for Action on Interprofessional Education and Collaborative Practice. This article introduces IPE/ICP in 5 phases of evolution, emphasizing dental influences and inclusion, from historical perspectives through current applications that are expanded on in the accompanying articles in this issue.

> Interprofessional collaboration in health has become essential to providing high-quality care, decreased costs, and improved outcomes. Patient-centered care requires synthesis of all the components of primary and specialty medicine to address patient needs. For individuals living with chronic diseases, this model is even more critical to obtain better health outcomes. Studies have shown that oral health and systemic disease are correlated as it relates to disease development and progression. Thus, inclusion of oral health in many of the existing and new collaborative models could result in better management of chronic illnesses and improve overall health outcomes.

> Interprofessional education (IPE) is a relatively new part of dental education. Its implementation is mandated by accreditation standards, but it is also essential to good patient care. Diverse dental schools from various regions of North America outline problems they have faced in IPE and the solutions that they have found to surmount these problems. Commonalities and unique features of these problems and solutions are discussed.

Lesbian, gay, bisexual and transgender (LGBT) persons are a diverse group who share a common need for competent, accessible healthcare, dispensed without intolerance and with an understanding of their unique health needs. Dental practitioners should recognize common issues shared by many LGBT persons yet understand specific oral health needs of each LGBT subgroup. This article reviews the literature on oral and overall health of LGBT persons in North America and discusses ways in which dentists might improve their care of this vulnerable population, including how interprofessional education and collaborative practice may help to reduce oral health disparities within this group.

Disaster and pandemic response events require an interprofessional team of health care responders to organize and work together in high-pressure, time-critical situations. Civilian oral health care professionals have traditionally been limited to forensic identification of human remains. However, after the bombing of the Twin Towers in New York, federal agencies realized that dentists can play significant roles in disaster and immunization response, especially on interprofessional responder teams. Several states have begun to incorporate dentists into the first responder community. This article discusses the roles of dental responders and highlights legislative advancements and advocacy efforts supporting the dental responder.

This article provides an example of interprofessional collaboration for policy development regarding environmental global health vis-à-vis the Minamata Convention on Mercury. It presents an overview of mercury and mercury-related environmental health issues; public policy processes and stakeholders; and specifics including organized dentistry's efforts to create global policy to restrict environmental contamination by mercury. Dentistry must participate in interprofessional collaborations and build on such experiences to be optimally placed for ongoing interprofessional policy development. Current areas requiring dental engagement for interprofessional policy development include education, disaster response, HPV vaccination, pain management, research priorities, and antibiotic resistance.

With the growing complexity of health care, interprofessional communication and collaboration are essential to optimize the care of dental patients,

DENTAL CLINICS OF NORTH AMERICA

THE CLINICS ARE AVAILABLE ONLINE!
Access your subscription at:
www.theclinics.com

Preface

The Alphabet Soup of Interprofessional Education and Collaborative Practice Acronyms with Dental Seasoning

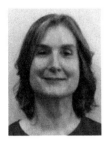   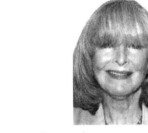

Linda M. Kaste, DDS, MS, PhD   Leslie R. Halpern, MD, DDS, PhD, MPH
Editors

In 2009, six health professional educational associations came together to enhance efforts to develop team-based approaches to health care and initiated the Interprofessional Education Collaborative (IPEC). IPEC awareness increased as its core competencies for interprofessional practice became disseminated.[1] The Collaborative continued to become incorporated in 2013 with Richard Valachovic, DMD, MPH (President and Chief Executive Officer of the American Dental Education Association) as its President (https://ipecollaborative.org/About_IPEC.html). Notably, while IPEC was in formation, the World Health Organization (WHO) released the report "Framework for action on interprofessional education and collaborative practice"[2] as a foundation for addressing the global health workforce crisis by having "collaborative practice-ready" graduates.[2]

IPEC's role and development are based upon Interprofessional Education (IPE) for preparing health care professional students to work in interprofessional collaborative practice (IPCP or IPC), also known as interprofessional practice (IPP) or collaborative care. An overarching view of IPE and IPCP may be seen as Interprofessional Education and Collaborative Practice (IPECP), which is directed at patient-centered care and the PCP (which might be used to represent either Primary Care Provider or Primary Care Physician).

In addition to IPEC and WHO's efforts, other entities and products have been developed as resources for IPECP. A current list in North America, albeit not remotely exhaustive, includes from the general health professional perspective: the American Interprofessional Health Collaborative (https://aihc-us.org/), National Center for Interprofessional Practice and Education (https://nexusipe.org/), and an increasing number

Dent Clin N Am 60 (2016) xiii–xvi
http://dx.doi.org/10.1016/j.cden.2016.07.001
0011-8532/16/© 2016 Published by Elsevier Inc.

of interprofessional centers at universities and agencies. Specific efforts have emerged to seek attention to the inclusion of oral health into the training of non-dental health care providers. Examples of these include "Smiles for Life" as a curricular product of the Society of Teachers of Family Medicine,[3] the Oral Health Nursing Education and Practice Interprofessional Oral Health Faculty Toolkit (www.OHNEP.org/faculty-toolkit), and "A User's Guide for Implementation of Interprofessional Oral Health Core Clinical Competencies"[4] directed by the National Network for Oral Health Access in response to the US Department of Health and Human Services Health Resources and Services Administration (HRSA)'s Integration of Oral Health and Primary Care Practice.[5] Haber and colleagues[6] recently emphasized the need for inclusion of oral health in traditional practice with their commentary, "Putting the Mouth Back in the Head: HEENT to HEENOT," where HEENOT becomes the examination "for assessment, diagnosis, and treatment of oral-systemic health" with "the addition of the teeth, gums, mucosa, tongue, and palate" to the "traditional head, ears, eyes, nose, and throat."

Due to a considerable list of interprofessional topics, this issue could not cover all and does not cover some of the more common collaborations. Existing papers providing additional examples include those out of the 2012 Symposium at Columbia University College of Dental Medicine[7] and the 2014 Conference on Interprofessional Education and Practice held by the California Dental Association and the American Dental Association. Topics from the symposia subsequently were published in the *Journal of the California Dental Association* across three issues in January, September, and October, 2014. The topics ranged from a background review of private practice and interdisciplinary collaboration[8] to a craniofacial perspective[9] and consideration given to influences from outside dentistry, such as by "The Patient Protection and Affordable Care Act."[10] Continuation of the foci was presented in the March 2016 issue of the *Journal of the California Dental Association* by showcasing case studies of integrated health systems.[11–13]

The first article in this *Dental Clinics of North America* issue provides further IPECP history and introductory aspects of the topics included in this issue. Dr Southerland and her team, in the second article, provide insight on approaches for chronic diseases, focusing on collaborative practice models not initiated in dentistry. The development of IPECP is a pivotal point for IPE, including dentistry. Drs Gordon and Donoff steer us through examples of challenges and solutions concerning IPE in North American dental schools in the third article.

The next four articles provide review of familiar topics in interprofessional collaborations. Dr Shaefer and coauthors provide insight into working collaboratively for patients needing chronic pain management and identify resources such as International Association for the Study of Pain (http://www.iasp-pain.org/) and NIH Pain Consortium Centers of Excellence in Pain Education (http://painconsortium.nih.gov/NIH_Pain_Programs/CoEPES.html). Dr Glassman and colleagues take us through interprofessional perspectives for collaboratively caring for patients with special needs. Dr Farmer-Dixon and team demonstrate advances on Women's Health, particularly for confronting issues of intimate partner violence and abuse. Dr Kaufman and colleagues share cases concerning examples of care for geriatric patients and benefits of effective interprofessional communication.

The next several articles of this *Dental Clinics of North America* issue present topics that may be less mainstream, but nonetheless important, in the education for and practice of general dentistry. Drs Russell and More examine a health disparities example concerning sexual minority patients and provide guidance through LGBT (lesbian, gay, bisexual, and transgender) and other sexual identities. Dr Colvard and colleagues update dentistry as a team member in emergency response as a DER (dental emergency responder) as part of TEMS (tactical emergency medical support). Dr Meyer and colleagues discuss interprofessional policy development using the example of the United Nations Environment Program Minamata Convention (www.mercuryconvention.org) on the path to a global treaty on mercury. Drs Regier and Hart orient us on interprofessional research collaboration, specifically concerning genetics and resources such as the Genetic and Rare Diseases Information Center (https://rarediseases.info.nih.gov/gard/).

HRSA, as the federal "Access to Care" agency, has been a major partner with IPEC and other entities working for implementation of IPE to IPP/CP. The HRSA Coordinating Center for Interprofessional Education and Collaborative Practice (http://bhpr.hrsa.gov/grants/interprofessional/) is a hub of resources concerning interprofessional relations, including the "Integrating Oral Health and Primary Care Practice Initiative." Further discussion of these efforts is presented in the final article of this issue by Dr Joskow.

These articles use an array of terms related to IPECP and aim to provide a taste of its history, present, and future. Clearly, the health professional workforce needs to be educated to work interprofessionally and must be welcomed to work interprofessionally when entering the constantly developing workforce. We hope this issue provides general dentists in private practice, community-based clinics, and academic and research centers a clear broth to which ingredients can be added to have substantial nourishment and flavor enhancement for continuing the enrichment of achieving optimal oral and general health for all using interprofessional teams for patient-centered care.

ACKNOWLEDGMENTS

This issue of *Dental Clinics of North America* was made possible by the support and encouragement of John Vassallo, Editor of *Dental Clinics of North America*, and his editorial staff. We wish to extend our special thanks to Kristen Helm, Developmental Editor, and all the authors in this issue. We are privileged that they shared their experience, expertise, and creative insight as trailblazers within their respective realms.

Linda M. Kaste, DDS, MS, PhD
Department of Pediatric Dentistry
College of Dentistry
University of Illinois at Chicago
801 South Paulina Street
MC 850, Room 563A
Chicago, IL 60612, USA

Leslie R. Halpern, MD, DDS, PhD, MPH
Department of Oral and Maxillofacial Surgery
Meharry Medical College
School of Dentistry
1005 DB Todd Jr Boulevard
Nashville, TN 37208, USA

E-mail addresses:
kaste@uic.edu (L.M. Kaste)
lhalpern@mmc.edu (L.R. Halpern)

REFERENCES

1. Interprofessional Education Collaborative Expert Panel (IPECEP). Core competencies for interprofessional collaborative practice: report of an expert panel. Washington, DC: Interprofessional Education Collaborative; 2011. Available at: http://www.aacn.nche.edu/education-resources/ipecreport.pdf. Accessed February 15, 2016.
2. World Health Organization (WHO). Framework for action on interprofessional education and collaborative practice. Geneva (Switzerland): World Health Organization; 2010. Available at: http://apps.who.int/iris/bitstream/10665/70185/1/WHO_HRH_HPN_10.3_eng.pdf. Accessed April 24, 2016.
3. Clark MB, Douglass AB, Maier R, et al. Smiles for Life: a national oral health curriculum. 3rd edition. Society of teachers of family medicine. 2010. Available at: www.smilesforlifeoralhealth.com. Accessed April 24, 2016.
4. NNOHA. A user's guide for implementation of interprofessional oral health core clinical competencies: results of a pilot project. Denver (CO): National Network for Oral Health Access; 2015. Available at: http://www.nnoha.org/nnoha-content/uploads/2015/01/IPOHCCC-Users-Guide-Final_01-23-2015.pdf. Accessed April 24, 2016.
5. HRSA. Integration of Oral Health and Primary Care Practice. Rockville (MD): U.S. Department of Health and Human Services Health Resources and Services Administration; 2014. Available at: http://www.hrsa.gov/publichealth/clinical/oralhealth/primarycare/integrationoforalhealth.pdf. Accessed April 24, 2016.
6. Haber J, Hartnett E, Allen K, et al. Putting the mouth back in the head: HEENT to HEENOT. Am J Public Health 2015;105(3):437–41.
7. Valachovic RW. Integrating oral and overall health care—on the road to interprofessional education and practice: building a foundation for interprofessional education and practice. J Calif Dent Assoc 2014;42(1):25–7.
8. Hilton IV. Interdisciplinary collaboration: what private practice can learn from the health center experience. J Calif Dent Assoc 2014;42(1):29–34.
9. Slavkin HC, Sanchez-Lara PA, Chai Y, et al. A model for interprofessional health care: lessons learned from craniofacial teams. J Calif Dent Assoc 2014;42(9):637–44.
10. Glassman P. Interprofessional practice in the era of accountability. J Calif Dent Assoc 2014;42(9):645–51.
11. Acharya A. Marshfield Clinic Health System: integrated care case study. J Calif Dent Assoc 2016;44(3):177–81.
12. Taflinger K, West E, Sunderhaus J, et al. Health partners of Western Ohio: integrated care case study. J Calif Dent Assoc 2016;44(3):182–5.
13. Gesko DS. HealthPartners: integrated care case study. J Calif Dent Assoc 2016;44(3):186–9.

The Barber Pole Might Have Been an Early Sign for Patient-Centered Care

What Do Interprofessional Education and Interprofessional Collaborative Practice Look Like Now?

Linda M. Kaste, DDS, MS, PhD[a],*, Leslie R. Halpern, MD, DDS, PhD, MPH[b]

KEYWORDS

- Interprofessional relations • Dentistry • Oral health • Dental education
- Professional practice • Interdisciplinary studies • Barber surgeon
- History of dentistry

KEY POINTS

- Interprofessional collaborative practice related to oral health has existed across dentistry's history and is recently reinforced by changes in the US health care system.
- The Interprofessional Education Collaborative and its core competencies facilitate dental awareness and participation in collaborative practice, particularly for North America.
- The World Health Organization supports interprofessional education and collaborative practice as means toward solving health care workforce shortages.
- The ongoing development of interprofessional education and collaborative practice, with academic and clinical applications, contributes to the creation of concepts and support designed to achieve optimal health status for individuals and populations.
- Topics selected for this issue review interprofessional history, models, education, clinical practices, emerging applications, and resources.

INTRODUCTION

The historical influences by oral health care providers on nonoral health care and by nonoral health care providers on oral health care, deserve attention in consideration of the routes of how clinicians in dentistry have got to where they are and how they move forward. In current advancements of interprofessional education (IPE) and

[a] Department of Pediatric Dentistry, College of Dentistry, University of Illinois at Chicago, 801 South Paulina Street, MC 850, Room 563A, Chicago, IL 60612, USA; [b] Department of Oral and Maxillofacial Surgery, Meharry Medical College, 1005 DB Todd Jr. Boulevard, Nashville, TN 37208, USA
* Corresponding author.
E-mail address: kaste@uic.edu

Dent Clin N Am 60 (2016) 765–788
http://dx.doi.org/10.1016/j.cden.2016.05.011   dental.theclinics.com
0011-8532/16/© 2016 Elsevier Inc. All rights reserved.

interprofessional collaborative practice (ICP), the inclusion and influences of dentistry seem logical, but this may not have always been the case.

The fundamental definitions of IPE and ICP come from the World Health Organization (WHO).[1] *Interprofessional Education* is "When students from two or more professions learn about, from and with each other to enable effective collaboration and improve health outcomes."[1] *Interprofessional Collaborative Practice* is "When multiple health workers from different professional backgrounds work together with patients, families, careers, and communities to deliver the highest quality of care."[1]

The evolution of IPE and ICP incorporates an extensive number of events and details. Hence, this article and the accompanying articles in this issue are selective. The aims are on positive aspects of collaborations, centered on dentistry and focus on the Interprofessional Education Collaborative (IPEC) health professional partners of dentistry, medicine, nursing, pharmacy, public health, and osteopathic medicine.[2] The structure of this article is on 5 phases of IPE/ICP history that emerged during the course of our study spanning from *Predentistry* to *Interprofessional Education/ Interprofessional Collaborative Practice with Dentistry*. The reader is referred to the accompanying **Figs. 1–5** as a timeline through this evolution of the respective phases for the topics discussed in the text as well as with a few additional items which were added to help with historical context.

PHASE 1. PREDENTISTRY

Reports of craniomaxillofacial abnormalities and the human desires to have them corrected have existed for a long time. These conditions earned attention in epic poetry, such as in Homer's *Iliad*, recounting craniomaxillofacial war injuries thousands of years ago[3] and in Gothic and Renaissance paintings depicting cleft lip repairs such as by Paré.[4]

Sometime between the actions of Homer[3] and Paré,[4] an interprofessional practice (albeit by an individual rather than within a team) occurred, as seen via accounts of

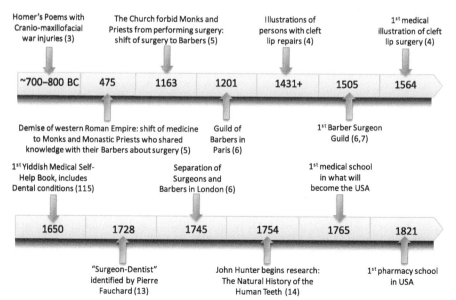

Fig. 1. Timeline of IPE/ICP milestones with oral health/dentistry significance, phase 1. Predentistry.

barber surgeons. The barber surgeon seems to have gained status as the unantici-pated consequence of the church removing the surgical roles of priests and monks in 1163.[5] Records of the first Guild of Barber Surgeons show its establishment in 1505,[6,7] an event that may represent the creation of the first professional health care providers, building on the founding of the Guild of Barbers in Paris in 1210.[6] Sub-sequently, physicians were recommended to not provide extractions but to leave such procedures laden with "unpleasant accidents"[6] to the barbers, hence contributing to the separation of barbers and surgeons, which might have raised expectations of defining scope of practice for health care professions. Concrete evidence of this occurrence can be seen in 1745, when a Great Britain Parliament bill called for the separation of the surgeons and barbers of London.[8]

Although it is perhaps commonly thought that the barber surgeon profession mainly existed outside the Americas, advertising by barber surgeons to have "teeth drawn, and old broken Stumps taken out very safely" have been found in North America.[9,10] Fascinating details have been captured about these self-contained practitioners of in-tegrated care,[6,10] including the advertising of their work via the barber pole, which might even "suspend a string of extracted teeth."[11] From the perspective of the bar-bers, an interesting synopsis exists from 1904 by William Andrews.[12] Andrews[12] in-cludes discussion of the derivation of the barber versus surgeon, and provides reports of barber surgeon performance conducted by both men and women.[12] A vali-dation exists for the importance of this group because PubMed (http://www.ncbi.nlm.nih.gov/) retains a MeSH (Medical Subject Headings of the National Library of Medi-cine) term of "Barber Surgeon" with the following definition:

> In the late Middle Ages barbers who also let blood, sold unguents, pulled teeth, applied cups, and gave enemas. They generally had the right to practice surgery. By the 18th century barbers continued to practice minor surgery and dentistry and many famous surgeons acquired their skill in the shops of barbers.
> —From Castiglioni, A. A History of Medicine, 2nd edition, pp 402, 568, 658[13]; http://www.ncbi.nlm.nih.gov/mesh/?term=barber+surgeon.

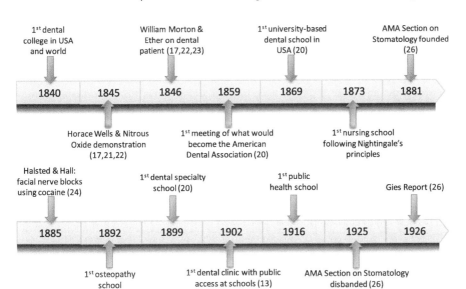

Fig. 2. Timeline of IPE/ICP milestones with oral health/dentistry significance, phase 2. Estab-lishing dental education.

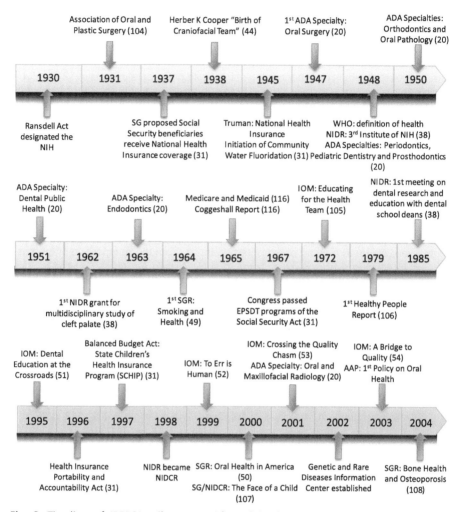

Fig. 3. Timeline of IPE/ICP milestones with oral health/dentistry significance, phase 3. Mature dental education.[104–108,116] IOM, Institute of Medicine; NIDCR, National Institute of Dental and Craniofacial Research; NIDR, National Institute of Dental Research; NIH, National Institutes of Health; SG, Surgeon General; SGR, Surgeon General's Report.

However, progress in scientific approaches, at least via published dissemination, to health care provision circa the mouth moved slowly. More than 200 years after the first establishment of a barber surgeons guild, John Hunter (http://library.uthscsa.edu/2015/03/the-natural-history-of-human-teeth-john-hunter/) in 1754 began assessing "the natural history of the human teeth,"[14] which led to publication in 1771 of "The Natural History of the Human Teeth: Explaining Their Structure, Use, Formation, Growth, and Diseases," which was republished with additional information in 1778.[14] His work contributed greatly to the understanding of the dentition and bone,[15,16] including his allotransplant of teeth from one person to another. There could be some debate about whether he was a surgeon or a dentist, which may be a moot point because he seems to have been on-the-job trained in an academic anatomy laboratory and in military service. His interest in teeth included the relationship of teeth to the digestive system.

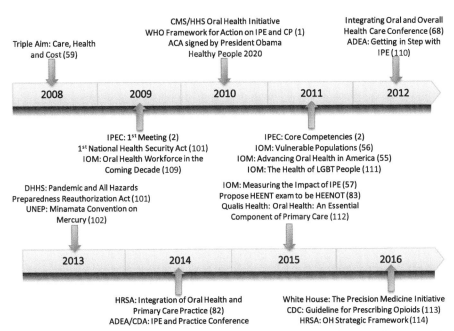

Fig. 4. Timeline of IPE/ICP milestones with oral health/dentistry significance, phase 4. Establishing IPE for ICP.[109–115] DHHS, Department of Health and Human Services; HEENT, head, ears, eyes, nose, and throat; HEENOT, HEENT plus teeth, gums, mucosa, tongue, and palate; HHS, Department of Health and Human Services; HRSA, Health Resources and Services Administration; UNEP, United Nations Environment Programme.

Much of his original work and specimen collection remains at the Hunterian Museum in London (http://www.hunterianmuseum.org/).

During Hunter's life, the first Medical School, in what was to become the United States of America, was opened in Philadelphia at the University of Pennsylvania (1765) (http://www.archives.upenn.edu/histy/features/1700s/medsch.html). Subsequently, the first pharmacy school was also placed in Philadelphia, at the Philadelphia College of Pharmacy (1821), now part of the University of Sciences in Philadelphia (http://www.usciences.edu/academics/collegesdepts/pcp). Continuance of accounting of the first of health professions schools is discussed later, starting with the opening of the first dental school.

PHASE 2. ESTABLISHING DENTAL EDUCATION

A notable unintended consequence happened when Chapin Harris' repeated attempts, in 1837 and 1838, to have the University of Maryland Medical College include dental studies were denied.[17] Hence, Harris organized the first dental school granting

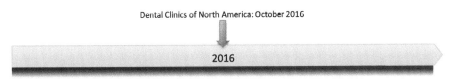

Fig. 5. Timeline of IPE/ICP milestones with oral health/dentistry significance, phase 5. IPE/ICP with dentistry.

the Doctor of Dental Surgery (DDS) in the United States and the world, which was chartered in 1840 as the Baltimore College of Dental Surgery (BCDS), which later merged with the University of Maryland[17–19] (http://www.dental.umaryland.edu/museum/index.html/about-us/). Also in 1840, the first dental organization and the first dental journal came to be, thus dentistry became a true profession based on the tripod of organization, education, and literature.[18] The first dental school associated with a university was at Harvard University, where, in choosing to keep with the Harvard tradition of awarding degrees in Latin, the granting of the Dentariae Mediciniae Doctoris (DMD) started in 1869.[20] The first US nursing school adhering to Florence Nightingale's nursing principles opened in 1873 as the Bellevue Hospital School of Nursing in New York City (https://archives.med.nyu.edu/collections/bellevue-school-nursing). The American School of Osteopathy in Kirksville, Missouri, opened in 1892 as the first school of osteopathy (https://www.atsu.edu/museum/). The first dental specialty school was opened in 1899: the Angle School of Orthodontia, in St Louis, Missouri.[20] The first school of public health did not open until 1916, when the Johns Hopkins School of Hygiene and Public Health was started in Baltimore, Maryland, with funding from the Rockefeller Foundation (http://rockefeller100.org/exhibits/show/education/medical-education/public-health-at-johns-hopkins). Given the 141-year spread of the creation of these first health professional educational institutions, it is reasonable to wonder whether the initiation of IPE would have been facilitated by simultaneous development of education for these and other health care professions.

Dentistry was involved, sometimes as the leader, with developments for the management and diagnosis of conditions of patients seen by multiple health care professionals. Several notable examples from the 1800s include the introduction of nitrous oxide in 1845,[17,21,22] ether in 1846 (by BCDS graduate William T.G. Morton),[17,22,23] nerve blocks in 1885,[24] and dental applications of radiographs in 1896.[25] However, these are select examples, and their histories show an often bumpy road to the development of dentistry with diversions into and from ICP.

During this period, organized dentistry was raised in America from several roots. The American Dental Convention, founded in 1855, encountered discontent that led to another effort to establish a dental association. In 1859, dentists from the American Dental Convention joined others, including dentists who had been members of the former American Society of Dental Surgeons (1840–1856), at a meeting in Niagara Falls, New York. This meeting of 26 dentists, from as far away as Illinois, Missouri, and Wisconsin, led to the formation of the American Dental Association (ADA).[20]

Notable diversity was added among the dental profession in the United States via the accomplishment of dental school graduation for individuals who were not white, European men. Examples of such diversity are the dental school graduation in 1866 of Lucy Hobbs Taylor, the first woman; in 1869 of Robert Tanner Freeman, the first African American man; and in 1890 of Ida Gray Nelson, the first African American woman.[20]

The Gies Report,[26] which is the familiar name for the *Dental Education in the United States and Canada: A report to the Carnegie Foundation for the Advancement of Teaching* by William J. Gies,[26] released in 1926, provides insight into interprofessional attitudes of the era, which amounted to clearer separation of the professions of medicine and dentistry. His summary of medical reaction is presented as:

> As a result of these unfounded assumptions and of such misapprehensions of the import of dental disorders, by physicians for centuries, medicine gave little attention to the health of the teeth. Although the advance of civilization has been accompanied by accentuation of dental abnormalities, medicine persistently

ignored the great desirability of careful observation in this field; and, sharing the popular belief that decay of teeth was unpreventable and loss of teeth unavoidable, physicians helped to bring about universal resignation to the supposedly inevitable incidence of dental imperfection and distress. Until recently, medicine viewed this situation with about as much concern as that excited by loss of hair from the scalp, and did little more to understand or to control the influences responsible for the one than for the other.[26]

Gies[26] went on in this report to provide evidence that dentistry merits a standing equivalent to a medical specialty. He recognized that local infections associated with oral disease may have consequences for other areas/systems of the body and recommended that both dentists and physicians need to be able to perform diagnosis and control "of numerous conditions of local or general disease."[26] Hence, "dentistry should no longer be ignored in medical schools, and its main health-service features should be given suitable attention in the training of general practitioners of medicine."[26] However, at the time of the report, the United States and Canada had statutes that would have required dental laws to be repealed if dentistry were to be moved into medicine as a specialty area, which was not welcomed by either medicine or dentistry. The Gies Report, which took 5 years to compile, has more than 600 pages and includes data on the US and Canadian dental schools, and the current (as of 1926) level of understanding of dental diseases, which suggested the need for research.[26] Gies made other major contributions to dentistry, including being the founder of the International Association for Dental Research (including the American Division, which subsequently became the American Association for Dental Research [AADR]) and the Journal of Dental Research.[27]

Also during this phase, the education of other health professionals went through initiation, evaluation, and modification. Abraham Flexner[28] produced a report on medical education, published in 1910, calling for reorganization of medical education to ensure its science base. The education of public health workers was proposed in 1915 to be conducted separately but in close proximity to medical education, in a report that came to be known as the Welch-Rose Report.[29] Nursing education was scrutinized by the Committee for the Study of Nursing Education, which yielded what was commonly called the Goldmark Report in 1923 and advocated the inclusion of university-level training for nursing.[30]

PHASE 3. MATURE DENTAL EDUCATION

Castiglioni[13] in his 1941 *A History of Medicine*, provided medical insight into the development of dentistry. He expressed his opinion that "The bonds between dentistry and medicine are steadily becoming closer and closer."[13] Moreover, he saw a major contribution from dentistry in the establishment of dental clinics in schools, a significant public health achievement, made by Ernest Jessen in 1902.[13]

During this phase, efforts to initiate National Health Insurance occurred, and selected highlights are presented here from the *Medicare & Medicaid Milestones: 1937-2015* report.[31] In 1937, the US Surgeon General proposed that Social Security beneficiaries receive National Health Insurance coverage. President Harry Truman lent support to National Health Insurance in 1945. Twenty years later, Medicare (Title XVIII) and Medicaid (Title XIX) were enacted as part of the Social Security Act in 1965.[31] Medicare and Medicaid provided specific health services to all Americans more than 65 years of age and options for states to gain federal funds for select population groups: low-income children, their caretaker relatives, the blind, and individuals with disabilities. In 1967, Early and Periodic Screening, Diagnosis, and Treatment (EPSDT) was provided for all children on Medicaid.[32] Fine tuning of these acts continues but the major involvement of dentistry remains with children who are Medicaid eligible. Although Federally Qualified Health Center (FQHC) became a term in 1986, clarification of this title was made with the Health Centers Consolidation Act of 1996 under Section 330 of the Public Health Service Act.[33] The child-specific focus was present again in the Balanced Budget Act of 1997, which created the Children's Health Insurance Program. Of these, the most clear, consistent, and comprehensive collaborative inclusion of dentistry/oral health has been through Medicaid/EPSDT.[34] The 2013 Centers for Medicare and Medicaid Services (CMS) report "Keep Kids Smiling: Promoting Oral Health Through the Medicaid Benefit for Children & Adolescents," including resources from the American Academy of Pediatrics,[35] showed a solid ICP effort.

The first community water fluoridation (CWF) project started in 1945 and CWF became recognized among the 10 great public health achievements of the century.[36,37] Perhaps an incentive for community-level prevention that had started before and was continuing during both World Wars, a leading cause of disqualification for entry to military service was failure to pass the entrance physical because of the poor condition of teeth.[20] World War II taught the United States much about its people's oral health status, which was poor. Missing teeth (attributed to dental caries) was the predominant reason for unfitness and rejection of entrance for military service. Hence, in 1948, the National Institute of Dental Research (NIDR) was created as the third institute of the US National Institutes of Health.[18,38]

The impact of oral and general health status during times of armed conflict[39] has been shown to be significant, for concerns ranging from the ability to consume sufficient nutrients (as simple as assurance of being able to chew rations of hard bread[40]) to having sufficient opposing teeth to be capable of tearing open and pulling closed weapon materials.[40] These accounts are clearly documented from the US Civil War for the purposes of recruitment and ability to function.[40,41] Statistics kept in the Civil War provided descriptive epidemiology of loss of teeth such as to prevent proper mastication,[41] showing tooth loss variation by age, geographic location, occupation, and county of origin,[41] and an overall 3.1% dental disqualification rate.[41] More recent engagements showed the need to measure and address oral health status differently, such as during the Vietnam War with the implementation of the Dental Combat Effectiveness Program to reduce rates of dental emergencies, and the Army Oral Health Maintenance Program to control caries risk attributable to military life.[42]

An orthodontist who practiced in Lancaster, Pennsylvania, studied the practice of dentistry and noted that, "in 1840 we separated the training of the dental student from that of the medical student. It seems we now try to separate the body because of that confusion in our thinking."[43] This thought seems to have arisen from the challenges of obtaining comprehensive care for "crippled children,"[44] as in his expression of "the realization that although orthopedics and orthodontics are so closely related, yet in the practical application of treatment of the deformities, orthodontics and orthopedics are completely severed."[45] Thus, Herbert Cooper, DDS, FACD, advocated for and used in his own practice the craniofacial team.[44] This team evolved to include surgeon, dentist, orthodontist, prosthodontist, speech therapist, pediatrician, psychologist, and social worker.[43,46] He postulated that, "a team can succeed only with smooth cooperation and men who, while feeling free and independent, are willing to fit or fill a position without friction. The team needs men who can be guided without force and prompted to go ahead in the greatest interest of the patient. The only way in my opinion to have this approach work satisfactorily lies in the three c's: communication, cooperation, and coordination of effort."[46] Henceforth, Dr Cooper and his work have been identified to "provide 'best practices' for the future of interprofessional education."[47]

Formal specialization in dentistry, as recognized by the ADA, started in 1947 with oral surgery. This event was followed by periodontics, pediatric dentistry, and prosthodontics in 1948; orthodontics and oral pathology in 1950; dental public health in 1951; endodontics in 1963; and oral and maxillofacial radiology in 2001.[20]

President John F. Kennedy signed the Health Professions Educational Assistance Act of 1963, which aided both dental and medical education.[20] The President relayed in his remarks about signing the Act: "The construction of urgently needed facilities for training physicians, dentists, nurses, and other professional health personnel can now begin. More talented but needy students will now be able to undertake the long and expensive training for careers in medicine, dentistry, and osteopathy."[48]

The first Surgeon General's report (SGR) was released in 1964 and focused on smoking and health, *Smoking and Health: Report of the Advisory Committee to the Surgeon General of the Public Health Service*.[49] Numerous SGRs, many focused on the ills of tobacco (more than two-thirds of the SGRs concern tobacco), have been published since (http://www.surgeongeneral.gov/library/reports/). However, not until 2000 was there an SGR specifically on oral health: *Oral Health in America: A Report of the Surgeon General*.[50] This SGR was compiled to convey why oral health is essential to general health and well-being.[50]

The 1995 Institute of Medicine (IOM) report *Dental Education at the Crossroads: Challenges and Change* was developed in reaction to challenges in dental education, often manifested in the closing and vulnerability to closure of multiple dental schools.[51] The committee that generated the report acknowledged 8 policy and strategic principles that give insight into perceptions of dental education at the end of the twentieth century, and these are presented in **Box 1**.[51] The committee, led by Dr. Marilyn Field,[51] generated 22 recommendations to provide guidance for dentistry to efficiently participate in the restructuring of health care. Numerous IOM reports reflect components of the need for restructuring of health care.[52–57]

PHASE 4. ESTABLISHING INTERPROFESSIONAL EDUCATION FOR INTERPROFESSIONAL COLLABORATIVE PRACTICE

A major recent motivator for IPE/ICP[58] has been the health care system's changes around the drive of outcomes assessment with the Triple Aim.[59] **Box 2** provides the components and outcomes of the Triple Aim.[59]

Dentistry and dental hygiene are not frequently included in the IPE/ICP literature.[58] An assessment of literature published between 2008 and 2013 found that dentistry was included only 6.4% of the time and dental hygiene 2.0%.[58] Concurrent work to assess the effects of IPE on professional practice and health care outcomes in the literature from 2006 to 2011, updating a 2008 Cochrane Collaborative report,[60] did not include any studies involving dental education.[61] Earlier work reinforces the rarity of integration of dentistry into health teams assessments. *Health Care Teams: An Annotated Bibliography*, published in 1974, includes only 2 examinations of teams considering dentistry.[62] A clinical example comes from 1970 in the United Kingdom and is interdisciplinary or intraprofessional (the team composition being only oral health care providers) rather than interprofessional.[63] A training example, also from around 1970, was from George Szasz of British Columbia, Canada, and provided insight into IPE with students in different health professions (medicine, nursing, dentistry, pharmacy, rehabilitation therapy, aspects of home economics, social work, and psychology) learning from each other.[64,65]

Box 1
Dental Education at the Crossroads: policy and strategic principles

1. Oral health is an integral part of total health, and oral health care is an integral part of comprehensive health care, including primary care.

2. The long-standing commitment of dentists and dental hygienists to prevention and primary care should remain vigorous.

3. A focus on health outcomes is essential for dental professionals and dental schools.

4. Dental education must be scientifically based and undertaken in an environment in which the creation and acquisition of new scientific and clinical knowledge are valued and actively pursued.

5. Learning is a lifelong enterprise for dental professionals that cannot stop with the awarding of a degree or the completion of a residency program.

6. A qualified dental workforce is a valuable national resource, and support for the education of this workforce must continue to come from both public and private sources.

7. In recruiting students and faculty, designing and implementing the curriculum, conducting research, and providing clinical services, dental schools have a responsibility to serve all Americans, not just those who are economically advantaged and in good health.

8. Efforts to reduce the wide disparities in oral health status and access to care should be a high priority for policymakers, practitioners, and educators.

From Field MJ, editor; Committee on the Future of Dental Education, Institute of Medicine. Dental education at the crossroads: challenges and change. Washington, DC: National Academy Press; 1995. Available at: http://www.nap.edu/catalog/4925.html. Accessed May 13, 2016; with permission.

Box 2
Defining and operationalizing the Triple Aim

Goals for improving US health and the health care system

- Improving the individual experience of care
- Improving the health of populations
- Reducing the per capita coasts of care for populations

Preconditions

- Recognition of a population as the unit of concern
- Externally supplied policy constraints
- Existence of an integrator able to focus and coordinate services

Functions of an integrator

- Partnership with individuals and families
- Redesign of primary care
- Population health management
- Financial management
- Macro system integration

From Berwick DM, Nolan TW, Whittington J. The Triple Aim: care, health, and cost: the remaining barriers to integrated care are not technical; they are political. Health Affairs 2008;27(4):760–65; with permission.

Dentistry's inclusion in IPE intensified, because the American Dental Education Association was one of 6 health professional educational associations that first met in 2009 to enhance efforts to develop team-based approaches to health care. The 5 other health care professional associations were the American Association of Colleges of Nursing, American Association of Colleges of Osteopathic Medicine, American Association of Colleges of Pharmacy, the Association of American Medical Colleges, and the Association of Schools of Public Health. This group adopted the name of the IPEC. The IPEC's identity, role, and development are based on IPE for preparing health care professional students to work in ICP. The awareness of IPEC increased with the dissemination of its core competencies for interprofessional practice in 2011.[2] The IPEC competencies are based in 4 domains[2] (**Box 3**). The collaborative's efforts continued and it became incorporated in 2013 with Richard Valachovic DMD, MPH (President and Chief Executive Officer of the American Dental Education Association [ADEA]), as its President (https://ipecollaborative.org/About_IPEC.html).

Concurrently, while the IPEC was in formation, the WHO released the report *Framework for Action on Interprofessional Education and Collaborative Practice* in 2010 as a foundation for addressing the global health workforce crisis by having collaborative practice–ready graduates.[1] The WHO framework premise was that, for IPE/ICP to succeed, there was a need for teamwork that highlighted curricular and educator mechanisms as well as "institutional support, working culture, and environmental elements that drive collaborative practice."[1] This framework was intended to gain innovative health policy and structures to bolster IPE/ICP for the improvement of health and

---

Box 3
IPEC: interprofessional collaborative practice competency domains

Competency domain 1
  Values/Ethics for Interprofessional Practice
  General competency statement: work with individuals of other professions to maintain a climate of mutual respect and shared values
  [10 specific competencies]

Competency domain 2
  Roles/Responsibilities
  General competency statement: use the knowledge of your own role and those of other professions to appropriately assess and address the health care needs of the patients and populations served
  [9 specific competencies]

Competency domain 3
  Interprofessional Communication
  General competency statement: communicate with patients, families, communities, and other health professionals in a responsive and responsible manner that supports a team approach to the maintenance of health and the treatment of disease
  [8 specific competencies]

Competency domain 4
  Teams and Teamwork
  General competency statement: apply relationship-building values and the principles of team dynamics to perform effectively in different team roles to plan and deliver patient-centered/population-centered care that is safe, timely, efficient, effective, and equitable
  [11 specific competencies]

From Interprofessional Education Collaborative Expert Panel. Core competencies for interprofessional collaborative practice: report of an expert panel. Washington, DC: Interprofessional Education Collaborative; 2011. Available at: http://www.aacn.nche.edu/education-resources/ipecreport.pdf. Accessed April 24, 2016; with permission.

health care via the encouragement of stakeholders by "examining their local context to determine their needs and capabilities, committing to building interprofessional collaboration into new and existing programs, and championing successful initiatives and teams."[1] Specific actions (**Box 4**) were suggested to advance IPE to gain better health outcomes.[1] Also in 2010, the *Education of Health Professionals for the 21st Century: A Global Independent Commission* set forth findings of a proposed way to look at the future of health professional education via a systems framework approach.[66] They saw 3 generations of reform in such education: (1) science-based reform located at universities with a scientific curriculum, (2) problem-based reform located at academic centers using problem-based learning, and (3) systems-based reform with health education systems with competency-driven instruction that spans local to global.[66]

After the efforts of IPEC and WHO, other entities and products have been developed as resources for IPE/ICP, including, for North America, from the general health professional perspective, the American Interprofessional Health Collaborative (https://aihc-us.org/), National Center for Interprofessional Practice and Education (https://nexusipe.org/), and an increasing number of interprofessional centers at universities and agencies. The Federation Dentaire Internationale (FDI; the World Dental Federation) advocates for IPE/ICP, as detailed in the 2015 *Optimal Oral Health through Inter-Professional Education and Collaborative Practice*[67] based on the WHO work.

Two symposia greatly contributed to the inclusion of dentistry in IPE/ICP: the 2012 Symposium at Columbia University College of Dental Medicine[68] and the 2014 Conference on Interprofessional Education and Practice held by the California Dental Association and the ADA. Topics from the symposia subsequently were published in the *Journal of the California Dental Association* across 3 issues in January, September, and October, 2014. The topics ranged from an explanation of background for ICP with private practice[69] to craniofacial teams.[47] Several topics concerning influences

---

Box 4
WHO: actions to advance IPE for improved health outcomes

1. Agree to a common vision and purpose for IPE with key stakeholders across all faculties and organizations

2. Develop IPE curricula according to principles of good educational practice

3. Provide organizational support and adequate financial and time allocations for:
   a. The development and delivery of IPE
   b. Staff training in IPE

4. Introduce IPE into health worker training programs:
   a. All prequalifying programs
   b. Appropriate postgraduate and continuing professional development programs
   c. Learning for quality service improvement

5. Ensure that staff responsible for developing, delivering, and evaluating IPE are competent in this task, have expertise consistent with the nature of the planned IPE, and have the support of an IPE champion

6. Ensure the commitment to IPE by leaders in educational institutions and all associate practice and work settings

From World Health Organization. Framework for action on interprofessional education and collaborative practice. Geneva (Switzerland): World Health Organization; 2010; with permission.

from outside of dentistry on ICP with dentistry were discussed and include the Affordable Care Act (ACA),[70] ICP as a means to address oral health needs,[71] integration of care between dentistry and medicine,[72] and innovation in IPE.[73] Continuation of the interprofessional applications was presented in the March 2016 issue of the *Journal of the California Dental Association* by showcasing case studies of integrated health systems[74–76] and furthering discussion of health care reform,[77] oral health education innovations,[78] and primary care/population health management collaboration regarding oral health.[79]

Specific efforts have emerged to support the inclusion of oral health into the training of nondental health care providers. Examples of these include Smiles for Life as a curricular product of the Society of Teachers of Family Medicine,[80] the Oral Health Nursing Education and Practice Interprofessional Oral Health Faculty Toolkit (www.OHNEP.org/faculty-toolkit), and *A User's Guide for Implementation of Interprofessional Oral Health Core Clinical Competencies* directed by the National Network for Oral Health Access[81] in response to the US Department of Health and Human Services Health Resources and Services Administration (HRSA) *Integration of Oral Health and Primary Care Practice*.[82] Haber and colleagues[83] recently emphasized the need for inclusion of oral health in traditional practice with their commentary "Putting the Mouth Back in the Head: HEENT to HEENOT," in which HEENOT is the assessment, diagnosis, and treatment of oral-systemic health after the addition of the teeth, gums, mucosa, tongue, and palate to the traditional head, ears, eyes, nose, and throat (HEENT) clinical examination.[83]

Previous Clinics issues have included reviews of topics relating oral health to interprofessional practice. This current issue builds on and broadens the vision of these earlier works to update with a focus on the impact and influences of dentistry on interprofessionalism. The most recent article[84] describes Bouvé College's Health Sciences curriculum inclusion of oral health. A 2009 DCNA focus was on access to care and provided a range of thought from the inclusion of social work in dental patient management[85] to the incorporation of nondental health providers[86] to impact of public policy.[87] Dental involvement in disaster response[88] and forensics[89] have also been discussed in earlier Clinics issues. Other related topics captured in Clinics included dentistry as a focal point on occupational exposures,[90] collaborative care for patients with facial injuries,[91] and the influences of dentistry on office-based anesthesiology.[17]

PHASE 5. INTERPROFESSIONAL EDUCATION/INTERPROFESSIONAL COLLABORATIVE PRACTICE WITH DENTISTRY

As discussed earlier, the relationship between dentistry and other health care professions has waxed and waned. However, it should now be expected that dentistry is included. The series of articles in this issue provides a range of perspectives on what can be learned from other health professions collaborations; current progress in topical areas in which dentistry is integrated with other professions; and areas in which integrations are just beginning in clinical applications, policy, and research.

Every dentist is aware of oral side effects from systemic diseases and associated treatments. It seems natural to work with other health care providers to tackle these issues together. However, more than half of the National Institutes of Health, National Cancer Institute–designated Comprehensive Cancer Centers were found to be lacking dental programs,[92] showing that inclusion of oral health cannot be assumed. Nonetheless, health care teams have been shown to be cost-effective and to aid in such areas as optimal prescription writing.[93] What can dentistry learn from collaborative practice models that were not driven by dentistry? The article by Southerland and colleagues,[94] of this DCNA issue, provide insight on approaches for chronic diseases focusing on such collaborative practice models.

The role of dental schools and their curricula is being broadened to be a foundational education/graduate educational springboard for preparation of dental students for ICP. Implications then exist for continuing professional development to update dentists as team players for enhancing the overall performance of the health team and patient outcomes in oral health. IPE must provide the focus on teams striving to improve the health of patients; that is, to be patient centered. Dental schools and their faculty must value the incorporation of IPE into their programs and find interprofessional collaborators, especially if other health care provider programs are not colocated with dental institutions. Different dental programs have different challenges, such as IPE proximity, and therefore have different needs and solutions for achieving IPE. Gordon and Donoff[95] discuss examples of challenges and solutions facing North American dental school regarding IPE in this issue.

By the nature of many of its conditions and treatments, dentistry has been at the forefront of pain management throughout its history, but has the profession been an optimal participant and partner in the intraprofessional and interprofessional sharing of common, basic knowledge regarding the management of pain? Is there sufficient consideration of how patients travel through the health care system to obtain resolution of pain? Dental students must be engaged in IPE for pain management for ICP. The management of temporomandibular disorders and orofacial neuropathic pain must be included, as well as general chronic pain and the consideration of opioids, currently at an epidemic level of concern, because their ICP colleagues will seek their advice in the management of these cases. Thus, predoctoral and postdoctoral dental education accreditation standards should be comparable to the standards recommendations of the International Association for the Study of Pain (IASP) to be united across health care professions. Shaefer and colleagues[96] provide insight into working collaboratively for patients needing chronic pain management and identify resources such as IASP (http://www.iasp-pain.org/) and the National Institutes of Health (NIH) Pain Consortium Centers of Excellence in Pain Education (http://painconsortium.nih.gov/NIH_Pain_Programs/CoEPES.html).

Extensive challenges exist concerning health care, especially oral health care, for people with complicated health conditions, who have the most significant oral health disparities of any group. The interprofessional team networking needs to be applied to integrate oral health services into social, educational, and general health systems. IPE/ICP, with the inclusion of caregivers and other supports, should work toward the prevention of oral diseases as an obvious way to help the general health of special populations. An infrequent dental office visit with unreinforced threats and information is not the way to ensure the behavior change. Behavior change accomplishment is multifactorial, necessitating the inclusion of positive reinforcement of good oral health behaviors across the full interprofessional team. Glassman and colleagues[97] discuss interprofessional perspectives for collaboratively caring for patients with special needs.

An essential component in the ICP approach is consideration of women's health, because major oral-systemic health consequences disproportionally affect women compared with men. Conditions specifically associated with women's health include intimate partner violence (IPV), poor oral health and low birth weight, and oral health in patients with osteoporosis. By providing models for an ICP approach to women's health both from oral and overall health care disciplines, a greater awareness of women's health needs across all health care disciplines will motivate the development of competencies focusing on women's health, and enhance public concern about the importance of women's health curricula in health professions education. Oral health concerns exist before and during pregnancy, thus the ICP team should include representation from obstetrics/gynecology. Women experience violence and other trauma at high rates, meriting the inclusion of trauma-informed care in ICP. Confusion remains about the impact of bisphosphonate use in relation to oral health and safety of aging women. Farmer-Dixon and colleagues[98] discuss advances in women's health, particularly for confronting issues of IPV and abuse.

Communication skills for bridging generations of families and health care providers are vital for catching elder patients' interest in and acceptance of health care. Awareness of and assistance with navigation of the nuances and challenges of the health care system is tricky for all people, but often especially so for geriatric patients whose complex health statuses may require someone to be designated to assist in the coordination of ICP. Kaufman and colleagues[99] share cases concerning examples of care for geriatric patients and the benefits of effective interprofessional communication.

A group of patients who, at least among some subsections, may be more likely to receive ICP are the lesbian, gay, bisexual, transgender and other sexual minority populations, who share common needs for competent, accessible health care with an understanding of their unique health requirements. Oral health care providers, as well as other health care providers, must recognize the heterogeneity of individuals with respect to distinctive preparation for best disease prevention and promotion of both systemic and oral health. IPE and ICP are very important but the preparation in dentistry seems low compared with other health care professions, with all having room for improvement. Progress is needed interprofessionally to reduce oral health disparities within this group. Russell and More[100] examine health disparities in sexual minority patients, and provide guidance through sexual identity; sexual orientation; and competent, accessible interprofessional health care.

Emergency response is a dynamic field in a demanding world. The capabilities of dental health professionals in this arena are in the process of being defined and implemented. Evidence supports the obvious: that dentists can do more in interprofessional response teams. Increasing numbers of opportunities for coordinated affiliations and advocacy for the inclusion of dentistry are being created. Colvard and colleagues[101] update dentistry by a team member in emergency response as a dental emergency responder, part of tactical emergency medical support.

Amalgam has been used as a dental restorative material for more than 100 years. In spite of safe use of mercury in the amalgam mixture, mercury has been identified by the United Nations Environmental Program as a global health hazard. Consequently, global action has been initiated to remove human-associated environmental exposure to mercury, with major interprofessional and industrial impacts. The lack of a directly interchangeable dental material to replace amalgam, which an especially challenging prospect for low-income countries, contributes to ongoing discussion of the role and responsibility of dentistry in environmental mercury contamination via production processes and waste management. Meyer and colleagues[102] discuss interprofessional policy development using this example of the United Nations Environment Program Minamata Convention (www.mercuryconvention.org) on progress toward a global treaty to protect the environment from human-associated mercury pollution.

Dental education traditionally has not included human genetics, especially as related to interprofessional implications of genetic conditions. Genetic advances are occurring such that the application of genetic knowledge is needed for collaborative practice including dentistry. Of particular concern is the misuse of genetic information leading to mismanagement of patients and potentially their family members, be it through clinical applications or in assisting on referral decisions. Regier and Hart[103] discuss interprofessional research collaboration, specifically concerning genetics and resources such as the Genetic and Rare Diseases Information Center (GARD). GARD was established in 2002 by the Office of Rare Diseases Research and the National Human Genome Research Institute, two agencies of the NIH, to help people find useful information about genetic and rare diseases (https://rarediseases.info.nih.gov/gard/. Accessed 5/6/16).

Gaps exist between identified needs and the ability to respond to collaborative practice and IPE. As the US health care system continues to evolve, there are many members of the US population for whom fully accessing and engaging the system is difficult. Training and improved resources are needed. HRSA, as the federal access to care agency, has been a major partner with IPEC and other entities working for implementation of IPE to ICP. The HRSA Coordinating Center for Interprofessional Education and Collaborative Practice (http://bhpr.hrsa.gov/grants/interprofessional/) is a hub of resources concerning interprofessional relations, including the Integrating Oral Health and Primary Care Practice Initiative. Further discussion of these efforts is presented by Joskow, in this issue.[117]

SUMMARY

The timeline presents the phases of evolution of oral health/dentistry within IPE/ICP, thus showing how specific actions and reactions have narrowed and widened coordinated, team-based, patient-centered health care. Often as a consequence of the actions of others, the development of knowledge and skills were captured in unplanned professions. Nonetheless, all health professions have grown to expect that scholarly activities must exist to provide the evidence base for making optimal health care decisions, whether for disease prevention or treatment. However, especially in the current health care environment, these separate efforts show inefficiencies in the health care system and suboptimal outcomes for patients. Therefore, many efforts from outside the professions have called for assessment of the health care systems. Consequently, change is being sought, with a general consensus that a paradigm shift is necessary for patient-centered care with ICP based on IPE.

Oral health is already familiar with such an approach, especially with the recognition that oral health affects overall health, as shown by the leadership in dental practice such as by the ADA, in dental education by the ADEA, and dental research by the National Institute of Dental and Craniofacial Research and the AADR. Correspondingly, clinicians in oral health care should not overlook the consequences of progress in medicine. The patient populations presenting for oral health care are becoming more diverse in health status as result of medical accomplishments increasing health status and life-span; for example, chronic management of patients with hemophilia, cystic fibrosis, diabetes, stroke, and human immunodeficiency virus and hepatitis C infections. Each article within this series suggests models of interdisciplinary approaches that solidify IPE and its use to form patient-centered health networks with oral health care providers as core elements to the well-being of patients in each community.

Oral health/dentistry have not been universally included in IPE/ICP, and recently have sought inclusion across the full spectrum of oral health care needs, going beyond the long and multiphased history of craniofacial repair. Consideration must be given to whether dentistry may be considered for IPE inclusion by other health care professionals during training, if such training opportunities are not colocated.

Modern dentistry has arisen from an interesting and colorful past. Pride can be taken in the pivotal ideas that have arisen from its self-assessment through such efforts as those that generated the Gies Report,[26] *Dental Education at the Crossroads*,[51] and *Advancing Oral Health in America*.[55] Societal changes and knowledge development continue to shape oral health status and the oral health care system. Dentistry needs to recall its history, including its previous assessments. Looking to the future, dentistry must strongly advocate on its own behalf for its inclusion in IPE/ICP efforts and to have its workforce be ready for IPE/ICP and participation in the continued evolution of patient-centered care. The articles in this issue help provide glimpses into the applications for that preparedness.

ACKNOWLEDGMENT

The authors would like to recognize Karolina Reitmajer, University of Illinois at Chicago College of Dentistry, research volunteer, for her efforts in assisting with the creation of this article.

REFERENCES

1. World Health Organization. Framework for action on interprofessional education and collaborative practice. Geneva (Switzerland): World Health Organization; 2010.
2. Interprofessional Education Collaborative Expert Panel. Core competencies for interprofessional collaborative practice: report of an expert panel. Washington, DC: Interprofessional Education Collaborative; 2011. Available at: http://www.aacn.nche.edu/education-resources/ipecreport.pdf. Accessed April 24, 2016.
3. Mylonas AI, Tzerbos FH, Eftychiadis AC, et al. Cranio-maxillofacial injuries in Homer's Iliad. J Craniomaxillofac Surg 2008;36:1–7.
4. Pirsig W, Haase S, Palm F. Surgically repaired cleft lips depicted in paintings of the late Gothic period and the Renaissance. Br J Oral Maxillofac Surg 2001;39: 127–33.
5. Koenig HG, King DE, Carson VB. Handbook of religion and health. 2nd edition. New York: Oxford University Press; 2012.
6. Wynbrandt J. The excruciating history of dentistry: toothsome tales & oral oddities from Babylon to braces. New York: St Martin's Griffin; 1998.
7. Fischer JE. On the uniqueness of surgery. Am J Surg 2005;189:259–63.
8. Great Britain. Parliament. A bill, intituled, An Act for making the Surgeons of London and the Barbers of London Two Separate and Distinct Corporations. London, 1745. CIC University of Illinois Chicago; 2016. Gale Document Number: CW107998949. Accessed via Eighteenth Century Collections Online. Gale. Accessed August 15, 2016.
9. Weinberger BW. An introduction to the history of dentistry in America, vol. 2. St Louis (MO): The CV Mosby Company; 1948. Available at: https://babel.hathitrust.org/cgi/pt?id=mdp.39015048689486;view=1up;seq=9. Accessed May 12, 2016.
10. Geshwind M. Wig-maker, barber, bleeder and tooth-drawer. J Hist Dent 1996; 44(3):125–7.
11. Campbell JM. Dentistry Then and Now. S.l.: s.n.; 1981.
12. Andrews W. At the sign of the barber's pole: studies in hirsute history. Cottingham (Yorkshire): JR Tutin; 1904. Available at: http://www.gutenberg.org/files/19925/19925-h/19925-h.htm. Accessed April 29, 2016.

13. Castiglioni A. A history of medicine. New York: A. A. Knopf; 1941.
14. Hunter J. The Natural History of the Human Teeth: Explaining Their Structure, Use, Formation, Growth, and Diseases, 2nd Edition. London: Printed for J Johnson, St Paul's Churchyard; 1778. Available at: http://library.uthscsa.edu/2015/03/the-natural-history-of-human-teeth-john-hunter/); https://babel.hathitrust.org/cgi/pt?id=ucm.5315916114;view=1up;seq=9. Accessed August 15, 2016.
15. Keith A. Bone growth and bone repair. I. The foundation of our knowledge of bone growth by Duhamel and Hunter. Br J Surg 1918;5:685–93.
16. Meikle MC. Control mechanisms in bone resorption: 240 years after John Hunter. Ann R Coll Surg Engl 1997;79:20–7.
17. Orr DL. The development of anesthesiology in oral and maxillofacial surgery. Oral Maxillofacial Surg Clin North Am 2013;25:341–55.
18. Ring ME. A thousand years of dentistry. N Y State Dent J 2000;66(2):39–41.
19. McCauley HB. The first dental college: emergence of dentistry as an autonomous profession. J Hist Dent 2003;51(1):41–5.
20. American Dental Association. 150 Years of the American Dental Association: a pictorial history, 1859–2009. Chicago: American Dental Association; 2009.
21. American Dental Association. Horace Wells dentist, father of surgical anesthesia, Proceedings of centenary commemorations of Wells' discovery in 1844. Harford; 1948. Available at: https://babel.hathitrust.org/cgi/pt?id=mdp.39015023441630;view=1up;seq=8. Accessed April 27, 2016.
22. Finder RL. The art and science of office-based anesthesia in dentistry: a 150-year history. Int Anesthesiol Clin 2003;41(3):1–12 [1844].
23. Morton EW. The discovery of anaesthesia: Dr. W.T.G. Morton and his heroic battle for a new idea – how pain-less surgery began fifty years ago. McClure's Magazine 1896;311–8. Available at: https://archive.org/stream/39002011124048.med.yale.edu#page/n1/mode/2up. Accessed April 27, 2016.
24. Lopez-Valverde A, De Vicente J, Cutando A. The surgeons Halsted and Hall, cocaine and the discovery of dental anaesthesia by nerve blocking. Br Dent J 2011;211:458–87.
25. Riaud X. First dental radiograph (1896). Dent Hist 2014;59(2):87–8.
26. Gies WJ. Dental education in the United States and Canada: a report to the Carnegie Foundation for the Advancement of Teaching. New York: The Carnegie Foundation for the Advancement of Teaching; 1926. Available at: http://www.adea.org/ADEAGiesFoundation/William-J-Gies-and-Gies-Report.aspx. Accessed May 1, 2016.
27. International Association for Dental Research History Ad hoc Committee, Burrill DY, Crabb HSM, et al. The first fifty year history of the International Association for Dental Research (IADR). Chicago: IADR; 1973. Available at: http://www.iadr.com/files/public/IADR_First_Fifty_Year_History_V.1.pdf. Accessed May 18, 2016.
28. Flexner A. Medical education in the United States and Canada: a Report to the Carnegie Foundation for the Advancement of Teaching. New York: Bulletin (Carnegie Foundation for the Advancement of Teaching); 1910. no. 4. Available at: http://archive.carnegiefoundation.org/pdfs/elibrary/Carnegie_Flexner_Report.pdf. Accessed May 11, 2016.
29. Welch WH, Rose W. Institute of Hygiene, presented to the General Education Board, May 27, 1915. RF, RG 1.1, series 200L, box 183, folder 2208, Rockefeller Archive Center. Discussed in The Rockefeller Foundation annual report 1916. Available at: https://www.rockefellerfoundation.org/app/uploads/Annual-Report-1916.pdf. Accessed May 12, 2016.

30. Goldmark J. Nursing and nursing education in the united states: report of the Committee for the Study of Nursing Education. New York: The Macmillan Company; 1923.

31. Centers for Medicare and Medicaid Services. Medicare & Medicaid milestones: 1937-2015. Department of Health and Human Services, Centers for Medicare and Medicaid Services; 2015. Available at: https://www.cms.gov/About-CMS/Agency-Information/History/Downloads/Medicare-and-Medicaid-Milestones-1937-2015.pdf. Accessed May 2, 2016.

32. Foltz AM. The development of ambiguous federal policy: early and periodic screening, diagnosis, and treatment (EPSDT). Milbank Mem Fund Q Health Soc 1975;53(1):35–64.

33. Goebel J. A brief history of federally qualified health centers (FQHC). 2013 notifymd. Available at: http://www.notifymd.com/author/jgoebel/. Accessed May 2, 2016.

34. Al-Tannir M. What practicing dentists should know about EPSDT. Early and periodic, screening, diagnosis and treatment. W V Dent J 1994;68(2):6–9.

35. CMS. Keep Kids Smiling: promoting oral health through the Medicaid Benefit for Children & Adolescents: Early and Periodic Screening, Diagnostic and Treatment (EPSDT). 2013. Available at: https://www.medicaid.gov/Medicaid-CHIP-Program-Information/By-Topics/Benefits/Downloads/Keep-Kids-Smiling.pdf. Accessed May 2, 2016.

36. Centers for Disease Control and Prevention (CDC). Ten great public health achievements – United States, 1990-1999. MMWR Morb Mortal Wkly Rep 1999;48(12):241–3.

37. Centers for Disease Control and Prevention. Achievements in Public Health, 1900-1999: Fluoridation of drinking water to prevent dental caries. MMWR Morb Mortal Wkly Rep 1999;48:933–40.

38. Sheridan PG. NIDR – 40 years of research advances in dental health. Public Health Rep 1988;103(5):493–9.

39. Hyson JM, Whitehorne JW, Greenwood JT. A history of dentistry in the US Army to World War II. Government Printing Office; 2008.

40. Ordronaux J. Manual of instructions for military surgeons on the examination of recruits and discharge of soldiers. New York: D Van Nostrand; 1863. Available at: http://resource.nlm.nih.gov/62430640R. Accessed May 12, 2016.

41. Bumgardner E. Disqualification for military service in the civil war on account of loss of teeth. The Dental Cosmos 1894;36(6):429–33. Available at: http://quod.lib.umich.edu/d/dencos/acf8385.0036.001/449:159?didno=ACF8385.0036.001;rgn=full+text;view=image. Accessed May 6, 2016.

42. King JE, Hynson RG. Highlights in the history of US Army dentistry. Falls Church (VA): Office of the Surgeon General, US Army; 2007. Available at: http://history.amedd.army.mil/corps/dental/general/highlights/Highlights.pdf. Accessed May 6, 2016.

43. Cooper HK. The responsibility of the orthodontist in the cleft palate problem. Surgery 1946;32(11):Λ675 83.

44. Long RE. Improving outcomes for the patient with cleft lip and palate: the team concept and 70 years of experience in cleft care. J Lancaster General Hospital 2009;4(2):52–6. Available at: http://www.jlgh.org/JLGH/media/Journal-LGH-Media-Library/Past%20Issues/Volume%204%20-%20Issue%202/v4_i2_Long.pdf. Accessed August 15, 2016.

45. Cooper HK. Crippled children? Am J Orthod Oral Surg 1942;28:35–8.

46. Cooper HK. Dental aspects (forward). In: Grabb WC, Rosenstein S, Bzoch KR, editors. Cleft lip and palate: surgical, dental, and speech aspects. Boston: Little, Brown and Company; 1971. p. xiv–xvi.

47. Slavkin HC, Sanchez-Lara PA, Chai Y, et al. A model for interprofessional health care: lessons learned from craniofacial teams. J Calif Dent Assoc 2014;42(9): 637–44.

48. Kennedy JF. Remarks upon signing the Health Professions Educational Assistance Act. September 24, 1963. Available at: http://www.presidency.ucsb.edu/ws/?pid=9425. Accessed May 6, 2016.

49. US Department of Health, Education, and Welfare. Smoking and health: report of the Advisory Committee to the Surgeon General of the Public Health Service. Public Health Service publication no. 1103. Washington, DC: US Government Printing Office; 1964. Available at: https://profiles.nlm.nih.gov/ps/retrieve/ResourceMetadata/NNBBMQ. Accessed May 13, 2016.

50. US Department of Health and Human Services. Oral health in America: a report of the Surgeon General. Rockville (MD): US Department of Health and Human Services, National Institute of Dental and Craniofacial Research, National Institutes of Health; 2000. Available at: https://profiles.nlm.nih.gov/ps/access/NNBBJT.pdf. Accessed May 6, 2016.

51. Field MJ, editor. Committee on the Future of Dental Education, Institute of Medicine. Dental education at the crossroads: challenges and change. Washington, DC: National Academy Press; 1995. Available at: http://www.nap.edu/catalog/4925.html. Accessed May 13, 2016.

52. Kohn LT, Corrigan JM, Donaldson MS, editors. Committee on Quality of Health Care in America, Institute of Medicine. To err is human: building a safer health system. Washington, DC: The National Academies Press; 2000. Available at: http://www.nap.edu/download.php?record_id=9728#. Accessed May 13, 2016.

53. Institute of Medicine. Crossing the quality chasm. Washington, DC: National Academy Press; 2001.

54. Institute of Medicine. Health professions education; a bridge to quality. Washington, DC: National Academy Press; 2003.

55. Institute of Medicine. Advancing oral health in America. Washington, DC: The National Academies Press; 2011.

56. IOM (Institute of Medicine), NRC (National Research Council). Improving access to oral health care for vulnerable and underserved populations. Washington, DC: The National Academies Press; 2011.

57. Institute of Medicine. Measuring the impact of interprofessional education on collaborative practice and patient outcomes. Washington, DC: The National Academies Press; 2015. Available at: http://www.nap.edu/download.php?record_id=21726#. Accessed May 13, 2016.

58. Brandt B, Lurfiyya MN, King JA, et al. A scoping review of interprofessional collaborative practice and education using the lens of the Triple Aim. J Interprof Care 2014;28(5):393–9.

59. Berwick DM, Nolan TW, Whittington J. The Triple Aim: care, health, and cost: the remaining barriers to integrated care are not technical; they are political. Health Aff 2008;27(4):759–69.

60. Reeves S, Zwarenstein M, Goldman J, et al. Interprofessional education: effects on professional practice and health care outcomes. Cochrane Database Syst Rev 2008;(1):CD002213.

61. Reeves S, Perrier L, Goldman J, et al. Interprofessional education: effects on professional practice and healthcare outcomes (update). Cochrane Database Syst Rev 2013;(3):CD002213.
62. Tichy MK. Health care teams: an annotated bibliography. New York: Praeger Publishers; 1974.
63. Craig JW. Teamwork in dentistry. Br Dent J 1970;128(4):198–202.
64. Szasz G. Interprofessional education in the health sciences: a project conducted at the University of British Columbia. Milbank Mem Fund Q 1969; 47(4):449–75.
65. Szasz G. Education for the health team. Can J Public Health 1970;61(5):386–90.
66. Frenk J, Chen L, Bhutta ZA, et al. Health professionals for a new century: transforming education to strengthen health systems in an interdependent world. Lancet 2010;376:1923–58.
67. FDI. Optimal oral health through inter-professional education and collaborative practice. FDI World Dental Federation. Version 5.1. 2015. Available at: http://www.fdiworldental.org/media/70740/collaborative-practice_digital.pdf. Accessed May 12, 2016.
68. Valachovic RW. Integrating oral and overall health care – on the road to interprofessional education and practice: building a foundation for interprofessional education and practice. J Calif Dent Assoc 2014;42(1):25–7.
69. Hilton IV. Interdisciplinary collaboration: what private practice can learn from the health center experience. J Calif Dent Assoc 2014;42(1):29–34.
70. Glassman P. Interprofessional practice in the era of accountability. J Calif Dent Assoc 2014;42(9):645–51.
71. Garland T, Smith L, Fuccillo R. Addressing oral health need through interprofessional education and practice. J Calif Dent Assoc 2014;42(10):701–9.
72. Mouradian WE, Lewis CW, Berg JH. Integration of dentistry and medicine and the dentist of the future: the need for the health care team. J Calif Dent Assoc 2014;42(10):687–96.
73. Friedrichsen S, Martinez TS, Hostetler J, et al. Innovations in interprofessional education: building collaborative practice skills. J Calif Dent Assoc 2014; 42(9):627–36.
74. Acharya A. Marshfield clinic health system: integrated care case study. J Calif Dent Assoc 2016;44(3):177–81.
75. Taflinger K, West E, Sunderhaus J, et al. Health partners of western Ohio: integrated care case study. J Calif Dent Assoc 2016;44(3):182–5.
76. Gesko DS, HealthPartners: integrated care case study. J Calif Dent Assoc 2016; 44(3):186–9.
77. Vujicic M. Can health care reform connect mouth and body? J Calif Dent Assoc 2016;44(3):163–4.
78. Brand MK, Slifkin R. Innovations in oral health education and practice. J Calif Dent Assoc 2016;44(3):165–6.
79. Hummel J, Phillips KE. A population health management approach to oral health. J Calif Dent Assoc 2016;44(3):167–72.
80. Clark MB, Douglass AB, Maier R, et al. Smiles for Life: A National Oral Health Curriculum. 3rd Edition. Leawood, KS: Society of Teachers of Family Medicine; 2010. Available at: www.smilesforlifeoralhealth.com.
81. National Network for Oral Health Access. A user's guide for implementation of interprofessional oral health core clinical competencies: results of a pilot project. Denver (CO): National Network for Oral Health Access; 2015. Available

at: http://www.nnoha.org/nnoha-content/uploads/2015/01/IPOHCCC-Users-Guide-Final_01-23-2015.pdf. Accessed April 24, 2016.

82. Health Resources and Services Administration. Integration of oral health and primary care practice. Rockville (MD): US Department of Health and Human Services Health Resources and Services Administration; 2014. Available at: http://www.hrsa.gov/publichealth/clinical/oralhealth/primarycare/integrationof oralhealth.pdf. Accessed April 24, 2016.

83. Haber J, Hartnett E, Allen K, et al. Putting the mouth back in the head: HEENT to HEENOT. Am J Public Health 2015;105(3):437–41.

84. Dolce MC, Aghazadeh-Sanai N, Mohammed S, et al. Integrating oral health into the interdisciplinary health sciences curriculum. Dent Clin North Am 2014;58: 829–43.

85. Doris JM, Davis E, DuPont C, et al. Social work in dentistry: the CARES model for improving patient retention and access to care. Dent Clin North Am 2009;53: 549–59.

86. Cohen LA. The role of non-dental health professionals in providing access to dental care for low-income and minority patients. Dent Clin North Am 2009;53: 451–68.

87. Gehshan S, Snyder A. Why public policy matters in improving access to dental care. Dent Clin North Am 2009;53:573–89.

88. Colvard MD. Dentistry's role in disaster response: preface. Dent Clin North Am 2007;52(4):xv–xvii.

89. Sweet D. Why a dentist for identification? Dent Clin North Am 2001;45:237–51.

90. Younai FS. Health care-associated transmission of hepatitis B and C viruses in dental care (dentistry). Clin Liver Dis 2010;14:93–104.

91. Shetty V, Marshall GN. Collaborative care of the facial injury patient. Oral Maxillofacial Surg Clin North Am 2010;22(2):iii–xii, 209–282.

92. Epstein JB, Parker IR, Epstein MS, et al. A survey of National Cancer Institute-designated comprehensive cancer centers' oral health supportive care practices and resources in the USA. Support Care Cancer 2007;15(4):357–62.

93. Crissinger ME, Marchionda KM, Dunlap ME. Adherence to clinical guidelines in heart failure (HF) outpatients: Impact of an interprofessional HF team on evidence-based medication use. J Interprof Care 2015;29(5):483–7.

94. Southerland JH, Webster-Cyriaque J, Bednarsh H. Interprofessional collaborative Practice models in Chronic Disease management. Dent Clin North Am 2016;60(4):789–809.

95. Gordon S, Donoff RB. Problems and Solutions for Interprofessional Education in North American Dental Schools. Dent Clin North Am 2016;60(4):765–87.

96. Shaefer J, Barreveld AM, Arnstein P, et al. Interprofessional education for the dentist in managing acute and chronic pain. Dent Clin North Am 2016;60(4): 825–42.

97. Glassman P, Harrington M, Namakian M, et al. Interprofessional collaboration in improving oral health for special populations. Dent Clin North Am 2016;60(4): 843–55.

98. Farmer-Dixon C, Thompson M, Young D, et al. Interprofessional collaborative practice: an oral health paradigm for women. Dent Clin North Am 2016;60(4): 857–77.

99. Kaufman LB, Henshaw MM, Brown BP, et al. Oral health and interprofessional collaborative practice: Examples of the team approach to geriatric care. Dent Clin North Am 2016;60(4):879–90.

100. Russell SL, More F. Addressing health disparities via coordination of care and interprofessional education: Lesbian, gay, bisexual, and transgender health and oral health care. Dent Clin North Am 2016;60(4):891–906.

101. Colvard MD, Vesper BJ, Kaste LM, et al. The evolving role of dental responders on interprofessional emergency response teams. Dent Clin North Am 2016; 60(4):907–20.

102. Meyer DM, Kaste LM, Lituri KM, et al. Policy development fosters collaborative practice: the example of the minamata convention on mercury. Dent Clin North Am 2016;60(4):921–42.

103. Regier DS, Hart TC. Genetics: The future is now with interprofessional collaboration. Dent Clin North Am 2016;60(4):943–9.

104. Deranian HM. The transformation of the American Association of Oral Surgeons into the American Association of Oral and Plastic Surgeons. J Hist Dent 2008; 56(2):79–86.

105. Institute of Medicine. Report of a conference: educating for the health team. Washington, DC: National Academy of Sciences; 1972. Available at: https://nexusipe-resource-exchange.s3.amazonaws.com/Educating_for_the_Health_Team_IOM_1972.pdf. Accessed May 20, 2016.

106. Institute of Medicine (U.S.). Healthy People: The Surgeon General's Report on Health Promotion and Disease Prevention: Background Papers : Report to the Surgeon General on Health Promotion and Disease Prevention. Healthy People: The Surgeon General's Report on Health Promotion and Disease Prevention. 1979. DHEW (PHC) Publication No. 79-55071. Washington, D.C.: U.S. Government Printing Office. Available at: https://profiles.nlm.nih.gov/ps/access/NNBBGK.pdf. Accessed August 15, 2016.

107. The Face of a Child: Surgeon General's Workshop and Conference on Children and Oral Health proceedings. 2000. Available at: http://www.nidcr.nih.gov/DataStatistics/SurgeonGeneral/Conference/ConferenceChildrenOralHealth/Documents/SGR_Conf_Proc.pdf. Accessed May 20, 2016.

108. Office of the Surgeon General (US). Bone Health and Osteoporosis: a report of the Surgeon General. Rockville (MD): Office of the Surgeon General (US); 2004. Available at: http://www.ncbi.nlm.nih.gov/books/NBK45513/?report=reader#!po=25.0000. Accessed May 13, 2016.

109. IOM (Institute of Medicine). The U.S. oral health workforce in the coming decade: workshop summary. Washington, DC: The National Academies Press; 2009.

110. Valachovic RW. Getting in step with interprofessional education. ADEA Charting Progress 2012. Available at: http://www.adea.org/uploadedFiles/ADEA/Content_Conversion_Final/about_adea/ADEA_CP_May_2012.pdf. Accessed May 20, 2016.

111. IOM (Institute of Medicine). The health of lesbian, gay, bisexual, and transgender people: building a foundation for better understanding. Washington, DC: The National Academies Press; 2011. Available at: http://www.nationalacademies.org/hmd/Reports/2011/The-Health-of-Lesbian-Gay-Bisexual-and-Transgender-People.aspx#sthash.9OreiG4k.dpuf. Accessed May 20, 2016.

112. Hummel J, Phillips KE, Holt B, et al. Oral health: an essential component of primary care. Seattle (WA): Qualis Health; 2015. Available at: http://www.safetynetmedicalhome.org/sites/default/files/White-Paper-Oral-Health-Primary-Care.pdf. Accessed May 18, 2016.

113. Dowell D, Haegerich TM, Chou R. CDC guideline for prescribing opioids for chronic pain - United States, 2016. MMWR Recomm Rep 2016;65(1):1–49.

Available at: http://www.cdc.gov/mmwr/volumes/65/rr/rr6501e1.htm. Accessed May 20, 2016.

114. US Department of Health and Human Services Oral Health Coordinating Committee. U.S. Department of Health and Human Services Oral Health Strategic Framework, 2014–2017. Public Health Rep 2016;131:242–57. Available at: http://www.publichealthreports.org/issueopen.cfm?articleID=3498. Accessed May 20, 2016.

115. Ring ME. Dental writings in a medical self-help book of 1650. J Hist Dent 2004; 52(3):125–9.

116. Coggeshall LT. Planning for Medical Progress through Education: A Report submitted to the Executive Council of the Association of American Medical Colleges. Evanston (IL): Association of American Medical Colleges; 1965.

117. Joskow RW. Integrating oral health and primary care: federal initiatives to drive systems change. Dent Clin N Am 2016;60(4):951–68.

Interprofessional Collaborative Practice Models in Chronic Disease Management

Janet H. Southerland, DDS, MPH, PhD[a],*,
Jennifer Webster-Cyriaque, DDS, PhD[b],
Helene Bednarsh, BS, RDH, MPH[c], Charles P. Mouton, MD, MS[d]

KEYWORDS

- Chronic disease • Health care reform • Interprofessional relations • Oral health
- Cooperative behavior • Mouth disease • Patient-centered care • Primary health care

KEY POINTS

- Collaborative models of care have been effective in improving health outcomes for those with chronic illness.
- Oral disease can impact development and progression of chronic disease.
- Interdisciplinary teams that include dental providers could further enhance oral and overall health outcomes for patients with chronic disease.

INTRODUCTION
History of Collaborative Practice in Chronic Disease Management

Chronic diseases affect a significant number of individuals nationally and internationally. A global report of the devastation of chronic disease on world health and economies by the World Health Organization entitled "Preventing Chronic Disease a vital investment", presented a goal in 2005 to reduce death rates by 2% over 10 years and anticipated that this would lead to prevention of 36 million chronic disease deaths by 2015.[1] In addition to the mortality associated with chronic disease experience, the aging of the population

[a] Department of Oral and Maxillofacial Surgery, Meharry Medical College, School of Medicine, 1005 Dr. D.B. Todd Jr. Boulevard, Nashville, TN 37208, USA; [b] Department of Dental Ecology, UNC School of Dentistry, 4506 Koury Oral Health Sciences Building, CB#7455, Chapel Hill, NC 27599, USA; [c] HASD/HIV Dental Program, Boston Public Health Commission, 1010 Massachusetts Avenue, Boston, MA 02118, USA; [d] Department of Family and Community Medicine, Meharry Medical College, School of Medicine, 1005 Dr. D.B. Todd Jr. Boulevard, Nashville, TN 37208, USA
* Corresponding author.
E-mail address: jsoutherland@mmc.edu

and development of chronic diseases that affect multiple systems have contributed significantly to disability in the population. Projections are that by year 2050 the number of individuals over 60 years of age in the world will double from 12.3% to over 20%.[2] The Centers for Disease Control and Prevention (CDC) suggests that about 117 million people had one or more chronic health conditions in 2012 and one of 4 adults had 2 or more chronic health conditions.[3] Seven of the top causes of death in 2013 were attributed to chronic diseases, such as heart disease and cancer, which together were responsible for nearly 65% of all deaths.[4] In 2001, the Institute of Medicine released a report "Crossing the Quality Chasm: A New Health System for the 21st Century" that described a disconnect between health care knowledge and practice.[5] Bringing together members of the health care team to coordinate care through reorganization of care delivery and utilization of improved systems of communication using clinical information systems, such as the electronic health record, seem to be significant components needed for improvement and management of chronic disease outcomes. Previously in 2000, the US Office of the Surgeon General released a report on the state of oral health and disparities in the nation.[6] As such, numerous studies that have documented oral health disparities across life cycles and the connection between poor oral health and progression of systemic disease have been documented.[7–9] Studies have indicated a relationship between severe periodontal disease or gum disease and worsening/progression in cardiovascular disease (CVD), end-stage renal disease, diabetes, pulmonary infections, human immunodeficiency virus (HIV)/AIDS, and numerous other disorders.[10–14] Oral health is recognized as an important part of overall health and well-being but is often overlooked as an important component of many interprofessional collaborative models of care.

The purpose of this article is to examine established models of interprofessional collaborative practice in the management of chronic diseases. Collaborative models of care specifically as they relate to diabetes, CVD, HIV/AIDS, and mental health are described. There are still significant challenges bringing all of the members of the health care team together leveraging adequate opportunities for communication and decision-making. Going forward, future models of care must require that the oral health care provider take a more prominent position in helping to develop strategies for chronic disease management.

Established Models of Chronic Disease Management in Medicine

Chronic care model

The most well-known and accepted model in chronic disease management is the Chronic Care Model (CCM).[15] The intent of the CCM was to transform the daily care for patients with chronic illnesses from acute and reactive to proactive, planned, and population based. An expanded version of the model has also been proposed that adds 3 additional strategies that includes patient safety, care coordination, and case management (**Boxes 1** and **2**).[16]

The CCM provided the framework for how we could approach morbidity in chronic disease management. Although it helped to improve health outcomes, the changes initially were small with many barriers identified. Specifically, there were definite challenges with organizational transformation of health care due to lack of specificity.[17] Since its inception, the CCM has been used to guide national quality improvement initiatives involving groups of primary care practices, such as the Health Disparities Collaborative (HDC) established by the Health Resources and Services Administration's (HRSA) Bureau of Primary Health Care. In addition to state-based and regional efforts, the CCM has been used in working with a significant number of physician practices in the United States and internationally.[18] The CCM is also an integral part of existing patient-centered medical home models. The model has also been

---

Box 1
Chronic care model

Organization of patient care

Formation of community linkages

Encouragement of patient self-management support

Maximize delivery system design

Provision of patient decision support

Improvement of patient sharing systems

Data from Wagner EH. Chronic disease management: what will it take to improve care for chronic illness? Eff Clin Pract 1998;1(1):2–4.

---

incorporated into several national initiatives aimed at minimizing disease progression and improving patient outcomes along with the Institute for Healthcare Improvement. The HDC relies on data and public health partnering to improve chronic disease care by improving health care delivery systems.[19,20]

Medical and dental home

The Medical and Dental Home Model represents innovation and opportunity to not only positively impact health outcomes but to also incorporate oral health into collaborative interdisciplinary practice.[20] Over the years, the American Academy of Pediatrics (AAP), the World Health Organization, the Institute of Medicine, the American Academy of Family Physicians (AAFP), Dr Edward Wagner (director of the W.A. MacColl Institute for Healthcare Innovation at the Center for Health Studies in Seattle), and others have honed this medical/health home model, expanding its scope and placing more emphasis on adults with chronic conditions.[21,22] In 2007, the AAFP, the AAP, the American College of Physicians, and the American Osteopathic Association issued principles defining their vision of a patient-centered medical home.[23] Also, other organizations along with health insurance purchasers created the Patient-Centered

---

Box 2
Expanded chronic care model

Organization of patient care

Formation of community linkages

Encouragement of patient self-management support

Maximize delivery system design

Provision of patient decision support

Improve of patient sharing systems

Patient safety

Care coordination

Case management

Data from Tsiachristas A, Hipple-Walters B, Lemmens KM, et al. Towards integrated care for chronic conditions: Dutch policy developments to overcome the (financial) barriers. Health Policy 2011;101:122–32.

Primary Care Collaborative to advocate for widespread implementation of the medical home model.[24] The core features include a physician-directed medical practice; a personal doctor for every patient; the capacity to coordinate high-quality, accessible care; and payments that recognize the medical home's added value for patients. The model has not been as widely disseminated currently; in most clinical practices in the United States it is unavailable, although it is more of a reality in many other industrialized countries.[25,26]

The Patient-Centered Medical-Dental Home (PCM-DH) has also been proposed. This model is an extension of the primary care medical home to include oral care. The goal of PCM-DH ensures patients have a personal physician or dentist who leads a team of clinical care providers and staff who take collective responsibility for delivering comprehensive, coordinated care that addresses all of a patient's health care needs including dental.[20] A more complete concept of the model has been further suggested by Northridge and colleagues[27] that identifies the model as the health home.

Interdisciplinary Collaborative Models for Chronic Disease

It is reported that nearly half of the US health care expenditure is incurred for the treatment of just 5 chronic conditions, namely, mood disorders, diabetes, heart disease, asthma, and hypertension.[28] The increasing prevalence, health burden, and cost of chronic diseases have increased interest in innovative care models that are able to incorporate community-based care and information technology into models to improve disease prevention, diagnosis, and treatment, particularly diseases that are multi-morbid.[28] Among chronic diseases that impact health outcomes, oral infection and inflammation are often overlooked, even though dental caries and periodontitis represent the first and sixth most prevalent global diseases.[29] Oral conditions have increased in prevalence because of significant population growth and aging. Oral diseases are largely preventable bacterial infections, opportunistic or viral in nature, and have reached epidemic proportions, particularly in underserved populations and countries. There are key reasons that oral health inequalities exist and are thought to contribute to poor health outcomes; these include gaps in knowledge and an insufficient focus on social policy, the separation of oral health from general health, and inadequate evidence-based data.[30]

Collaborative care models that involve patient-centered as well as community-based preventive interventions and include oral health, have the ability to increase access to care, improve health outcomes, and reduce the burden of disease and the costs of care for those living with chronic disease.[31] Additionally, the attention to how oral health may contribute to better overall health outcomes should be evaluated and made a part of innovation in chronic disease care management. The bidirectional impact of oral and systemic health has been extensively reported in the literature suggesting oral health has significant influence on quality of life and disease progression in those who are most vulnerable in the population.[32] Understanding this relationship and development of models that will accommodate oral health outcomes as a measure of improvement in management of chronic diseases will be important to improved overall health outcomes in this group.

The following models describe an interprofessional paradigm to manage chronic illnesses, some of which include an oral health perspective.

Diabetes collaborative models

Diabetes is the seventh leading cause of death based on US death certificates in 2010.[33] The division of Diabetes Translation at the CDC and HRSA have worked collaboratively since 1999 to provide guidance on management and treatment of diabetes. This chronic disease has reached epidemic proportions affecting more than 29.1 million, representing 9.3% of the population. Approximately 8.1 million individuals with diabetes are undiagnosed. Globally, 387 million individuals are thought to have diabetes.[34,35] Several large randomized controlled trials nationally and internationally have confirmed that lifestyle interventions can be successful in reducing the incidence of diabetes from 29% to 58% in populations with the highest risk and good maintenance for up to 20 years.[36,37]

Major complications and comorbid illnesses result from diabetes, including blindness and vision problems, nervous system disorders, kidney disease, amputations, periodontal disease, heart disease, stroke, and oral health disparities, that is, periodontal disease.[38] With respect to periodontal disease, our current understanding of the relationship between diabetes and periodontal disease is based on epidemiologic studies that have clearly observed that diabetes is a major risk factor for periodontitis, increasing the risk approximately 3-fold compared with nondiabetic individuals with poor glycemic control.[39] A report from a consensus workshop on periodontitis and systemic disease, indicates that severe periodontitis adversely affects blood glucose levels expressed as hemoglobin A1c (HbA1c) in individuals with and without diabetes.[40] Also, moderate to severe periodontitis is associated with an increased risk for the development of diabetes.[40] A recent Danish study sought to identify individuals presenting for dental care with undiagnosed diabetes or prediabetes. Participants had no history of diabetes and were placed in 2 groups: those with periodontal disease and those without. HbA1c levels were also measured at baseline. Investigators found that more patients with undiagnosed diabetes and prediabetes were observed in the periodontitis group than in the control group with 32.7% versus 17.4%, $P>.054$, respectively. The investigators concluded that routine evaluation of HbA1c in dental offices may help identify individuals with diabetes and prediabetes at early stages of disease and could potentially prevent future diabetes complications.[41]

The report discussed earlier suggests recommendations for not only dental providers managing oral health for those with diabetes but also guidelines for physicians and individuals with diabetes/patients, *thereby suggesting the need for an interprofessional collaborative (IPC) practice approach*. The complex nature of diabetes prevention requires a multidisciplinary approach because diabetes affects all organ systems. Prevention/treatment strategies require collaboration among many health care professionals, especially those in oral health disciplines. Physicians and other health professionals, however, do not receive adequate training in oral health and do not feel comfortable performing periodontal examinations or advising patients on their oral health care needs.[42,43] A survey by Kunzel and colleagues[44] showed that similar to the medical counterparts, general dentists did not think that they had mastery of the knowledge or behavioral areas involved in management of patients with diabetes and viewed these activities as peripheral and did not think that their colleagues or patients expected them to perform such assessment activities. The need for team care for people with diabetes that include dental professionals as well as other health care providers is essential to improve outcomes for those with this chronic illness.

An innovative example of a model that includes dental and other health care professionals, such as pharmacists, podiatrists, and optometrists, has already been implemented by the National Diabetes Education Program (NDEP).[45] The program is a joint effort of the CDC and the National Institutes of Health (NIH). The NDEP work group of pharmacists, podiatrists, optometrists, and dentists (PPOD) exist under the umbrella and has more than 200 public and private partners from multiple sectors that encompass public health, health systems, community programs especially targeting populations with a large burden of diabetes. The group is involved in the development and dissemination of evidence-based, focused, group-tested materials that include diabetes control and prevention messages.[46] The NDEP has produced several resources, particularly the PPOD Primer tool. The tool is written for the other providers to read and educates each provider about the role that other professions play on the diabetes care team. Emphasis is placed on the importance of conducting routine examinations for complication prevention, recognizing danger signs, making recommendations regarding referrals, reinforcing among patients the need for self-examinations, and, of course, the importance of metabolic control. The goal of the PPOD Primer tool is to provide consistent messages across the disciplines and to encourage collaboration and a team approach in the caring for people with diabetes.[45,47] The International Diabetes Federation's (IDF) "IDF Guideline on Oral Health for People with Diabetes" is another good example of a collaborative model that recommends that diabetes care providers incorporate oral health into diabetes education and refer patients to dental health professionals annually for oral health care.[48] The Building Community Supports for Diabetes Care program of the Robert Wood Johnson Foundation Diabetes Initiative works through clinic-community partnerships. Several projects demonstrate how various clinic-community partnerships promote diabetes self-management better than any organization could do so alone.[49] This diabetes initiative was able to demonstrate that effective self-management programs and supports can be implemented in clinical and community settings.[50] This model could easily integrate oral health care as a component. Provision of training for oral self-examination and educational materials designed to provide information on the relationship to diabetes and dental infection would greatly enhance the benefits communities receive to improve the health of patients who have diabetes.

Cardiovascular collaborative models
CVD is one of the leading causes of morbidity and mortality in the United States. The chronicity of CVD requires an interdisciplinary team to address the care of patients over a range of practice settings, including inpatient, outpatient, inner city, rural, and suburban.[51,52] This interdisciplinary approach to the care of individuals with CVD has several advantages versus traditional models of care. Advantages of interprofessional team care exist for patients and providers. For patients, interprofessional teams improve care by increasing the coordination of services; integrating health care for a wide range of health needs; empowering patient/clients as active partners in care; orienting to serving patients of diverse cultural backgrounds; and allowing for more efficient use of time between patients and providers.[53,54] For providers, interprofessional care increases professional satisfaction because of clearer, more consistent goals of care and facilitates a shift in emphasis from acute, episodic care to long-term preventive care and chronic illness management. The collaborative experience enables the provider to learn new skills and approaches to care, provides an environment for innovation, and allows providers to focus on individual areas of expertise. For health profession educators and health career students, interprofessional collaborative models for CVD offers multiple health care approaches to care and new models for training, fosters appreciation and understanding for other health care disciplines, demonstrates models for future practice, and breaks down outdated norms and values of a traditional discipline-centric approaches to care.[55]

Studies have shown that the aforementioned approaches have been effective in CVD management. Teams with dense interactions among all team members were associated with fewer hospital days (rate ratio [RR] = 0.62; 95% confidence interval

[CI], 0.50–0.77) and lower medical care costs (–$556; 95% CI, –$781 to –$331) for patients with CVD.[56] Teams with more members reporting daily interactions with a greater number of team members showed better quality of care, as measured by a 38% reduction in hospital days and $516 less spent on average per patient in the previous 12 months. Furthermore, results suggest that teams with more daily face-to-face interactions had a 66% reduction in urgent care visits, a 73% reduction in emergency department visits, and $594 less spent in medical costs per patient in the previous 12 months.

This finding suggests that teams that overcome the limitation around communication between team members may be the most successful in the management of CVD. Models range from small teams of primary care physicians and a pharmacist working together to optimize hypertension management to non–physician-led provider teams. Other models are broader in their approach, using a team of primary care physicians, cardiologists, nursing, pharmacists, exercise physiologists or physical therapists, and social workers to care for patients with a variety of cardiac conditions.

Although these results seem encouraging, major challenges to their success include the lack of prominence of the dental care provider in the IPC framework for CVD treatment. Periodontal and now endodontic infections have been linked to CVD, including atherosclerosis and systemic inflammation, extensively in the literature.[57–61] The incorporation of oral health care professionals in strategies to identify individuals at risk for coronary heart disease and diabetes will compliment preventive and screening efforts necessary to decrease the progression and development of these chronic illnesses and provide a portal for individuals who do not see a physician on a regular basis to gain access to the general health care system.[62] The dental practitioner sees these patients on a regular basis for oral health needs and can more readily monitor CVD status, that is, blood pressure status.[63]

Hypertension Team-based care to improve blood pressure control is a health systems-level, organizational intervention that incorporates a multidisciplinary/interprofessional team to improve the quality of hypertension care for patients. Each team should include the patients, the patients' primary care provider, and other professionals, such as nurses, dentists, pharmacists, dietitians, social workers, and community health workers. Team members provide process support and share responsibilities of hypertension care to complement the activities of the primary care provider. These responsibilities include medication management, patient follow-up, and adherence and self-management support.[64] Patients are also central to their care and supplementing their knowledge with education about hypertension medication, adherence support, and tools and resources for self-management (including health behavior changes associated with oral health). The Community Preventive Services Task Force provided recommendations for team-based care to improve blood pressure control from strong evidence of effectiveness in improving the proportion of patients with controlled blood pressure and in reducing systolic and diastolic blood pressure. Evidence was considered strong based on findings from 80 studies of team-based care organized primarily with nurses and pharmacists working in collaboration with primary care providers, patients, and other professionals.[65]

The economic evidence indicates that team-based care is cost-effective. Collaborative, team-based hypertension management interventions have shown the largest effects in blood pressure reduction in contrast with other tested interventions, such as patient education, clinician education, promotion of self-management, facilitated relay of clinical data, and financial incentives. Some of these approaches have been as simple as a primary care physician and pharmacist review of antihypertensive medication selection to optimize dosing and drug selection. Other approaches have added nursing to provide home blood pressure monitoring and medication adherence. The oral health care provider is essential to monitoring blood pressure on a regular basis with routine patient visits.[66,67]

Congenital heart disease Because of the advances in cardiac and pediatric care, greater numbers of children with congenital heart disease (CHD) are surviving into adulthood; now 85% to 90% of those born with CHD grow up to become adults.[68] With the increasing survival, there has been an increasing number of adults who require special medical management given their congenital disease. These individuals are transitioned from pediatric to adult cardiology care, and their needs are typically different from patients with adult-onset CVD. Therefore, because of the complex nature, a team approach is necessary to provide optimal care for these patients.[69] Some have suggested that the interprofessional teams for adult patients with CHD, including adult CHD specialists, adult and pediatric cardiologists and cardiovascular surgeons, specialized nurses, and other specific disciplines, are fundamental features in care facilities for adult CHD.[68] Additional support from primary care medicine, psychology, and social work is necessary but often overlooked in the description of the multidisciplinary centers caring for these adults.

Adults with CHD (ACHD) carry lifelong emotional, psychological, and financial concerns in addition to cardiac structural, electrical, and mechanical issues. An expert consensus panel suggests that a system of lifelong preventative care by a qualified health care team of providers with knowledge both of CHD and age-related systemic health issues will ensure that early warning signs of impending problems are identified and appropriate intervention is initiated.[69] The role of psychology, social work, and primary care should be considered as an additional key component of the team. This team, regardless of patients' age, should include those with the best working knowledge of structural congenital heart anatomy and physiology. Adding a broader array of health professionals beyond the typical team of a qualified, board-certified pediatric cardiologist, including any of the subspecialties (electrophysiology, catheter intervention, echocardiography), as well as a certified congenital heart surgeon, is important to providing a comprehensive and invaluable service to the management and treatment of patients of any age with CHD. This combination allows a lifelong working association to optimize care.

The usefulness of the interprofessional team approach to the care of ACHD can be seen by the development of centers for ACHD. A Resource for ACHD is the Adult Congenital Health Association (http://www.achaheart.org/). The complexity of clinical issues to be addressed within ACHD centers points directly toward establishment of clinical care teams as an ideal method to provide shared expertise to care for patients. Each team must include at least one individual who can be considered a CHD expert as well as a specialist in adult cardiology. Other personnel include surgeons, anesthesiologists, nurses and technicians, social and financial counselors, coordinators, and subspecialty physicians, particularly geneticists and obstetricians/gynecologists. A comprehensive collaborative care team can improve results for mother and child through a concerted collaborative approach that relies on a thorough understanding of patients' underlying cardiac pathology and its anticipated interaction with the pregnancy and ongoing close evaluation and communication with a team of trained and experienced specialists, including (but not limited to) cardiologists, obstetricians, anesthetists, pediatricians, clinical nurse specialists, and clinical geneticists.[70] Although data are limited, a collaborative interprofessional approach to care of ACHD has shown good outcomes. Based on information available concerning oral infection and bacterial endocarditis as well as CVDs in general, it is important that the oral health provider be considered as a valuable member.

Congestive heart failure management Congestive heart failure (HF) is one of the major chronic diseases in the United States, with more than 5.1 million people affected, and accounts for 1 in 9 deaths.[71] As part of the constellation of conditions known as heart disease, it is the number one cause of death in the United States. To meet the challenge of managing HF, multiple health professionals need to be involved; interprofessional models of care are proving to be useful. Teams consisting of several health professionals, including primary care medicine, cardiology, pharmacy, nursing, and exercise physiology, have been shown to be effective in providing quality care for patients with congestive HF. In a study of collaboration in the Veterans Affairs system to reduce HF hospitalization, a collaborative model with a primary physician and pharmacist performing medication reviews, the unadjusted results showed a 37% reduction in the rate of hospitalization for HF at any time (hazard ratio, 0.63; 95% CI, 0.44–0.89). Adjusted results showed a 45% reduction (hazard ratio, 0.55; 95% CI, 0.39–0.77) among those who had received a home medicine review. Unadjusted results showed a 37% reduction in rate of hospitalization for HF at any time (hazard ratio, 0.63; 95% CI, 0.44–0.89). Adjusted results showed a 45% reduction (hazard ratio, 0.55; 95% CI, 0.39–0.77) among those who had received home medicine reviews compared with controls.[72]

Additionally, a retrospective chart review was performed on adult patients with an ejection fraction of 40% or less and a diagnosis of congestive HF. They were seen by a single provider type (HF team, cardiologist, or primary care physician) at least twice within a 12-month period at an academic county hospital. Utilization rates of any angiotensin-converting enzyme inhibitor/angiotensin receptor blocker (ACEI/ARB) and any beta-blocker were robust across provider types, though evidence-based ACEI/ARB and beta-blocker were greatest from the HF team. Doses of evidence-based therapies decreased markedly in the non-HF team groups. The percent of patients prescribed optimal doses of an evidence-based ACEI/ARB and beta-blocker was 69%, 33%, and 25% for the HF team, cardiologists, and primary care providers, respectively ($P < .0167$).

Patients followed by the HF team were more frequently prescribed evidence-based medications at optimal doses. This finding supports using specialized interprofessional HF teams to attain greater adherence to evidence-based recommendations in treating systolic HF.[73] Finally in a study to determine whether the management of HF by specialized multidisciplinary HF disease-management programs was associated with improved outcomes, subgroup analysis of the 9 studies using specialized follow-up by a multidisciplinary team showed similar results (summary RR = 0.77; 95% CI, 0.68–0.86; test of heterogeneity, $P > .50$). Seven of the 9 studies did not show any significant association between intervention and reduced hospitalization, but the 2 studies that used follow-up by primary care physicians and telephone failed to show any significant reduction in hospitalization (summary RR = 0.94; 95% CI, 0.75–1.19). In fact, one of the studies demonstrated a higher risk of hospitalization for patients receiving intervention (RR = 1.26; 95% CI, 1.04–1.52). Of the 11 studies, only 6 reported mortality as an outcome. None of these studies found any association between intervention and mortality (summary RR = 1.15; 95% CI, 0.96–1.37; test of heterogeneity, $P > .15$).[74]

Human immunodeficiency virus/acquired immunodeficiency syndrome collaborative models

As discussed, the CCM is a widely adopted approach for ambulatory care improvement in the setting of chronic diseases like HIV. HIV disease is now a chronic illness requiring lifelong therapy. This therapy often prevents AIDS and results in rapid control of HIV viral replication but only partially restores immune function resulting in inflammation-associated and/or immunodeficiency-associated complications. HIV-infected adults with suppression of HIV replication remain at risk for progressive serious non-AIDS events that include CVD, cancer, kidney disease, liver disease, osteopenia/osteoporosis and neurocognitive disease, metabolic disturbances, and end-organ damage. This population is at greater risk than the general population of developing clinical manifestations of early aging.[75]

The need for oral health care is at least twice as prevalent as the unmet need for medical care among people living with HIV.[76,77] Within this chronically infected population, oral health is among the highest unmet need and the least federally funded.[78] In 2011, Gardner and colleagues[79] observed that "for individuals with human immunodeficiency virus (HIV) to fully benefit from potent combination antiretroviral therapy, they need to know that they are HIV infected, be engaged in regular HIV care, and receive and adhere to effective antiretroviral therapy" and based on these observations developed a treatment cascade. Optimally, the CCM for HIV occurs within the context of this "treatment cascade", a commonly used conceptual model targeted largely toward medicine that quantifies the delivery of services to persons living with HIV across the entire continuum of care.[80] Along this cascade, there are many opportunities for the oral health care team to provide appropriate interventions.

The PCM-DH represents a team-based enhanced health care model that could also work well in the setting of HIV. It has been suggested that in the setting of HIV, the health care team would be composed of the HIV/primary care provider, specialty medical care, clinical pharmacist, care coordinator, dentists, and nursing. This team would work closely with support services to ensure service delivery and integration.[80] This combination would touch on multiple elements of the CCM model: self-management support, clinical information systems, health care organization, and community resources. Optimally, patients would have a trusted relationship with their physician and dentist, each of whom leads a team of clinical care providers and staff who take collective responsibility for delivering comprehensive, coordinated care that addresses all of a patients' health care needs. Compassionate, culturally competent, comprehensive, prevention-based care is provided by both the medical and dental homes. Together this health home delivers comprehensive preventive care and broad-based multi-disease management within a multidisciplinary team-based setting. The importance of this collaboration is emphasized in the curriculum recently developed by the US Department of Health and Human Services HRSA HIV/AIDS Bureau on HIV oral health for primary care providers.[81] Information technology, promotion of an active partnership with educated patients, and coordination of care are central tenants of the PCM-DH. It has been shown by the Institute of Medicine that this infrastructure helps reinforce patients' compliance with prescribed treatments and behavioral interventions.[82]

As a part of the health care team, the oral health provider is well positioned to impact the HIV epidemic across the continuum of care. The AIDS Care Cascade begins with knowledge of HIV status. Knowledge of status is critical. It has been demonstrated that individuals who are aware of their status are less likely to engage in risky behaviors.[83] The oral health care team (OHCT) could advise individuals on the CDC's current recommendations on routine testing, conduct a salivary rapid test, or refer for testing.[84,85] The OHCT can ensure patients are linked to or retained in medical care and can inquire about adherence and compliance. Oral examination reveals oral mucosal manifestations of HIV in more than 50% of HIV-infected individuals who are not on antiretroviral therapy and in greater than 20% of those on antiretroviral therapy. These lesions may be a presenting sign of HIV infection and are often detected with lack of adherence, development of resistance, or incomplete immune reconstitution. This information is critical to the health of patients and to their health care team. Medical-dental interactions can have a significant local and potentially systemic impact within the HIV-infected individual.

The Special Project of National Significance (SPNS) Oral Health Initiative parent study, conducted by the HRSA, was intended to increase access to and promote retention in oral health for persons living with HIV through replicable and sustainable, delivery models.[86] This initiative embodied multiple elements of the CCM. The data set (N = 2469) covered 12 US states, including rural and urban districts, and one US territory.[87] Fifteen sites were located in New York, New York; San Francisco, California; Miami, Florida; New Orleans, Louisiana; Chapel Hill, North Carolina; Eugene, Oregon; US Virgin Islands; Lane County, Oregon; Norwalk, Connecticut; Hyannis, Massachusetts; Chester, Pennsylvania; Jefferson, South Carolina; Tyler, Texas; and Green Bay, Wisconsin. The sites delivered various models of oral health care in university hospital dental clinics, community health centers, private dental offices, mobile dental units, and AIDS service organizations. A recent analysis of SPNS data determined that oral intervention in chronically HIV-infected individuals could decrease oral morbidity. Among the 2178 HIV-seropositive individuals from the US-based SPNS study, chronically HIV-infected individuals were more likely to report oral problems, toothaches, tooth decay or cavities, and/or dental sensitivity in the 12 months before baseline data collection compared with newly diagnosed individuals. Chronically HIV-infected subjects were also more likely to require oral surgeries, restorative treatments, endodontic treatments, and more than 10 clinic visits as compared with newly diagnosed subjects. Subjects had worse oral health compared with newly HIV-diagnosed subjects. Overall, findings based on both self-perceived oral health and service utilization data suggested that oral health care delivery within the first year of HIV diagnosis may protect HIV-positive individuals from declining oral health as one moves to chronic infection (R Burger-Calderon, JS Smith, K Ramsey, J Webster-Cyriaque. SPNS Innovations in Oral Health Care Initiative Team, Oral Health Outcomes in Relation to Time Since HIV Diagnosis: The Potential Impact of Early Oral Care. 2016, unpublished).

Interactions at the University of North Carolina, Chapel Hill site incorporated several CCM principles. The team included infectious disease experts, dentists, a dental case manager/hygienist, and community partners. The dental case manager/hygienist worked closely with social workers and nurses to coordinate dental care and appointments with medical care clinical case management to ensure regular follow-up by the care team. Electronic patient records accessible to both the treating physicians and dentists meant that clinical information systems were available to ensure ready access to patient data. Aggressive patient education about oral manifestations of HIV and oral hygiene facilitated effective self-management support for patients. Provider education on oral health and HIV/AIDS oral manifestations through Area Health Education and local community health care centers facilitated building partnerships with community programs to promote referral for comprehensive dental care and allowing for the building of medical-dental homes. At baseline, subjects received comprehensive examination and treatment plan. Participants were seen at least every 6 months for dental prophylaxis/debridement, oral HIV education, and oral self-care instruction; information was collected including periodontal metrics. Comprehensive dental care included dental prophylaxis at least every 6 months, scaling and root planing, oral hygiene instruction, extractions, and restorative and prosthetic dental treatment. Although at baseline periodontal inflammation was prevalent regardless of antiretroviral therapy status, the intervention resulted in improved oral and systemic health outcomes. In virologically suppressed subjects, the intervention decreased periodontitis with concomitant interleukin 6 decrease and CD4 increase. These findings suggest a relationship between periodontal inflammation, oral microbial translocation, and HIV status.[88] Recognizing that the control of oral infection and inflammation is critical to the HIV chronic disease model, collaboration between medical and dental professionals is important to achieve the goals of increasing access to care, reducing new infections, and most importantly improving health outcomes.[89]

Mental health collaborative models

Interprofessional care is useful in mental health because of its capacity to provide and coordinate a variety of responses to individuals with complex health and social care needs.[90] Health care providers, such as psychologists, mental health nurses, pharmacists, occupational therapists, social workers, and case managers, play increasingly important roles in the delivery of mental health services.[91] As part of the National Mental Health Strategy developed by the Commonwealth of Australia, the National Standards for Mental Health Services in Australia provide guiding principles to mental health service providers on the delivery of services, treatment, care, and support to mental health consumers.[91]

In the United States, interprofessional collaboration has been used to manage a variety of mental health disorders. In the mental health setting, interprofessional collaboration was perceived to facilitate shared decision-making by addressing time barriers and providing more opportunities for patients to discuss their medical-related concerns. Some health care providers also perceived that mental health patients may be more comfortable in discussing certain treatment concerns with nonmedical providers (such as pharmacists) compared with their medical practitioners. Examples of interprofessional collaborative care for alcohol/substance abuse, schizophrenia/psychosis, and dementia is provided next.

Alcohol/substance abuse In the area of alcohol and substance abuse, there are currently several approaches to collaborative interdisciplinary education, practice, and/or research referred to as *interdisciplinary collaborative addiction education* (ICAE). The ICAE movement is still in the early stages of development. The Substance Abuse and Mental Health Service Administration (SAMHSA) is facilitating the evaluation and adoption of the best of these practices through various grant programs. These programs have focused on teams of trained health professionals from medicine (particularly primary care, psychiatry, and emergency medicine), nursing, psychology, pharmacology, and social work.[92] Community health centers have also become a major location of care. These community settings use a variety of health care professionals (eg, advanced practice nurses, physicians, dentists, social workers, counselors, and pharmacists). The patient population in these settings is largely underserved, disenfranchised, and of low income. They commonly present with chronic social and health-related problems. Providing effective quality care for these patients is a constant challenge for health professionals, and team support is a key factor in maintaining workplace harmony and satisfaction for team members.[92] As mentioned, to promote collaboration in alcohol and substance abuse, the SAMHSA has awarded grants to promote the Screening, Brief Intervention, and Referral for Treatment (SBIRT) approach with adults in primary and community health settings to intercede in the problem of alcohol and substance abuse as early as possible.

The promotion of ICAE initiatives is essential for implementing SBIRT in individuals with potential or actual alcohol and other drug abuse problems. Interprofessional collaboration in addictions has the promise of using team models to implement SBIRT as appropriate depending on the professional role. At the University of Pittsburgh, SBIRT uses collaborative groups by impacting risks associated with substance abuse, which is an ideal health issue for interprofessional collaborative practice because substance abuse is an individual patient and overall community health concern.[93] Bringing together the health disciplines in collaborative practice helps to deconstruct stereotypes associated with substance use and facilitates linkages between fragmented health care sectors.

Schizophrenia/psychosis Psychotic disorder, one of the most debilitating mental conditions, requires a coordinated approach to provide the best outcomes of care. The ability to find effective methods to involve a variety of health care disciplines in the clinical decision-making processes for the management of psychotic disorders can improve care and yield benefits for patients.[94] An interprofessional approach that involves the collaborative efforts of psychiatry and pharmacy services can be vital in achieving positive therapeutic outcomes within an inpatient care setting.[95] The collaboration between psychiatrists and pharmacists in the inpatient psychiatric setting has the potential to reduce the incidences of polypharmacy and lead to effective patient care as a result of (1) obtaining an accurate medication and physical history, (2) linking each prescribed medication to the psychiatric condition, (3) identifying medications that are being used to treat side effects, (4) initiating interventions to ensure medication compliance or adherence, and (5) prevention by regularly considering the appropriateness of the medication for the condition.[96] Additionally, the side effects of many antipsychotic medications result in development of a dry mouth or xerostomia that could lead to severe dental caries. The inclusion of an oral health care provider to this team could help to significantly improve oral health outcomes as well as overall health and well-being.

Dementia The management of patients with dementia requires a multifaceted approach as well as multi-professional collaboration of key health care disciplines to ensure a high-quality outcome for this devastating and debilitating disease.[97] The ability to achieve a positive therapeutic outcome with patients with dementia generally involves the active participation of multiple disciplines given the complex and progressive nature of dementia. The quality of individualized treatment revolves around the interprofessional relationship that exists among the disciplines of psychiatry, pharmacy, and psychology with geriatrics/primary care medicine and nursing as it relates to the management of the observable behavioral and psychological disturbances of the disorder. Again, patients with dementia may lack the ability to effectively maintain adequate oral hygiene and access routine dental care. It is important that an oral health provider is knowledgeable and skilled in caring for the special needs population, including those with mental health challenges.

Cancer
Care of patients with cancer has a long-standing tradition of collaborative practice, particularly across multiple subspecialties in medicine. Tumor boards (or cancer committees) that bring together health professionals from a broad a range of medical professions have been the standard of care for patients with cancer for 4 decades.[98] More recently, these models have incorporated dental, nursing, pharmacology, and social work professionals to bring their professional expertise to cancer care. Collaborative research across multiple clinical centers has been the mainstay of improvements in cancer treatment with the Cooperative Group Program (Eastern Cooperative Oncology Group, the Southwest Oncology Group, and so forth) that has now evolved

into the National Clinical Trials Network, providing many of the latest advances in chemotherapy protocols for patients with cancer. Even surveillance of cancer survival has involved a collaborative process through Surveillance, Epidemiology, and End Results programs.

Thus, cancer treatment has had a long-standing history of a collaborative approach to care of patients with cancer. However, this approach has been relatively slow to incorporate other health professionals outside of medicine. More than 55% of the National Cancer Institute (NCI)–designated comprehensive centers (the high level of designation for cancer treatment) did not have a dental program. At these centers, two-thirds of patients with head and neck cancer had a dental evaluation with oral assessment before receiving radiation therapy.[99] None of the centers in this survey of NCI-designated cancer centers had standard protocols in place for preventive dental care to prevent oral complications from cancer treatment.[99]

In a study to evaluate the effect of the intensity of interprofessional collaboration on hospitalized patients with cancer, the analysis revealed the existence of significant differences between patients who are cared for by teams operating with a high intensity of collaboration and those who are cared for by teams operating with a low intensity of collaboration, as measured by the mean satisfaction ($P<.001$) among a specific group of patients (patients who have a high level of education and perceive their state of health as poor), mean uncertainty ($P = .047$), and adequacy of pain management ($P = .047$). The analysis also found no significant difference ($P = .217$) in their length of hospital stay.[100]

Despite the deliberate pace of progress, education and training for health professionals caring for patients with cancer has led to collaborative models for training health professionals. Building on the Interprofessional Education Collaborative Expert Panel's recommendations, oral health has been used as one exemplar of interprofessional cancer education.[101,102] Also, the Transforming HEENT to HEENOT program at New York University has incorporated oral cancer screening and oral assessment into nurse practitioner, physician, physician assistant, and nurse-midwife training.[101]

In another example, the National Center for Integrative Primary Healthcare was launched as a collaboration between the University of Arizona Center for Integrative Medicine and the Academic Consortium for Integrative Health and Medicine to develop a core set of integrative health care competencies and educational programs that embraces interprofessional primary care training and practice, has become a required part of primary care education. As part of this program, primary care screening and management of patients with cancer is part of the core competencies. The program has developed a shared set of 10 "meta-competencies" involving a diverse interprofessional team. Team members represent nursing, the primary care medicine professions, pharmacy, public health, acupuncture, naturopathy, chiropractic, nutrition, and behavioral medicine.[103] Also, the University of Massachusetts Medical School implemented the Cancer Prevention and Control Education initiative, an interdisciplinary curriculum focusing on behavioral and psychosocial aspects of cancer prevention, control, and research. This curriculum uses an interdisciplinary operations committee that developed courses, clerkships, and programs. Each education program stressed the team approach. The evaluation of this curriculum demonstrates its potential for shaping a collaborative attitude among health care providers.[104]

Models of interprofessional education have also extended to various service learning activities for health care profession students. The University of Texas at San Antonio has developed an interprofessional care program for refugees in the San Antonio area. The use of this interprofessional model has resulted in holistic and accessible health care for the refugees in San Antonio. Patients receive complimentary comprehensive care, and students benefit from development of cultural competence reinforcement of humanitarian values. As the dental students reflected, "We started attending the clinic as a service learning project. We then became their advocates, treated them at our dental school, and became knowledgeable about our community's dental clinics while offering tailored referrals."[105]

Discussion/Future Direction

The collaborative models that involve patient-centered as well as community-based preventive interventions have the ability to increase access to care, improve health outcomes, and reduce the burden of disease and the cost of care for those living with chronic disease, "a perfect storm" for the Triple Aim of Berwick.[106] Understanding of this relationship and development of interprofessional models that will accommodate oral health outcomes as a measure of improvement in management of chronic disease will be important to improved overall health outcomes in this group of patients. As stated earlier, challenges exist that have impeded integration of oral health into team-based models of care, keeping this concept from being fully implemented. In order to improve integration of oral health care into chronic disease management models, there will need to be continued growth and development in reorganization of health care systems as well as reimbursement systems that cover oral screening or preventive serves for other nondental providers and electronic records that allow access for all health providers. Using a combination of these approaches, some groups have been able to innovate and demonstrate improvement using a variety of theories and models and advances in technology aimed at chronic diseases that are most devastating and debilitating among citizens nationally and globally. Although there has been implementation of models and systems that will enhance the collaborative model and interdisciplinary practice, there are still significant challenges in bringing all of the members of the health care team together leveraging adequate opportunities for communication and decision-making. Additionally, the attention to how oral health may contribute to better overall health outcomes should be evaluated and made a part of innovation in chronic disease management.

The challenges discussed earlier only muddy the waters because the health care system is a very confusing and complex entity that has not adequately addressed the needs of those who are chronically ill. In order to reverse this trend, we all must learn to embrace models that address all facets of health care, all members of the health care team, and technology that will facilitate better communication and more effective and efficient management for those who fall into this group of patients. Additionally, the oral health care provider must take a more prominent place in model evolution for chronic disease management. Inclusion will inevitably bring about a more comprehensive approach and better disease outcomes.

REFERENCES

1. World Health Organization. Preventing chronic diseases: a vital investment. Geneva (Switzerland): WHO Press; 2005. Available at: http://www.who.int/chp/chronic_disease_report/full_report.pdf. Accessed March 27, 2016.

2. United Nations, Department of economic and social affairs, population division. World Population Ageing. 2015. Available at: Esa.un.org/unpd/popdev/Profilesofaging/index.html. Accessed March 27, 2016.

3. Ward BW, Schiller JS, Goodman RA. Multiple chronic conditions among US adults: a 2012 update. Prev Chronic Dis 2014;11:E62.

4. Xu J, Murphy SL, Koschanek KD, et al. Deaths: final data for 2013. Natl Vital Stat Rep 2016;64(2):1–119. Available at: http://www.cdc.gov/nchs/nvsr/nvsr64/nvsr64_02.pdf. Accessed March 27, 2016.

5. Committee on Quality of Health Care in America, Institute of Medicine. Crossing the quality chasm: new health system for the 21st century. Washington, DC: National Academies Press; 2001.

6. US Department of Health and Human Services. Oral health in America: a report of the surgeon general. Rockville (MD): US Department of Health and Human Services; National Institute of Dental and Craniofacial Research; National Institutes of Health; 2000.

7. Sharma P, Dietrich T, Ferro CJ, et al. Association between periodontitis and mortality in stages 3-5 chronic kidney disease: NHANES III and linked mortality study. J Clin Periodontol 2015;43(2):104–13.

8. Madianos PN, Bobetsis YA, Offenbacher S. Adverse pregnancy outcomes (APOs) and periodontal disease: pathogenic mechanisms. J Periodontol 2013;84(4 Suppl):S170–80.

9. Southerland JH, Taylor GW, Moss K, et al. Commonality in chronic inflammatory diseases: periodontitis, diabetes, and coronary artery disease. Periodontol 2000 2006;40:130–43.

10. Southerland JH, Moss K, Taylor GW, et al. Periodontitis and diabetes associations with measures of atherosclerosis and CHD. Atherosclerosis 2012;222(1):196–201.

11. Ariyamuthu VK, Nolph KD, Ringdahl BE. Periodontal disease in chronic kidney disease and end-stage renal disease patients: a review. Cardiorenal Med 2013;3(1):71–8.

12. Tsai C, Hayes C, Taylor GW. Glycemic control of type 2 diabetes and severe periodontal disease in the US adult population. Community Dent Oral Epidemiol 2002;30(3):82–92.

13. Shen TC, Chang PY, Lin CL, et al. Risk of periodontal diseases in patients with chronic obstructive pulmonary disease: a nationwide population-based cohort study. Medicine (Baltimore) 2015;94(46):e2047.

14. Salas JT, Chang TL. Microbiome in human immunodeficiency virus infection. Clin Lab Med 2014;34(4):733–45.

15. Wagner EH. Chronic disease management: what will it take to improve care for chronic illness? Eff Clin Pract 1998;1(1):2–4.

16. Tsiachristas A, Hipple-Walters B, Lemmens KM, et al. Towards integrated care for chronic conditions: Dutch policy developments to overcome the (financial) barriers. Health Policy 2011;101:122–32.

17. Hroscikoski MC, Solberg LI, Sperl-Hillen JM, et al. Challenges of change: a qualitative study of chronic care model implementation. Ann Fam Med 2006;4(4):317–26.

18. Coleman K, Austin BT, Brach C, et al. Evidence on the chronic care model in the new millennium. Health Aff (Millwood) 2009;28(1):75–85.

19. Landon BE, Hicks LS, O'Malley AJ, et al. Improving the management of chronic disease at community health centers. N Engl J Med 2007;356:921–34.

20. Coming home: the patient-centered medical-dental home in primary care training. Advisory Committee on Training in Primary Care Medicine and Dentistry; Seventh annual report to the Secretary of the US Department of Health and Human Services and Congress. 2008. Available at: http://www.hrsa.gov/advisorycommittees/bhpradvisory/actpcmd/Reports/seventhreport.pdf. Accessed October 25, 2015.

21. Iglehart JK. No place like home — testing a new model of care delivery. N Engl J Med 2008;359(12):1200–2.
22. National network for health access oral health and the patient centered health home. Available at: nnoh.org/nnoha-content/uploads/2013/09/PCHH Action guide 02.12_final.pdf. Accessed January 05, 2016.
23. Aysola J, Rhodes KV, Polsky D. Patient-centered medical homes and access to services for new primary care patients. Med Care 2015;53(10):857–62.
24. American Academy of Family Physicians, American Academy of Pediatrics, American College of Physicians, American Osteopathic Association. Joint principles of the patient-centered medical home. 2007. Available at: http://www.pcpcc.net/content/joint-principles-patientcentered-medical-home. Accessed September 2, 2008.
25. Moore D. Effect of an enhanced medical home on cost and outcomes. AAP Grand Rounds 2015;33:4–40.
26. Mosquera RA, Avritscher EB, Samuels CL, et al. Effect of an enhanced medical home on serious illness and cost of care among high-risk children with chronic illness: a randomized clinical trial. JAMA 2014;312(23):2640–8.
27. Northridge ME, Glick M, Metcalf SS, et al. Public health support for the health home model. Am J Public Health 2011;101(10):1818–20.
28. Druss BG, Marcus SC, Olfson M, et al. Comparing the national economic burden of five chronic conditions. Health Aff (Millwood) 2001;20(6):233–41.
29. The Challenge of Oral Disease – A call for global action. The Oral Health Atlas. 2nd ed. Geneva: FDI World Dental Federation; 2015. Available at: http://www.fdiworldental.org/media/77552/complete_oh_atlas.pdf.
30. William DM. The research agenda on oral health inequalities: the IADR-GOHIRA initiative. Med Princ Pract 2014;23(Suppl 1):52–9.
31. Niederman R, Feres M, Ogunbodede E. Chapter 10. Dentistry. In: Debas HT, Donkor P, Gawande A, et al, editors. Disease control priorities, vol. 1, 3rd edition. Washington, DC: World Bank; 2015. p. 173–95. Essential surgery.
32. World Health Organization. Oral health: action plan for promotion and integrated disease prevention (EB120/10). 120th session, provisional agenda item 4.6. Geneva (Switzerland): WHO; 2006. issue date 2007.
33. Narayan KM, Boyle JP, Thompson TJ, et al. Lifetime risk of diabetes mellitus in the United States. JAMA 2003;290(14):1884–90.
34. American Diabetes Association. Statistics about diabetes data from the national diabetes statistics report. 2014. Available at: http://www.diabetes.org/diabetes-basics/statistics/#sthash.sBhNOd93.dpuf. Accessed February 1, 2016.
35. International Diabetes Federation. IDF diabetes atlas. 6th edition. Brussels (Belgium): International Diabetes Federation; 2013. Available at: http://www.idf.org/diabetesatlas.
36. Knowler WC, Barrett-Connor E, Fowler SE, et al. Diabetes prevention program research group. Reduction in the incidence of type 2 diabetes with lifestyle intervention or metformin. N Engl J Med 2002;346(6):393–403.
37. Diabetes Prevention Program Research Group, Knowler WC, Fowler SE, et al. 10-year follow-up of diabetes incidence and weight loss in the diabetes prevention program outcomes study. Lancet 2009;374(9702):1677–86.
38. National diabetes statistics. Available at: http://diabetes.niddk.nih.gov/DM/PUBS/statistics: Accessed February 4, 2016.
39. Mealey BL, Ocampo GL. Diabetes mellitus and periodontal disease. Periodontol 2000 2007;44:127–53.

40. Chapple IL, Genco R. Working group 2 of the joint EFP/AAP workshop. Diabetes and periodontal diseases: consensus report of the Joint EFP/AAP workshop on periodontitis and systemic diseases. J Periodontol 2013;84(4 Suppl):S106–12.

41. Holm NR, Belstrøm D, Østergaard JA, et al. Identification of individuals with undiagnosed diabetes and pre-diabetes in a Danish cohort attending dental treatment. J Periodontol 2016;87(4):395–402.

42. Al-Habashneh R, Barghout N, Humbert L, et al. Diabetes and oral health: doctors' knowledge, perception and practices. J Eval Clin Pract 2010;16:976–80.

43. Al-Khabbaz AK, Al-Shammari KF, Al-Saleh NA. Knowledge about the association between periodontal diseases and diabetes mellitus: contrasting dentists and physicians. J Periodontol 2011;82:360–6.

44. Kunzel C, Lalla E, Lamster IB. Dentists' management of the diabetic patient: contrasting generalists and specialists. Am J Public Health 2007;97:725–30.

45. National Diabetes Education Program. Redesigning the health care team diabetes prevention and lifelong management. 2013. Available at: http://ndep.nih.gov/media/NDEP37_RedesignTeamCare_4c_508.pdf?redirect=true. Accessed February 4, 2016.

46. National Diabetes Education Program. Collaborative care in practice. Available at: http://www.niddk.nih.gov/health-information/health-communication-programs/ndep/health-care-professionals/team-care/collaborative-care-practice/Pages/publicationdetail.aspx. Accessed February 1, 2013.

47. Piccinino L, Griffey S, Gallivan J, et al. Recent trends in diabetes knowledge, perceptions, and behaviors: implications for national diabetes education. Health Educ Behav 2015;42(5):687–96.

48. International Diabetes Federation Clinical Guidelines Task Force: IDF guideline on oral health for people with diabetes. Brussels (Belgium). 2009. Available at: https://www.idf.org/guidelines/diabetes-and-oral-health/guideline. Accessed March 31, 2016.

49. Brownson CA, O'Toole ML, Gowri S, et al. Clinic-community partnerships: a foundation for providing community supports for diabetes care and self-management. Diabetes Spectr 2007;20(4):209–14.

50. Fisher EB, Brownson CA, O'Toole ML, et al. The Robert Wood Johnson Foundation Diabetes Initiative: demonstration projects emphasizing self-management. Diabetes Educ 2007;33(1):83–4, 86–8, 91–2, 94.

51. Mayberry RM, Nicewander DA, Qin H, et al. Improving quality and reducing inequities: a challenge in achieving best care. Proc (Bayl Univ Med Cent) 2006;19(2):103–18.

52. Dracup K, Debusk RF, De Mots H, et al. Task force 3: partnerships in delivery cardiovascular care. J Am Coll Cardiol 1994;24(2):275–328.

53. Bridges DR, Davidson RA, Odegard PS, et al. Interprofessional collaboration: three best practice models of interprofessional education. Med Educ Online 2011;16. http://dx.doi.org/10.3402/meo.v16i0.6035.

54. Jaarsma T. Inter-professional team approach to patients with heart failure. Heart 2005;91(6):832–8.

55. Webb CL, Jenkins KJ, Karpawich PP, et al. Collaborative care for adults with congenital heart disease. Circulation 2002;105:2318–23.

56. Mundt MP, Gilchrist VJ, Fleming MF, et al. Effects of primary care team social networks on quality of care and costs for patients with cardiovascular disease. Ann Fam Med 2015;13(2):139–48.

57. Boillot A, Demmer RT, Mallat Z, et al. Periodontal microbiota and phospholipases: the Oral Infections and Vascular Disease Epidemiology Study (INVEST). Atherosclerosis 2015;242(2):418–23.

58. Cotti E, Mercuro G. Apical periodontitis and cardiovascular diseases: previous findings and ongoing research. Endod J 2015;48(10):926–32.

59. Shetty D, Dua M, Kumar K, et al. Oral hygiene status of individuals with cardiovascular diseases and associated risk factors. Clin Pract 2012;2(4):e86.

60. Lee YL, Hu HY, Chou P, et al. Dental prophylaxis decreases the risk of acute myocardial infarction: a nationwide population-based study in Taiwan. Clin Interv Aging 2015;10:175–82.

61. Dave S, Batista EL Jr, Van Dyke TE. Cardiovascular disease and periodontal diseases: commonality and causation. Compend Contin Educ Dent 2004;25(7 Suppl 1):26–37.

62. Greenberg BL, Glick M. Assessing systemic disease risk in a dental setting: a public health perspective. Dent Clin North Am 2012;56(4):863–74.

63. Jowett NI, Cabot LB. Patients with cardiac disease: considerations for the dental practitioner. Br Dent J 2000;189(6):297–302.

64. The Guide to Community Preventive Services What Works to Promote Health. Cardiovascular disease prevention and control: team-based care to improve blood pressure control. Available at: http://www.thecommunityguide.org/cvd/teambasedcare.html. Accessed February 5, 2016.

65. Walsh J, McDonald KM, Shojania KG, et al. Quality improvement strategies for hypertension management: a systematic review. Med Care 2006;44:646–57.

66. Health Resources and Services Administration. Integration of oral health and primary care practices. Rockville (MD): U.S. Department of Health and Human Services; 2014.

67. Qualis health. Oral health: an essential component of primary care. Available at: https://dphhs.mt.gov/Portals/85/publichealth/documents/OralHealth/White-Paper-Oral-Health-Primary-Care.pdf. 2015. Accessed November 12, 2015.

68. Niwa K. Adults with congenital heart disease transition. Curr Opin Pediatr 2015; 27(5):576–80.

69. Katerndahl D. Providing complex (rather than complicated) chronic care. J Am Board Fam Med 2014;27(1):6–7.

70. Kafka H, Johnson MR, Gatzoulis MA. The team approach to pregnancy and congenital heart disease. Cardiol Clin 2006;24(4):587–605.

71. Go AS, Mozaffarian D, Roger VL, et al. Heart disease and stroke statistics—2013 update: a report from the American Heart Association. Circulation 2013; 127:e6–245.

72. Roughead EE, Barratt JD, Ramsay E, et al. The effectiveness of collaborative medicine reviews in delaying time to next hospitalization for patients with heart failure in the practice setting: results of a cohort study. Circ Heart Fail 2009;2:424–8.

73. Crissinger ME, Marchionda KM, Dunlap ME. Adherence to clinical guidelines in heart failure (HF) outpatients: impact of an interprofessional HF team on evidence-based medication use. J Interprof Care 2015;29(5):483–7.

74. Ahmed A. Quality and outcomes of heart failure care in older adults: role of multidisciplinary disease-management programs. J Am Geriatr Soc 2002; 50(9):1590–3.

75. Deeks SG, Lewin SR, Havlir DV. The end of AIDS: HIV infection as a chronic disease. Lancet 2013;382(9903):1525–33.

76. Jeanty Y, Cardenas G, Fox JE, et al. Correlates of unmet dental care need among HIV-positive people since being diagnosed with HIV. Public Health Rep 2012;127(Suppl 2):17–24.

77. Lennon CA, Pellowski JA, White AC, et al. Service priorities and unmet service needs among people living with HIV/AIDS: results from a nationwide interview of HIV/AIDS housing organizations. AIDS Care 2013;25:1083–91.

78. Benjamin RM. Oral health care for people living with HIV/AIDS. Public Health Rep 2012;127(Suppl 2):1–2.

79. Gardner EM, McLees MP, Steiner JF, et al. The spectrum of engagement in HIV care and its relevance to test-and-treat strategies for prevention of HIV infection. Clin Infect Dis 2011;52(6):793–800.

80. Gallant JE, Adimora AA, Carmichael JK, et al. Essential components of effective HIV care: a policy paper of the HIV Medicine Association of the Infectious Diseases Society of America and the Ryan White Medical Providers Coalition. Clin Infect Dis 2011;53(11):1043–50.

81. Implementing Oral Health Care into HIV Primary Care Settings. U.S. Department of Health and Human Services Health Resources and Services Administration HIV/AIDS Bureau Special Projects of National Significance Program. 2013. Available at: http://hab.hrsa.gov/abouthab/files/cyberspns_ihip_2013.pdf. Accessed January 12, 2016.

82. Smedley BD, Stith AY, Nelson AR. Unequal treatment: what health care system administrators need to know about racial and ethnic disparities in healthcare, committee on understanding and eliminating racial and ethnic disparities in health care. Washington, DC: Institute of Medicine of the National Academies; The National Academies Press; 2003.

83. Novitsky V, Bussmann H, Okui L, et al. Estimated age and gender profile of individuals missed by a home-based HIV testing and counselling campaign in a Botswana community. J Int AIDS Soc 2015;18(1):19918.

84. Branson BM, Handsfield HH, Lampe MA, et al. Revised recommendations for HIV testing of adults, adolescents, and pregnant women in health-care settings. MMWR Recomm Rep 2006;55(RR-14):1–17.

85. Centers for Disease Control and Prevention. Revised guidelines for HIV counseling, testing, and referral. MMWR Recomm Rep 2001;50(No. RR-19):1–57.

86. Fox JE, Tobias CR, Bachman SS, et al. Increasing access to oral health care for people living with HIV/AIDS in the US: baseline evaluation results of the Innovations in oral health care initiative. Public Health Rep 2012;127(Suppl 2):5–16.

87. HRSA HIV/AIDS Program, US Department of Health and Human Services. Available at: http://hab.hrsa.gov/data/index.html. Accessed February 8, 2016.

88. Valentine J, Saladyanant T, Ramsey K, et al. Impact of periodontal intervention on local inflammation, periodontitis, and HIV outcomes. Oral Dis 2016; 22(Suppl 1):87–97.

89. Shiboski CH, Chen H, Secours R, et al. High accuracy of common HIV-related oral disease diagnoses by non-oral health specialists in the AIDS Clinical Trial Group. PLoS One 2015;10(7):e0131001.

90. Onyett S, Ford R. Multidisciplinary community teams: where is the wreckage? J Ment Health 1996;5:47–55.

91. Milnes A, Pegrum K, Nebe B, et al. Australian Institute of Health and Welfare 2011. Young Australians: their health and wellbeing 2011. Cat. no. PHE 140 Canberra: AIHW. p. 1–246

92. Broyles LM, Conley JW, Harding JD, et al. A scoping review of interdisciplinary collaboration in addictions education and training. J Addict Nurs 2013;24(1): 29–36.

93. Interprofessional practice: collaborative practice targeting substance use in rural populations. University of Pittsburgh School of Nursing. Available at: http://www.nursing.pitt.edu/continuing-education/sbirt-teaching-resources. Accessed January 05, 2016.

94. Makoul G, Clayman ML. An integrative model of shared decision making in medical encounters. Patient Educ Couns 2006;60(3):301–12.

95. Hahn RK, Albers LJ, Reist C. Psychiatry. Blue Jay (CA): Current Clinical Strategies Publishing; 2008.

96. De las Cuevas C, Sanz E. Polypharmacy in psychiatric practice in the Canary Island. BMC Psychiatry 2004;4(18):1–8.

97. Farinde A. The Interprofessional Management of Dementia-Related Behavioral and Psychological Disturbances. Health and Interprofessional Practice2(2):eP1064. Available at: http://dx.doi.org/10.7772/2159-1253.1064

98. Keating NL, Landrum MB, Lamont EB, et al. Tumor boards and the quality of cancer care. J Natl Cancer Inst 2013;105(2):113–21.

99. Epstein JB, Parker IR, Epstein MS, et al. A survey of National Cancer Institute-designated comprehensive cancer centers' oral health supportive care practices and resources in the USA. Support Care Cancer 2007;15(4):357–62.

100. San Martin-Rodriguez L, D'Amour D, Leduc N. Outcomes of interprofessional collaboration for hospitalized cancer patients. Cancer Nurs 2008;31(2):E18–27.

101. Haber J, Harnett E, Allen K, et al. Putting the mouth back in the head: HEENT to HEENOT. Am J Public Health 2015;105(3):437–41.

102. Interprofessional education collaborative expert panel core competencies for interprofessional collaborative practice: report of an expert panel. 2011. Available at: http://www.aacn.nche.edu/education-resources/ipecreport.pdf. Accessed March 20, 2016.

103. Kligler B, Brooks AJ, Maizes V, et al. Interprofessional competencies in integrative primary healthcare. Glob Adv Health Med 2015;4(5):33–9.

104. White MJ, Zapka JG, Coughlin-Storm J, et al. Interdisciplinary collaboration for health professional education in cancer control. J Cancer Educ 2004;19(1): 37–44.

105. Farokhi MR, Glass BJ, Gureckis KM. A student operated, faculty mentored dental clinic service experience at the University of Texas Health Science Center at San Antonio for the underserved refugee community: an interprofessional approach. Tex Dent J 2014;131(1):27–33.

106. Berwick DM, Nolan TW, Whittington J. The triple aim: care, health, and cost. Health Aff 2008;27(3):759–69.

Problems and Solutions for Interprofessional Education in North American Dental Schools

Sara C. Gordon, DDS, MS, FRCD (Canada), FDSRCS (Edinburgh)[a,*],
Robert Bruce Donoff, DMD, MD[b]

KEYWORDS

- Interprofessional relations • Interprofessional education • Professional education
- Professional education, dental • Patient care team • Professional competence
- Education, dental • Patient-centered care

KEY POINTS

- Interprofessional education (IPE) must be clinically relevant to our students. Therefore, IPE cases must promote teamwork, be applicable to dental care, and be authentic.
- Relevance and learning are enhanced by moving from the classroom to clinical care and by the use of actual or simulated cases.
- There is no need to reinvent the wheel, but assessments should be calibrated and evidence based. Learning objectives and assessments can be adapted from high-quality preexisting resources.
- Learning in a community setting promotes recognition of discipline-specific biases and can help to create sustainable interprofessional resources.
- Sustainability is enhanced by an effort to overcome institutional barriers and by embedding IPE/interprofessional collaborative practice in the fabric of the institution.

INTRODUCTION

Interprofessional education (IPE) and interprofessional collaborative practice (ICP) are relatively new to most health professional schools in North America. Dental accreditation authorities in Canada and the United States recognize their importance to good patient care and in 2013 adopted new accreditation standards, which mandate that IPE be part of dental education. Standard 2-19 of the 2016 Predoctoral Accreditation Standards of the USA Commission on Dental Accreditation states, "Graduates must

[a] Department of Oral Medicine, University of Washington, School of Dentistry, 1959 Northeast Pacific Street, HSB B-530F, Box 357480, Seattle, WA 98195-7480, USA; [b] Department of Oral and Maxillofacial Surgery, Harvard School of Dental Medicine, 188 Longwood Avenue, Boston, MA 02115, USA
* Corresponding author.
E-mail address: gordons@uw.edu

Dent Clin N Am 60 (2016) 811–824
http://dx.doi.org/10.1016/j.cden.2016.05.002
0011-8532/16/$ – see front matter © 2016 Elsevier Inc. All rights reserved.

dental.theclinics.com

be competent in communicating and collaborating with other members of the health care team to facilitate the provision of health care."[1] Dental schools face some unique problems because unlike MDs or nurses, most dentists do not participate in hospital-based practice, and many IPE activities simulate hospital scenarios. Furthermore, in North America, oral health care often follows a different track from general health care, including practice locations, practitioner attitudes, and billing practices, reinforcing the false impression that the mouth is not part of the body. Oral health can be fully integrated into ICP only if all providers fully understand its importance to our patients' overall health.

Just as graduate dentists concentrating on treatment of dental disease may need to be reminded about basic medical science, general physicians and other health care professionals need to be reminded about the oral cavity's place in the body and to think of the teeth as well as the toes[2] when they consider patient health. All health care workers, not just dentists, need to change the conversation from *oral health is connected to systemic health* toward *oral health is integral to overall* health because characterizing it as a connection rather than a synthesis is an understatement.

We also need to change the culture of dentistry from only addressing the *what* (the procedure to be done) at the exclusion of the *why* (the diagnosis and reason for treatment). It could be argued that attempts to simply integrate oral health into primary care via nurse practitioners (NPs) and physician assistants (applying fluoride varnish, learning to do oral examinations, and so forth) is detrimental to ICP because it does little to alter the reciprocal education needed to truly understand and respect each other's roles. The dental team needs education, collaboration, and practice with other health care professionals; other health care professionals need education, collaboration, and practice with us.

Palatta and colleagues[3] say "IPE and collaborative practice have surfaced as among the most significant changes to health care education and delivery in the 21st century." Nonetheless, its implementation in dental schools faces numerous hurdles. Palatta and colleagues[3] surveyed dental schools and found the most important perceived barriers to IPE implementation include funding limitations, lack of curricular time, and assessment of student learning. Rafter and colleagues[4] found similar results when they interviewed leaders at 7 key academic health centers who stated that the major hurdles include lack of curricular time, funding limitations, lack of scientific evidence for effectiveness of IPE, and lack of support by faculty and administration, including poor communication between health profession schools and the perception that IPE is a fad. Dental hygiene schools seem to face similar barriers. Furgeson and colleagues[5] surveyed US dental hygiene schools and identified that the most important anticipated future barriers are scheduling and logistics, lack of programs with which to collaborate, and lack of administrative support.

This article attempts to turn the conversation toward solutions. Diverse Canadian and US dental schools report the range of problems that they have faced during their introduction of IPE and discuss the solutions that they have found in a brief format. These contributions are shown next.

PROBLEM 1: HOW DO WE MAKE INTERPROFESSIONAL EDUCATION CLINICAL REQUIREMENTS MORE RELEVANT AND FLEXIBLE?
Karen Burgess DDS, MSc, FRCD (Canada) and Sylvia Langlois MSc, OT Reg (Ontario), University of Toronto

The University of Toronto (UT) IPE curriculum for 11 health profession programs requires students to interact with each other's professions. The IPE component in clinical placements typically occurs in hospital inpatient units, where many of the university health programs work side by side. Because clinical experiences for dentistry students are completed within the faculty patient clinics, dental students do not have a hospital placement where they interact with students from the other health professions. Dental students also report that some IPE activities do not apply to them and they cannot participate fully in the discussions, particularly when activities relate to inpatients and topics like discharge planning.

Solutions

UT faculty from dentistry and the Center for IPE jointly designed community IPE activities that were more relevant and flexible for dental students. The resulting Flexible Model enables dental students to complete core requirements, yet permits enough flexibility to ensure that learning opportunities meet student learning needs and faculty requirements. Dental students participate in each of the 3 learning activities in the Flexible Model. Each activity involves at least one other profession and is structured to include a briefing, an experience, a formalized debriefing, and a reflective writing assignment. Learning experiences for students in each of these activities are as follows:

- Participation in interprofessional team education: When a medical emergency occurs at the dentist's office, the team must call 911. This time is one of the most stressful times in practice. Dental students and paramedics work together to find the best ways to manage medical emergencies in practice and learn about 911 calls at the Toronto 911 Call Center. Dental students learn how to deal with 911 calls effectively and efficiently and to develop an appreciation of patients' needs. This experience promotes an understanding of how dentists should communicate and collaborate with paramedical staff to ensure efficient and effective responses.
- Interviewing/shadowing a team member: Dental students shadow dental laboratory technologists at a community dental laboratory. They develop an appreciation of the laboratory technologists' roles and responsibilities and what is required to interact as team members. Together, they find ways to enhance communication to benefit patients.
- Participation in team meetings: Dental students participate with other students in team meetings with registered nurses, patients, and families to plan and then provide care.

Discussion

Dental students want experiences that expand on existing dental training but will also help them in their professional life after graduation. These learning activities are highly valued by dental students who need to be engaged in some learning activities with professions that will be their partners in future practice. As future practitioners in a community office, students need to consider unique competencies required to address patient concerns in a comprehensive and collaborative manner. Interactions with paramedics and dental laboratory technologists promote an appreciation of scope of practice, roles and responsibilities of these community-based professions, and how to communicate and collaborate to enhance best practices in patient care. Dental students also are exposed to a traditional team meeting with involvement of both patients and family members. Flexibility in the original design of the mandatory structured IPE clinical experience enables full participation of dental students so they can develop needed collaborative competencies.

PROBLEM 2: HOW DO WE MOVE BEYOND THE CLASSROOM TO THE CLINICAL ENVIRONMENT?

Kenneth Allen DDS, MBA and Judith Haber PhD, APRN, BC, FAAN, New York University

Identifying effective strategies for teaching health professions students how to collaborate as effective team members is a challenge. The transformation of health care delivery will occur in clinical settings at the point of care. Providers across disciplines will be expected to transcend traditional professional silos, partnering to achieve the outcomes for which they are accountable.[6]

Solutions

New York University (NYU) has developed a large interprofessional clinical simulation and case study experience, embedding the Interprofessional Education Collaborative (IPEC) competencies and creating a relevant clinical focus for 3 different health professions. Oral-systemic health is the perfect clinical exemplar to bring together 168 medical (Doctor of Medicine [MD]), 84 dental (Doctor of Dental Surgery [DDS]), and 100 NP students. The New York Simulation Center for the Health Sciences has 14 glass-enclosed, fully-equipped examination rooms with video recording capabilities and conference rooms for case study sessions. Faculty members trained in IPE facilitate collaboration using a brief-and-debrief approach to begin and close each session. Using standardized patients, students collaborate to teach each other to complete oral, cardiac, and respiratory assessments. Teach back demonstrations provide evidence of clinical competence. The interprofessional case study experience, focused on a patient with symptoms of diabetes and periodontal disease, requires NP, DDS, and MD students to integrate the IPEC competencies and clinical assessment, diagnosis, and management competencies to develop a management plan.[7]

Discussion

Transcending schedules of 330 students in 3 different schools, each with a different course and credit configuration, required weeks of advanced planning and flexibility. Developing a faculty leadership team committed to transcending professional silos was an evolutionary process. Now in its third year, the Teaching Oral-Systemic Health experience has become a standardized component of the curriculum in all 3 professional schools. Faculty development continues to be an essential ingredient for success. More than 90% of faculty members evaluate the experience very positively as a valuable interprofessional experience for faculty and students. Using the Interprofessional Collaborative Competency Attainment Survey, a 20-item valid and reliable tool that aligns with the IPEC competencies, students complete pre-event and post-event surveys that assess the degree to which they change their attitudes and perceptions of the importance of interprofessional experiences. Evaluation data reveal a statistically significant change from before to after the test ($P<.001$) across the dental, medical, and nursing professions.[8]

It is essential to have support from leaders of the academic units; it is they who commit to allocating the resources integral with successful interprofessional initiatives. Engaging faculty champions is important; whether faculty are formal or informal leaders, their buy-in will be important in growing a critical mass of early adopters.[9] Exposing students to interprofessional clinical experiences provides an opportunity for future health professionals to learn from and about each other's roles and responsibilities as well as how to communicate and collaborate. The aim is that positive student interprofessional clinical experiences will prepare graduates to join clinical teams as effective collaborators. The success of this program has provided a catalyst for developing interprofessional live clinical experiences involving smaller groups of NP, DDS, and MD students. The authors' goal is to acquire more curricular resources to expand the program so that it includes every student and, ideally, does this more than once per year.

PROBLEM 3: HOW DO WE INTEGRATE ORAL HEALTH INTO INTERPROFESSIONAL EDUCATION/INTERPROFESSIONAL PRACTICE PROGRAMS?
A. Conan Davis DMD, MPH and Stephen C. Mitchell DMD, University of Alabama

Physicians, nurses, and physician assistants have collaborated together through IPE activities for years. Oral health was considered a critical health care component for inclusion in IPE only in recent years. Physicians and dentists have been taught basic sciences together but have never received integrated IPE clinical training.

Solutions

The DentaQuest Foundation funded a pilot interprofessional training program in which University of Alabama (UAB) medical, nursing, optometry, physician assisting, and dental students collaborate to learn how to perform baseline screenings. These screenings identify when a patient should be referred to another discipline. All participating students are required to review the *Smiles for Life* curriculum,[10] and each participating health school is encouraged to incorporate it into their standard curriculum. UAB health school students are then assigned to interdisciplinary teams that provide holistic health screenings at monthly events organized by community partners in elementary schools and child care centers. Each discipline is charged with not only screening patients but also teaching their methods to the other disciplines. Members are encouraged to then perform screenings outside their domain. Students are surveyed after each session to gauge interest and degree of learning through the experience.

Discussion

The online *Smiles for Life*[10] modules allow students to work through the curriculum at their own convenience. Student feedback suggests that the oral health knowledge acquired through the curriculum will impact their future practices as licensed health care providers. Additionally, students value the interprofessional (IPE) nature of the project, which exposes them to other health professions and allows students from each field the opportunity to reciprocally educate their fellow students about their professions. Unlike IPE simulation activities, our structured screenings horizontally integrate IPE learning experiences around live patients, creating an environment that allows students to intermingle and develop collegial relationships that often result in students leaving the event as interprofessional groups, rather than with their own colleagues as when they arrived. The authors think the great collegiality developed among the students results from shared treatment of live patients and is critical to the project's success.

PROBLEM 4: HOW DO WE MASTER INSTITUTIONAL BARRIERS?
Blase P. Brown DDS, MS, Jennifer O'Rourke RN, PhD, and Anne Koerber DDS, PhD, University of Illinois at Chicago

The established structure of major teaching/research institutions, many with independently functioning programs and colleges, creates a framework of barriers to the implementation of IPE. These barriers are found in every level of organization within various institutions and include physical, administrative, faculty, student, and financial barriers.

Solutions

Overcoming institutionalized barriers at the University of Illinois in Chicago (UIC) began as a grass-root effort of individual faculty and staff within the 7 health science colleges, which created the Collaborative for Excellence in Interprofessional Education (CEIPE). CEIPE successfully garnered internal support from the UIC Provost's office and the health sciences colleges' administration. The CIEPE has created an annual campus-wide UIC IPE Immersion Day since 2012, using external funding from the Health Resources Services Administration, the Josiah Macy Jr Foundation, and an internal university grant. At the same time, students promote IPE norms through an Institute of Healthcare Improvement Open School Chapter and through activities of the Health Professions Student Council. This intersection of faculty, staff, and student engagement in IPE, together with individual college IPE accreditation challenges, has been the impetus for the creation of a salaried IPE administrative position within the provost's office and the recent creation of a university strategic plan for IPE.

Discussion

UIC has seen the beginning of campus-wide cultural change that includes a shift in how administrators view the value of IPE. The high level of support from stakeholders and administration for the strategic plan are part of an initial framework for building a competency model for the health science college programs. The 5-year strategic plan depends on integrated support from the UIC Provost and Vice-Chancellor for Health Affairs for the following activities:

- Design UIC IPE curriculum encompassing prelicensure and postlicensure learners' needs.
- Develop a sustainable financial model for IPE at UIC (tuition/fees), including faculty time, and support for infrastructure.
- Establish units to support IPE on all UIC campuses.
- Design a faculty development plan.
- Create a clinical placement database to support development of clinically based IPE learning experiences.
- Review and modify UIC policies to create structure for IPE and remove barriers to participation.
- Develop needs-based and sustainable training plan for UIC.

Anticipated outcomes from these planned actives are based on assumptions closely linked to high-level administrative support. These assumptions are as follows:

- IPE at UIC will include academic programs on all 6 campuses.
- IPE will be centrally coordinated from the Vice-Chancellor for Health Affairs' office.
- Most IPE learning experiences will be developed by colleges collaborating locally.
- Funding will include tuition, graduate research fellowships, and other sources.
- Continuing education will be financially self-sustaining.

Significant barriers to the continuity and sustainability of IPE at UIC remain (fiscal, budget models, faculty workloads, student diversity and volume, curricula coordination) that can only be overcome by continual administrative support and leadership outlined in the assumptions discussed earlier. The 7 health colleges have logistical barriers that intersect space and schedules, dense and rigid curricula, and faculty workforce/workload concerns that cannot be changed solely within each unit. Administrative intervention has been defined and articulated in the strategic plan to include the attainment of proper financial resources, the support of faculty development and incentive pay, and the facilitation of cooperation between health care educational programs.

PROBLEM 5: HOW DO WE OVERCOME DISCIPLINE-SPECIFIC BIASES?
Gerald Davis II DDS, MA and Jacinta Leavell PhD, MS, Meharry Medical College

Students at Meharry had not communicated at length with peers from other health professions and had not taken the time to research the core practices and values of the various other disciplines. Consequently, students had general concepts of each health profession but were typically unaware of which concepts were biased generalizations.

Solutions

This project pairs diverse teams of students from 5 institutions and 10 disciplines with designated community partners who provide services for adults with financial and/or health limitations. All 6 teams consist of at least 5 of the represented disciplines. Each team engages community partners and those they serve by investigating community-specific needs. Students are informed of the expected learning outcomes based on the IPE collaboration objectives. Each team initially receives cultural competency training and protocols on how to foster positive relationships within groups. The Meharry-Vanderbilt IPE Faculty Collaborative (see *Acknowledgements*), composed of faculty from 5 institutions and a diverse array of health-based fields, provides guidance for project activities, addresses student concerns, and provides clarification throughout the project. If students encounter challenges, faculty members encourage open dialogue but avoid solving the problem. For 6 months, each team works to find the best way to create a sustainable interprofessional resource that will address the needs of their assigned community. It was originally estimated that students would spend a total of 26 hours from project onset to completion.

Discussion

By the end of the 6-month project, each group has spent 32 to 42 hours working together, including training, role playing different disciplines, conducting focus groups for their assigned community partner, and creating a sustainable solution to meet community needs. The students present an overview of their proposed resource/solution and demonstrate their cohesive team dynamics. Each student expounds on previous assumptions made regarding other disciplines and how his or her opinions have evolved. During their presentations, students relay a more accurate view of each other, including the discipline-specific education process, types of specialties, and patient care.

Exposing students to interprofessional/interdisciplinary processes in a community setting promotes student interactions that aid them in recognizing discipline-specific biases. As time progresses, students begin working towards overcoming their biases to better serve the needs of the community partners through the development of community-specific solutions and tangible products meant to be used as resources or supplement existing resources.

There are some limitations to this pilot project. Every group does not have the same number of disciplines represented. Some groups are paired with communities whose needs are centered around a specific health care issue, whereas others are not. The current data are limited to students self-reporting. However, further analysis is currently underway for assessing students' IPE competency using the Core Competencies of Interprofessional Collaborative Practice. The authors are also in the process of analyzing a pre-evaluation, midevaluation, and postevaluation using the Interprofessional Socialization and Valuing Scale,[11] a validated instrument for measuring student attitudes toward IPE.

PROBLEM 6: HOW DO WE ASSESS COMPETENCY?
Amy S. Kim DDS, Sandra Phillips MPA, and Joel H. Berg DDS, MS, University of Washington

Health professional students have been colearning for decades; however, their learning and competence have not been assessed in a repeatable way. This is compounded by other factors, including difficulty of measuring mastery of soft sciences and emotional quotient types of learning.

Solutions

Although IPE/ICP is a new element of most health science curricula, components that lead to successful learning in this area are not new. Therefore, the authors' strategy includes exploring skills and learning assessments that are already in place within the existing curricular infrastructure at the University of Washington School of Dentistry (UWSOD). They include metrics around problem-based learning, critical thinking, self-assessment, multicultural competence, and effective communication. Disciplines that apply to the needs of assessing competence in IPE/ICP include

- Principles and philosophies of practice management
- Ethics and professionalism
- Safety and compliance
- Comprehensive treatment planning

UWSOD has also focused on learning objectives for IPE that are based on industry standards with preexisting guidance documents. For example, the authors discovered verbiage regarding IPE in self-study documents from the American Dental Association's Commission on Dental Accreditation (CODA) as well as publications coming out of the IPEC.

Discussion

UWSOD, as a forerunner in dental education, already had learning objectives and competence assessments pertinent to assessing competence in IPE/ICP. The authors have incorporated relevant material from CODA self-study documents and IPEC recommendations into their overall assessment plan.

UWSOD has determined that a practical way to indicate proficiency in IPE/ICP is through students preparing a reflection paper discussing insights into their colearning with other professional students through the IPE/ICP curriculum. The reflection process is a good tool for assessing curricular elements that may have been deemed difficult to ascertain in traditional ways. Health professional programs, including schools of dentistry, have used it successfully. Several resources refer to use of student reflections for IPE/ICP on MedEd Online, including a best practices model piece by Bridges and colleagues.[12] Reflection papers also offer the added benefit of providing insight to educators on areas in need of further development in their educational programming.

Institutions with well-established educational infrastructures can look within and adapt what is currently in use for metrics for assessing IPE/ICP competence. Not all elements will apply; thus, it is important to choose wisely and modify to serve the specific needs of the curriculum area to be assessed. The authors look forward to gaining insight into what students gained from the IPE/ICP program as well as what they could improve on as educators through the reflections process.

PROBLEM 7: HOW DO WE OVERCOME THE IMPACT OF TIME AND ATTITUDES?
Elizabeth Andrews DDS, MS, Jenny Sun Tjahjono DMD, and Elizabeth Maugh MS, PAC, DFAAPA, Western University of Health Sciences

In 2014, when the Health Resources and Services Administration proposed integrating oral health into primary care practice, Western University of Health Sciences College of Dental Medicine (WesternU CDM) spearheaded an Interprofessional Collaborative Practice Curriculum (IPCP), partnering with WesternU's Physician Assistant Program. The authors faced 2 major hurdles: lack of shared value towards IPE and lack of student time in already full curricula.

Solutions

Addressing the lack of shared value towards IPE, the authors have designed a clinically relevant IPE with real-world applications. WesternU CDM has embraced an integrated IPE preclinical curriculum, in which case studies include basic sciences, preclinical/clinical, and IPE concepts for preclinical students. Examples of pertinent, realistic clinical information include review of systemic conditions requiring dental treatment modifications, incorporation of antibiotic prophylaxis and hypertension protocols, and construction of referral letters to other health care providers.

Following didactic IPE, students participate in IPCP. Dental and physician assistant students pair up to work simultaneously on patients during regular allotted clinic sessions. The pairs discuss medical considerations, perform oral cancer screenings, identify oral diseases, and provide health education to their common patients. Students help patients identify a medical and dental home and draft consultation letters to appropriate health care professions. Assessments are designed and used to test students' ability to apply newfound knowledge in both IPE and IPCP.

Discussion

Clinically relevant IPE cases help students to increase acceptance and understanding of IPE. These cases reinforce preclinical students' didactic knowledge, increase clinical exposure, and lead to smoother clinical care transitions. Students apply the didactic knowledge in real clinical situations and are more prepared as beginning providers on the clinic floor. In IPCP, the importance of oral health and overall health connections is reinforced for dental and PA students. By interacting directly with students from different professions, students increase their understanding of the scope of practice of other professions, decrease anxiety when working in an unfamiliar clinical setting, and develop better communication techniques by composing referral letters to other health professions. Students appreciate the direct benefits and see immediate results in this integrated curriculum during regular clinical sessions. Therefore, students are ready for the real world in which the health care system is shifting toward collaborative care.

Making IPE clinically relevant by using already allotted lecture or clinical time is an innovative method to carry out IPE programs in curricula that are already full. IPE can be discretely incorporated into case-based studies in conjunction with already taught material. This incorporation seamlessly allows for understanding of IPE concepts and knowledge, with little or no increase in curriculum time. IPCP can be built into existing clinical sessions for further application of the IP collaborative patient care skills.

Faculty and students have higher acceptance and better understanding of the concept and importance of IPE, if it is relevant and practical without demanding additional curriculum time. With the health care delivery system gearing toward more patient-centered team-based care, this innovative IPE curriculum helps to foster and mold fledgling future clinicians into confident team members who will lead health care into the future and to better patient outcomes.

DISCUSSION

There are more than 70 dental schools in Canada and the United States, too many to fit in one article. This article has included a mixture of some schools that are well known in IPE as well as some that have not previously had a chance to speak up. It is important for educators to understand the barriers faced by dental schools who are not recognized as the gold standard of IPE. The resulting diverse conversation shows that reported barriers in IPE education include making it relevant and flexible, assessing IPE activities efficiently and effectively, overcoming institutional barriers, and making programs sustainable. These barriers are similar to those pointed out by Palatta and colleagues[3] and Rafter and colleagues.[4]

Providing Relevancy and Flexibility

UT, NYU, WesternU, and UAB offer their diverse solutions to integrate dentistry with other health professions in a realistic and feasible manner that captures the interest of the learners while working with available resources. Teaching teamwork early can be a catalytic mechanism for collaboration in the future. These solutions all demonstrate that relevance and learning can be enhanced by moving from the classroom to clinical care and by the use of actual or simulated cases.

Burgess and Langlois' UT vignette poses a common dilemma faced by dental educators: *How do we make IPE clinical requirements more relevant and flexible?* Seeking to increase the applicability of the IPE experience, yet fit it into a busy curriculum, they have arranged for dental students to shadow 911 call station staff, spend time with dental technologists, and participate in team meetings with nurses, patients, and families. Their success underlines the point that IPE/ICP cases must promote teamwork, be applicable to dental care, and be authentic. Sutherland and Moline,[13] also of UT, describe their similar solution for authenticity in the Appreciating Roles and Collaboration to Improve Care (ARCTIC) Workshop: "Using the compelling narrative of a patient's journey through cancer treatment in our center, we sought to engage the students to discover and appreciate the interventions provided by their colleagues and to recognize the importance of interprofessional care for complex patients."

Allen and Haber at NYU also recognize the need for authenticity in IPE/ICP. Their solution is to use standardized patients to provide a case study experience on oral and systemic health. In this solution, they seek to break down the silos between NP, medical, and dental students and to improve other health professions' understanding of oral health. Anders and colleagues[14] at the University of Buffalo use standardized patients as well; theirs have multiple chronic medical diagnoses, including an oral-systemic component, to provide an interprofessional experience for NP and dental students.

Andrews, Sun Tjahjono, and Maugh at WesternU report time constraints and seek to increase participant enthusiasm. Their solution is to provide real-world experience. They pair dental and physician assistant students to help real patients together. Davis and Mitchell at UAB similarly team health profession students (medical, nursing, optometry, physician assisting, and dental) to provide holistic screenings and referrals for real patients. They use the *Smiles for Life* curriculum to help teach other health professions about oral health.

Gandara and colleagues[1] at UW join dentistry, medicine, and nursing students together to provide foot and oral health care to underserved populations at Teeth and Toes clinics in the Seattle area. Dolce and colleagues[15] at Bouvé College in Boston promote team-based practice several ways, including participation in the Program of All-inclusive Care for the Elderly (PACE), a national program that provides multidisciplinary community health care (including dentistry) in at least 31 US states. Dolce notes, "Transformation of health professions education necessitates innovative models linking interprofessional education (IPE) and collaborative practice." ICP, simulated or real, is the choice of many institutions seeking to maximize the fidelity of the interprofessional learning experience.

Assessing Competency

Kim, Phillips, and Berg at UWSOD needed to establish clear learning objectives and to assess learning. They discovered that many useful resources are already in place at UWSOD and in industry standards, including preexisting guidance documents. They indicate that self-reflection papers can be a particularly powerful way to assess changing attitudes and knowledge.

The Institute of Medicine Report[6] points out the difficulty in finding assessment metrics for the impact of IPE. Emmert and Cai[16] of WesternU underline that "research should continue to focus on testing and refining methodologically sound assessment tools at the graduate and post-graduate level." There is no need to reinvent the wheel, but assessments should be calibrated and evidence based. Learning objectives and assessments can be adapted from high-quality preexisting resources.

Overcoming Institutional Barriers and Making Programs Sustainable

At UIC, institutional barriers have been tackled head-on, as described by Brown, O'Rourke, and Koerber. UIC achieved a campus-wide change by centralizing the CEIPE in the Office of the Provost. This vibrant collaborative group meets regularly, holds a campus-wide IPE event annually, and has fostered institutional changes in attitude that have been accompanied by the growth of student organizations and other projects, including some with external funding. Sustainability is enhanced by an effort to overcome institutional barriers and by embedding IPE/ICP in the fabric of the institution.

Davis and Leavell at Meharry Medical College take a different direction to foster sustainability. They team with community partners who provide services for adults with financial and/or health limitations, thereby addressing community needs and improving cultural competency in students at the same time as providing a rich multidisciplinary team experience. Doris and colleagues[17] at the University of Buffalo also provide an interprofessional social services perspective with the Counseling, Advocacy, Referral Education, and Service model. This model provides social work services at the dental school and has demonstrated its sustainability since 1999.

Doris and colleagues[17] point out "Few of the social work initiatives that have been implemented in dental schools have survived after initial grant funding ran out, or the institutional supporters of the program moved on." The Meharry program shows that learning in a community setting promotes recognition of discipline-specific biases and can help to create sustainable interprofessional resources.

SUMMARY

Noted management consultant Jim Collins coined the term *catalytic mechanisms* to describe initiatives that have unexpected outcomes yet strengthen progress towards goals, especially what he calls "Big Hairy Audacious Goals"[18] like putting the mouth back in the body. Individual efforts like student reflections seem so straightforward but can be so powerful in creating a culture change for all of the students involved. The simple interaction of emergency 911 providers and students makes emergency management real and creates lasting impressions.

The concept of *consilient thinking* refers to bringing together data from different disciplines that reach similar findings, thereby strengthening confidence in the resulting conclusion. Steven Johnson's book *The Ghost Map*[19] shows how the consilient thinking of a physician and a preacher helped change our understanding of the spread of disease and checked the cholera epidemic in London in the mid-1800s. Medical thinking tempered by social thinking worked then. The ability for combining insights from a diversity of disciplines and cultures and experiences to create connections not previously conceived, the so-called aha moment, is still possible. This is the essence of IPE, ICP, and teamwork in health care. It is about the best care of patients.

ACKNOWLEDGMENTS

The authors would like to sincerely thank the contributors of the Problems and Solutions for their generous contributions to the development of this article: *K Burgess* and *S Langlois* of the University of Toronto; *K Allen* and *J Haber* of New York University; *AC Davis* and *SC Mitchell* of the University of Alabama; *B Brown, J O'Rourke*, and *A Koerber* of the University of Illinois at Chicago; *G Davis II* and *J Leavell* of Meharry Medical College; *A Kim, S Phillips*, and *J Berg* of the University of Washington; and *E Andrews, J Sun Tjahjono*, and *E Maugh* of Western University of Health Sciences. The Meharry Medical College School of Dentistry project was made possible through the collaborative efforts of the following departments and institutions: Meharry-Vanderbilt Alliance; Meharry Medical College (School of Dentistry, School of Medicine, School of Graduate Studies and Research); Belmont University (Tennessee Simulation Alliance, School of Occupational Therapy, and the School of Nursing [undergraduate]); Lipscomb University (College of Pharmacy); Tennessee State University (College of Public Service and Urban Affairs); Vanderbilt University and Medical Center (Divinity School, School of Medicine, Dietetic Internship Program, Department of Hearing and Speech Sciences, and the School of Nursing [advanced practice]).

REFERENCES

1. American Dental Association, Commission on Dental Accreditation. Accreditation Standards for Dental Education Programs. Available at: http://www.ada.org/~/media/CODA/Files/2016_predoc.pdf?la=en. Assessed June 15, 2016.

2. Gandara B, Overstreet F, Murphy N, et al. From teeth to toes, interprofessional education in community outreach settings. Seattle, WA: University of Washington; 2015. Available at: http://69.59.162.218/ADEA2013/Washington State CC/3.18.13_Mon/WSCC 609/Mon_1530/791_Beatrice_Gandara_WSCC 609/FINAL_Teeth_and_Toes_Presentation_Gandara March 18 2013.pdf. Accessed January 18, 2016.

3. Palatta A, Cook BJ, Anderson EL, et al. 20 years beyond the crossroads: the path to interprofessional education at U.S. dental schools. J Dent Educ 2015;79(8):

982–96. Available at: http://www.jdentaled.org/content/79/8/982.full. Accessed January 18, 2016.

4. Rafter ME, Pesun IJ, Herren M, et al. A preliminary survey of interprofessional education. J Dent Educ 2006;70(4):417–27.

5. Furgeson D, Kinney JS, Gwozdek AE, et al. Interprofessional education in U.S. dental hygiene programs: a national survey. J Dent Educ 2015;79(11):1286–94. Available at: http://www.jdentaled.org/content/79/11/1286.long. Accessed January 18, 2016.

6. Institute of Medicine (IOM). Measuring the impact of interprofessional education on collaborative practice and patient outcomes. Washington, DC: The National Academies Press; 2015. Available at: http://www.nap.edu/catalog/21726/measuring-the-impact-of-interprofessional-education-on-collaborative-practice-and-patient-outcomes. Accessed January 18, 2016.

7. Haber J, Spielman A, Wolff M, et al. Interprofessional education between dentistry and nursing: the NYU experience. CDA J 2014;42(1):44–51.

8. Haber J, Hartnett E, Allen K, et al. Putting the mouth back in the head: HEENT to HEENOT. Am J Public Health 2015;105(3):437–41.

9. Interprofessional Education Collaborative Expert Panel (IPEC). Core competencies for interprofessional collaborative practice: report of an expert panel. Washington, DC: Interprofessional Education Collaborative; 2011. Available at: https://www.aamc.org/download/186750/data/core_competencies.pdf. Accessed February 8, 2016.

10. STFM Group on Oral Health. Smiles for life curriculum. Leawood, KS: Society of Teachers of Family Medicine; 2015. Available at: http://www.smilesforlifeoralhealth.org/. Accessed January 18, 2016.

11. King G, Shaw L, Orchard CA, et al. The interprofessional socialization and valuing scale: a tool for evaluating the shift toward collaborative care approaches in health care settings. Work 2010;35(1):77–85. Available at: https://www.researchgate.net/profile/Carole_Orchard/publication/41466173_The_Interprofessional_Socialization_and_Valuing_Scale_A_tool_for_evaluating_the_shift_toward_collaborative_care_approaches_in_health_care_settings/links/00b7d51c9b6dd6de6c000000.pdf. Accessed January 19, 2016.

12. Bridges DR, Davidson RA, Odegard PS, et al. Interprofessional collaboration: three best practice models of interprofessional education. Med Educ Online 2011;16. http://dx.doi.org/10.3402/meo.v16i0.6035. Available at: http://www.ncbi.nlm.nih.gov/pmc/articles/PMC3081249/. Accessed January 19, 2016.

13. Sutherland SE, Moline KA. The ARCTIC workshop: an interprofessional education activity in an academic health sciences center. J Dent Educ 2015;79(6):636–43. Available at: http://www.jdentaled.org/content/79/6/636.long. Accessed January 18, 2016.

14. Anders PL, Scherer YK, Hatton M, et al. Using standardized patients to teach interprofessional competencies to dental students. J Dent Educ 2016;80(1):65–72. Available at: http://www.jdentaled.org/content/80/1/65.long. Accessed January 18, 2016.

15. Dolce MC, Aghazadeh-Sanai N, Mohammed S, et al. Integrating oral health into the interdisciplinary health sciences curriculum. Dent Clin North Am 2014;58(4):829–43. Available at: http://www.dental.theclinics.com/article/S0011-8532%2814%2900065-2/pdf. Accessed January 18, 2016.

16. Emmert MC, Cai L. A pilot study to test the effectiveness of an innovative interprofessional education assessment strategy. J Interprof Care 2015;29(5):451–6.

Available at: http://www.tandfonline.com/doi/full/10.3109/13561820.2015. 1025373. Accessed January 18, 2016.

17. Doris JM, Davis E, DuPont C, et al. Social work in dentistry: the CARES model for improving patient retention and access to care. Dent Clin North Am 2009; 53:549–59. Available at: http://www.dental.theclinics.com/article/S0011-8532% 2809%2900021-4/pdf. Accessed January 18, 2016.

18. Collins J. Turning goals into results: the power of catalytic mechanisms. Brighton, MA: Harvard Business Review; 1999. Available at: https://hbr.org/1999/07/turning-goals-into-results-the-power-of-catalytic-mechanisms/ar/1. Accessed February 8, 2016.

19. Johnson S. The ghost map: the story of London's most terrifying epidemic and how it changed science, cities and the modern world. New York: Riverhead Books; 2006.

Interprofessional Education for the Dentist in Managing Acute and Chronic Pain

Jeffry Shaefer, DDS, MS, MPH[a,*], Antje M. Barreveld, MD[b,c],
Paul Arnstein, RN, PhD, FNP-C, ACNS-BC[d], Ronald J. Kulich, PhD, MS[e,f]

KEYWORDS

- Interprofessional relations • Pain management • Opioid analgesics
- Dental education • American board of pain medicine • Chronic pain • Acute pain
- Pain clinics

KEY POINTS

- A symbiotic relationship exists between control of chronic disease and dental health, especially pain management; neither can be achieved without the other.
- Health care members in collaborative practice must understand the diagnosis and evidence-based treatment standards for patients and the roles of fellow health care collaborators in meeting those standards.
- The treatment standards for pain management build on educational standards, such as those of the Commission on Dental Accreditation, to create collaborative practice standards, such as those of the International Association for the Study of Pain.
- Faculty development is necessary for teaching effective pain management skills in an interprofessional education program.
- Licensure and accreditation requirements should reinforce an interprofessional focus for pain management education in preparation for collaborative practice of patient-centered care.

[a] Department of Oral and Maxillofacial Surgery, Harvard School of Dental Medicine, 188 Longwood Ave, Boston, MA 02115, USA; [b] Department of Anesthesiology, Newton-Wellesley Hospital, Tufts University Medical School, 2014 Washington Street, Newton, MA 02462, USA; [c] Department of Anesthesiology, Perioperative and Pain Medicine, Brigham and Women's Hospital, Harvard Medical School Teaching Affiliate, Boston, MA, USA; [d] Nurse Practitioner Program, MGH Institute for Health Professionals, Massachusetts General Hospital (MGH), Boston, MA, USA; [e] Tufts School of Dental Medicine, 1 Kneeland St Boston, Boston, MA 02111, USA; [f] Department of Anesthesia, Critical Care and Pain Medicine, Massachusetts General Hospital, 15 Parkman St Boston, Boston, MA 02114, USA
* Corresponding author.
E-mail address: Jeffry_Shaefer@HSDM.Harvard.edu

Dent Clin N Am 60 (2016) 825–842
http://dx.doi.org/10.1016/j.cden.2016.05.003
0011-8532/16/$ – see front matter © 2016 Elsevier Inc. All rights reserved.

Collaborative practice in health care occurs when multiple health workers from different professional backgrounds provide comprehensive services by working with patients, their families, insurance carriers, communities, and each other to deliver the highest quality of care across clinical settings. Interprofessional education (IPE) is defined as 2 or more professions learning from and about each other to improve collaboration and the quality of care.[1,2] IPE is in contrast with a more traditional model involving different departments within the same profession (eg, medical departments of surgery, anesthesia, neurology; or dental departments of oral surgery, restorative dentistry, and periodontics) potentially teaching the same subject but from different disciplinary perspectives.[3]

IPE is today's buzzword in health care education.[3] At a time when effective collaborative practice is a target for addressing the opioid crisis. Pain management is complex, often requiring collaborative approaches that exceed the expertise of any single profession.[4] As such, IPE is a critical advancement for effective pain management education and practice.[3] Guidelines for pain management education to prepare health professionals to function in a collaborative practice are available and summarized in **Box 1.**[5]

This article reviews how national, state, and local institutions are influencing pain management standards and the teaching of these standards, specifically in response to the opioid crisis, for dentistry and other health care disciplines. Innovations in IPE pain management education at Boston-based health care institutions are presented. In addition, current and proposed accreditation standards and their influence on the preparation of health care providers to implement effective pain management are discussed as supportive evidence for an IPE collaboration to manage pain.

FROM WHERE DOES THIS MOVEMENT FOR INTERPROFESSIONAL EDUCATION IN PAIN MANAGEMENT ARISE?

Standards for both acute and chronic pain management are being reviewed and updated at the national, state, and local level. The Federal Drug Administration, National Institutes of Health (NIH), and organizations such as the International

---

Box 1
Interprofessional collaborative practice competencies

1. Work with individuals of other professions to maintain a climate of mutual respect and shared values.

2. Use the knowledge of one's own role and the roles of other professions to appropriately assess and address the health care needs of the patients and populations served.

3. Communicate with patients, families, communities, and other health professionals in a responsive and responsible manner that supports a team approach to maintaining health and treatment of disease.

4. Apply relationship-building values and the principles of team dynamics to perform effectively in different team roles to plan and deliver patient-centered care that is safe, timely, efficient, effective, and equitable.

Data from Barr H, Freeth D, Hammick M, et al. Evaluations of interprofessional education: a United Kingdom review for health and social care. London: Centre for the Advancement of Interprofessional Education with the British Educational Research Association; 2000. Available at: http://caipe.org.uk/silo/files/evaluations-of-interprofessional-education.pdf. Accessed March 30, 2016.

Association for the Study of Pain (IASP), the American Academy of Pain Medicine (AAPM), and the American Dental Association (ADA), have outlined goals for pain management education involving IPE.[6–11]

At the national level, and in response to the Institute of Medicine (IOM) 2011 report[7] calling for a transformation in pain prevention, care, education, and research, the NIH commissioned a National Pain Strategy report that was released in 2015 (http://iprcc.nih.gov/docs/drafthhsnationalpainstrategy.pdf). In particular, this report outlines professional education and training principles in pain management, as well as highlights the core competencies in pain education developed by an interprofessional consensus summit in 2013.[9] As stated in the National Pain Strategy draft report, "The intent of the professional education and training component of the National Pain Strategy is to anchor an attitudinal transformation toward pain and a reorganization of pain management by the health care system, in the education… and training of health professionals. The mission includes grounding the pain-related education and training of physicians, nurses, clinical pharmacists, dentists, clinical health psychologists, physician's assistants, nurse practitioners, and other health professionals in core competencies, and making available easily accessible, evidence based information for educators to work toward this goal."[9]

On a state level, one can appreciate recent changes in such guidelines when comparing the Washington State Guidelines of 2015 to those of 2010 (**Table 1**).[6] The guidelines now refer to management of all phases of pain (eg, acute, perioperative, chronic, special populations) and stress a diagnosis-based pharmacotherapy for pain treatment. The state of Massachusetts also updated its advisory for dentists prescribing controlled medications in 2011[12] and issued a *Special Report on Prescribing in Dentistry* in 2015.[13] The advisory stresses the principles associated with effective pain management, identification of patients at risk for misuse of controlled medications, and informed consent for the use of opioids in the patient's treatment plan. The special report[13] outlines the Massachusetts Prescription Monitoring Program. The Massachusetts Boards of Medicine and Dentistry now require continuing education in pain management for license renewal (**Box 2**). The goals and objectives are given in a lecture that fulfills this licensure requirement. Recently, the governor of Massachusetts convened a working group of educators, *Governor's Medical Education Working Group on Prescription Drug Misuse,* and tasked them to develop improved pain education standards for the states' medical schools.[14] Dental educators from the Boston dental schools also contributed to this effort.

WHY IS UNDERSTANDING THE MANAGEMENT OF THE CHRONIC PAIN PATIENT IMPORTANT FOR DENTISTS?

Opioid treatment is an increasingly common form of therapy for patients with a history of chronic pain.[4,7] Ninety percent of physicians who specialized in pain medicine (pain physicians) reportedly maintain patients with nonmalignant pain on opioids.[15] As many as 40% of patients with temporomandibular disorder (TMD) seen in a tertiary care setting can be refractive to treatment.[16] This compares with 30% to 40% of facial neuralgia patients who do not respond to medical management with medications and/or surgery.[17] Providers, with the goal of improving function and quality of life for these patients, must consider the use of opioids in the patient's management regimen.

Dentists are in a unique position to have an impact on managing chronic disease because they have regular contact with their patients and commonly address issues of preventive health and wellness.[18] This places the dental provider in a critical decision-making role for the treatment of these patients[19] because oral health care

Table 1
Comparison of Washington state agency medical directors' group's interagency opioid guidelines from 2010 to 2015

2010 Guideline	2015 Guideline
Primary focus on chronic noncancer pain	Expands focus to include opioid use in acute, subacute, and perioperative pain phases, and in special populations Includes sections on tapering and opioid use disorder

2 main sections
I. Initiating, transitioning, and maintaining patients on COAT with principles of safe prescribing
II. Optimizing treatment of patients on >120 mg daily MED with brief sections on getting consultations, aberrant behaviors, tapering, and discontinuing COAT
	New and modified sections
	1. Recommendations for all pain phases
	  a. Clinically meaningful improvement in function
	  b. Expanded discussion on dosing threshold
	  c. Nonopioid options for pain management
	2. Opioids in the acute and subacute phases
	3. Opioids for perioperative pain
	4. Opioids for chronic noncancer pain (similar to previous guideline)
	5. New section on reducing or discontinuing COAT
	6. New section on recognition and treatment of opioid use disorder
	7. New sections on opioid use in special populations (during pregnancy and neonatal abstinence syndrome, in children and adolescents, in older adults, and in cancer survivors)

Appendices A. Opioid dose calculations & calculator B. Screening tools C. Tools to assess pain and function D. Urine drug testing for COAT E. Consultative assistance for Washington state payers F. Patient education resources G. Sample doctor-patient agreement for COAT H. Additional resources to streamline clinical care I. Emergency department opioid guidelines	Appendices A. Opioid dose calculations & calculator B. Renamed: Validated risk factor screening tools and combined former appendices B and C C. How to use the prescription monitoring program D. Urine drug testing for COAT E. Chronic pain syndromes in cancer survivors F. Diagnosis-based pharmacotherapy for pain G. Patient education resources (updated) H. Renamed: Clinical tools and resources and combines former appendices G, H, and I I. Guideline development and Agree II criteria
Recommended 120 mg daily MED as a yellow-flag dose as a strategy to prevent adverse events and overdose by advising providers to seek a consultation with a pain specialist	Remains the same, plus adds guidance for safe prescribing at any dose, based on new studies showing significant risks occurring at lower doses
Organized as narrative information and recommendations with evidence in citations	Organized with each section having specific clinical recommendations with supporting narrative evidence sections with citations

Abbreviations: COAT, chronic opioid analgesic therapy; MED, morphinr equivalent dose.
From Washington State agency medical directors' group's interagency opioid guidelines (AMDGO). Available at: http://www.agencymeddirectors.wa.gov/guidelines.asp.

Box 2
Goals and objectives for mandatory dental pain management continuing education

The attendee should

1. Understand the principles of acute pain management

2. Understand how to recognize the problem patient (drug seeker, at-risk patient)

3. Be able to address acute pain for a patient with chronic pain

4. Understand principles of pain management for the elderly and pediatric dental patient

From O'Neal M, editor. The ADA practical guide to substance use disorders and safe prescribing. Hoboken (NJ): Wiley-Blackwell; 2015; with permission.

---

is intimately associated orofacial pain diagnosis and treatment. They must advise the pain physician; the rheumatologist; the ear, nose, and throat surgeon; and/or the primary care provider (PCP) on appropriate interventions. They must provide care and management as necessary and decide when maximum medical benefit of physical treatments for these patients is reached. PCPs, pain physicians, and other medical providers often do not have the dental and facial pain expertise to properly evaluate these patients. Dental providers with appropriate training in pain management are best positioned to provide the service of assessment for opioid therapy on orofacial pain patients not responsive to treatment.

Chronic opioid prescribing for nonmalignant pain is controversial. The arguments for and against are compelling. However, even though a provider is not prescribing controlled medications to the patient, all providers must understand the current standards of care for opioid prescribing, the use of screening devices to identify those at risk for substance abuse, and the protocols for getting an at-risk patient the treatment needed. Following these standards of care for opioid prescribing can give confidence to the provider and remove the angst associated with treating patients who are on these medications.

Therefore, dentists have a prominent role in managing a significant part of society's pain burden; in particular, the diagnosis and treatment of acute dental pain and chronic orofacial pain problems, such as TMDs, trigeminal neuralgia, tension headaches, and neuropathic pain affecting oral tissues. Dental education must promote the ability for both students and graduates to function in today's collaborative practice, with the goal that all health care providers will have confidence when treating patients who suffer from these dental pain problems. An IPE approach in the principles of pain management allows this goal to be achieved.

WHAT CAN BE LEARNED FROM CASE-BASED EXAMPLES FROM BOSTON-BASED INSTITUTIONS IN DEVELOPING INTERPROFESSIONAL PAIN MANAGEMENT EDUCATION INNOVATIONS?
Dental

Despite its importance in clinical practice, pain management is not prominent in the curricula of most prelicensure health care professional education programs.[19–28] An assessment of teaching related to pain, TMDs, and orofacial pain diagnosis and management in the United States reveals that few dental schools are adequately providing their students with the experience necessary to effectively manage these cases.[29] Recent curriculum changes at dental schools in Boston, however, are addressing these discrepancies. The Harvard School of Dental Medicine (HSDM) is the lead institution in the Boston-based NIH Consortium Centers of Excellence in Pain Education (CoEPE).[30] At HSDM, with support from a 5-year contract from the NIH National Institute of Drug Addiction (NIDA), educators are collaborating to teach appropriate controlled substance prescribing via both intradisciplinary (dentistry) and interprofessional (medical, dental, nursing, pharmacy, and psychology) education.[30]

Under the new CoEPE NIDA-NIH contract, HSDM educators are implementing the IASP curriculum,[3,28] as well as the AAPM Core Competencies in Pain Management,[5,29] to guide students' learning objectives for pain management. At all of the NIH 11 CoEPEs, Web-based case modules will be used as the primary method for teaching pain management principles. At the HSDM, these modules will be used initially for second-year and third-year students' self-directed learning. Then, to address contemporary concern for opioid prescribing practices, small group sessions (third year) and interprofessional workshops (fourth year) that follow the use of these independent case-based modules will place a particular emphasis on specific topics (**Box 3**).[30]

The HSDM students are introduced to pain diagnosis and management concepts in the current problem-based learning curriculum, which gradually builds the student's knowledge foundation so they can eventually be able to diagnose and to treat (or refer) a complex dental patient. The new resources generated under the NIDA-NIH contract will be used to supplement the existing case-based, small-group tutorial curriculum (8–10 students with 1 tutor). Each case will have levels of difficulty and complexity to be used at the appropriate time in student development, allowing the case to be used to teach anatomy and clinical examination skills in the first 2 years (data gathering), diagnosis and treatment in the third year, and management of the patient in the fourth year.

Acute and chronic pain issues will be identified in the first 2 years, diagnoses and treatment in the third year, and long-term management addressed in the fourth year. In addition, these cases will be used for the problem-based learning curriculum during the fourth year as a conduit to discuss pain management principles during their HSDM clinical rotation and before clerkships in oral surgery and orofacial pain clinics.

Box 3
Harvard School of Dental Medicine Consortium Centers of Excellence in Pain Education goals for opioid prescribing

After completing this training, students will understand

1. Safe and effective opioid-based management

2. Recognition and assessment of risk factors and signs of potential abuse, addiction, or diversion

3. Management of patients with evidence of, or risk factors for, opioid misuse

4. Adjunct (nonopioid) treatments

5. Barriers to effective pain control

6. Biopsychosocial approaches and coping strategies for living with pain

7. Communication and teamwork in understanding and managing patients' suffering

From NIH Pain Consortium Centers of Excellence in Pain Education sponsored by the National Institute on Drug Abuse, NIH, Contract # HHSN271201500075C. Centers of Excellence in Pain Education (CoEPEs). Reference #: NO1DA-15-4427, 2015. Available at: http://painconsortium.nih.gov/NIH_Pain_Programs/CoEPES.html. Accessed March 22, 2016.

The fourth-year pain rotation in the orofacial pain clinic should become a required part of the dental school curriculum and these cases will be used to prepare the students for these rotations. Clinic directors at the community health centers at which the fourth-year dental students rotate for refining their clinical skills will find these cases excellent resources to enhance student learning and patient management.

The importance of these cases, developed to teach pain management principles, is that they be used at all levels of dental school training to develop an understanding of inflammatory pain, neuropathic pain, arthralgia, myalgia, management of acute pain, management of chronic pain, avoidance and recognition of substance abuse problems, use of physical therapy, dental appliance therapy, behavioral therapy, and alternative therapy to promote pain control and optimize patient function. These cases will be designed to fit into any dental school curriculum and be tailored to supplement pain education at various levels of student expertise, allowing the same cases to be used to teach pain management principles to medical, nursing, pharmacy, and psychology students. As such, the dental students should become confident in teaching the diagnosis and management principles for acute dental pain, TMDs, and orofacial neuropathic pain to students in other health professions.

The case modules will eventually be available to educators and students everywhere on an NIH Web site.[30] The reader should find the first 2 cases developed under the CoEPE program interesting because they show the potential for IPE module approaches in improving the care for patients suffering from orofacial (dental-related) pain. The first case involves an oral pharyngeal patient who has cancer with recurrent disease, dental pain, and limited jaw opening. The dental student teaching this case must explain the diagnosis and standard of care for treating these problems, as well as outline the dental protocol for preparing this patient for head and neck radiation. The second case involves a patient with TMD with masticatory muscle pain and the comorbidity of fibromyalgia. One can appreciate the benefit that the IPE student will receive while studying and teaching this case with his or her fellow health care students. They will learn and teach TMD anatomy, jaw function, and diagnosis; standards for care of both fibromyalgia and TMD; use of nonopioid medications; alternative treatments; and, most important, how to manage such a patient on opioids.

The concept behind the NIH promoting the creation of a multiple of cases concerning specific pain diagnosis is to support the principal goals of IPE: (1) diagnosis of the pain disorder, (2) knowledge of evidenced-based treatment of the disorder, (3) providers understanding their own role and the roles of all team members when treating the disorder, and (4) communication between health care professionals.[15,31]

Educators at Tufts School of Dental Medicine currently conduct weekly Interprofessional Pain and Headache Rounds with participation by students, faculty, and regional experts in the areas of pain and addiction. In addition, the school is in the process of developing and evaluating a protocol for integrating the Massachusetts Prescription Monitoring Program into the dental curriculum.[14]

A collaborative effort between educators (referred to as pain champions) at Boston-based health care institutions of medicine, nursing, pharmacy, psychology, and dentistry led to this team's distinction as an NIH CoEPEs.[30] Each of the pain champions at these institutions will insure the effectiveness of the intraprofessional pain management education at their schools, using the cases described. Roadblocks exist, however, to promote an IPE initiative due to scheduling a balanced curriculum timeframe for teaching IPE approaches in pain management. Sufficient time must be scheduled to allow students from each institution to work together. For this initiative to be successful it must have support at every level of each institution, from the deans down to the students. Faculty development for IPE and pain management education is required and must be supported.[31] The eventual reward of this support will be that students will develop confidence when communicating with other health professions, while understanding their and the other members' roles in providing appropriate pain management for the patients in a collaborative practice.

Medical

Harvard Medical School (HMS) students have access to many of the best educators and leaders in pain management. Their educational resources on pain management are sparse, however, and can be improved by a more directed, informative, creative, and thought-provoking curriculum, especially during students' clinical training years. Although the medical school's third-year clerkships have a session that briefly addresses the basics of pain management, this has been the only limited instruction that medical students have in this important field. The HMS educators recognize the importance of pain management, as well as IPE, and are eager to see an improvement in students' instructions and to incorporate a new pain education curriculum.

At HMS, the NIDA-NIH CoEPE curriculum resources will be first integrated into the Anesthesia-Surgical and Internal Medicine Clerkships. The goal is to use the subsequent evaluations to improve the formats of the case-based modules to develop the additional cases and implement them throughout the students' third-year clerkships. Because students have not had any regular or dedicated preclinical courses on pain management at HMS, and there is no formalized IPE, the CoEPE initiative promises to serve as a pioneer program in IPE pain education for medical students.

In response to the Massachusetts governor's request to update medical school training for pain management, HMS has recently added a new class combining neuroscience, psychiatry, and human development, while revamping the second-year Introduction to Psychiatry course to better address the opioid abuse crisis.[14] Other case-oriented experiences, such as the CoEPE's case-based modules, will also be added to the curriculum. The other Boston-based medical schools have responded to the governor's initiative with curriculum changes.

The Boston University School of Medicine has developed a course on the biology of addiction and its treatment strategies.[14] The fourth-year student Scope of Pain Program teaches pain management principles and appropriate opioid prescribing.[14] The University of Massachusetts Medical School is incorporating the core competencies from the governor's working group into its curriculum, actually hiring actors to make their case simulations more realistic.[14] The Tufts University School of Medicine's Curriculum Committee approved all 10 of the core competencies. In addition to having their students take an addiction course, third-year students will be tested throughout the year on the core competencies.[14]

Nursing

Pain is the most common nursing diagnosis that is used across the continuum of care in inpatient, rehabilitation, outpatient, and home settings.[32–34] As such, every nurse needs to have a working understanding of the assessment, prevention, and management of pain. There is an appreciation that nurses have both a duty to act independently to comfort patients and do not manage pain in isolation from other professionals. Instead, they work together as part of a patient-centered team to better understand and relieve it. Pain relief is an essential part of nursing practice. Every nurse, regardless of his or her role, has a responsibility to alleviate suffering; prevent complications that may result from unrelieved pain; and advocate and work collaboratively with patients, families, and other health care professionals to provide patient-centered care. To fulfill these responsibilities, the nurse must be knowledgeable and skilled in the assessment and management of pain. This involves developing and maintaining a working knowledge of pain assessment; pharmacologic and nondrug interventions; and the use of medications, equipment, and resources needed to promote safe, effective relief.[35–37]

As with all health professionals, nurses need to be trained in the multidimensional nature of pain; how to assess pain in a reliable, measurable way; and to manage pain in a collaborative way across the lifespan and the continuum of care. When the usual pain treatment fails or interferes with biopsychosocial functioning, nurses seek help by expanding the treatment team. They may seek refinement of the medical treatment plan, engage physical therapists, psychologists, social workers, chaplaincy, and/or other team members as appropriate to the setting and circumstance.[38]

This approach recognizes the limits of their scope of practice and the value-added contribution of an interdisciplinary framework to work collaboratively to best serve patients suffering from pain. The American Association of Colleges of Nursing and the National League for Nursing that accredits schools of nursing recognizes the value and supports the need to adopt evolving approaches to IPE, academic-service partnerships, and clinical and scientific learning to stimulate innovative thinking about turning today's challenges into opportunities to improve team-based pain treatment in the future.[39,40]

The Joint Commission that accredits many of the organizations in which nurses work has standards that require the assessment and management of pain is an important component of patient-centered care. Their standards further require patient involvement in their treatment planning that is based on clinical judgment, while taking into account the risks and benefits of available treatments, including the potential risks of dependency, addiction, and abuse when opioids are used.[41] The Joint Commission also recognizes that interprofessional communication is necessary for the development of trust among team members and the need for a variety of forums to proactively develop these skills. The complexities and interprofessional duty to assess and manage pain regardless of discipline makes this an excellent opportunity to develop the requisite interprofessional communication and collaboration skills.

With the Boston-based CoEPE, the Massachusetts General Hospital Institute for Health Professions and Regis College Nursing School recognize the importance of this endeavor and have signed on to be a setting for advanced practice nurse training. The shared goals are to promote interprofessional knowledge, skill, and dialogue about the importance of effectively alleviating pain and preventing, while identifying and treating substance use disorders. Case-based modules and group sessions or workshops will be integrated into the second year of courses and clinical rotations, and into their advanced nursing degree programs

Barriers to improving pain management education in nursing school include

- A packed curricula of study with little room for added content
- Scheduling conflicts across professional programs for the interprofessional dialogue component
- Faculty teaching loads and research interests
- Gaining cooperation of administration within the various programs when there is limited financial incentive to do so
- The reluctance of faculty to adopt new paradigms for education.

Psychology

The William James College of Graduate Psychology, formerly the Massachusetts School of Professional Psychology, also Boston-based, supports a commitment to experiential education combining rigorous academic instruction with diverse clinical experiences. An interprofessional pain management curriculum mirrors their educational mission to provide a diversified learning environment to allow students exposure to different disciplines. The use of the CoEPE's case-based modules, small group sessions, and interprofessional workshops will be dispersed throughout the 4-year clinical psychology doctorate program to enhance the student's pain management education.[42,43]

Pharmacy

Students at the Massachusetts College of Pharmacy and Health Sciences are provided with minimal pain management education within the current curriculum. With the evolving role of pharmacists, it is imperative that students be educated on pain management principles across various health care settings through a case-based approach that emphasizes collaborative care. With pharmacists being some of the most accessible health care providers, education on pain assessment and management becomes paramount to improve patient access to proper care. The leadership and administration personnel are dedicated to collaborating with the other health care institutions in Boston to provide students with innovative, evidence-based, and practical knowledge that will serve to improve patient outcomes. At the College, the CoEPE's case-based modules will be shared with students during their third professional year and will be discussed in a small group setting during the required Pharmacotherapeutics Seminar course. These modules will also be implemented for students on clinical clerkship at the Brigham and Women's Hospital.

Summary

A collaborative effort between pain champions at Boston-based health care institutions led to the collaboration's distinction as 1 of NIH 11 CoEPEs.[30] Each of the pain champions at these institutions will insure the effectiveness of the intraprofessional pain management education at their schools, using the cases described. Once trained, students at these institutions will participate in elective interprofessional workshops, applying the pain management principles they have learned in a collaborative practice setting.

WHAT ARE THE ACCREDITATION STANDARDS?

Are predoctoral and postdoctoral accreditation standards for IPE and pain management education (**Tables 2–5**[44]) consistent with the national, state, and local guidelines for effective pain management? Such an analysis is critical for predicting the ability of dental graduates to function effectively as an integral member of an interprofessional collaborative practice. (see **Table 3**)[44] details the predoctoral standards related to pain management and to the assessment of complex patients, such as TMD and/or chronic pain patients. These are general nonspecific standards but they do promote the competencies necessary for the new dental graduate to function in a collaborative practice. More specific education or knowledge, however, is required to meet the postdoctorate standards (see **Tables 4** and **5**,[44]). The postgraduate periodontal and prosthodontics standards specifically dictate understanding of orofacial pain, whereas standards for the discipline of prosthodontics also include the need to understand TMDs. Oral and maxillofacial surgery standards require an understanding of temporomandibular joint disease.

Table 2
Dental interprofessional education accreditation standards

Standard 1	Institutional Effectiveness
1–9	The dental school must show evidence of interaction with other components of the higher education, health care education, and/or health care delivery systems
Standard 2	Educational program Practice management and health care systems
2–19	Graduates must be competent in communicating and collaborating with other members of the health care team to facilitate the provision of health care
Intent	Students should understand the roles of members of the health care team and have educational experiences, particularly clinical experiences that involve working with other health care professional students and practitioners Students should have educational experiences in which they coordinate patient care within the health care system relevant to dentistry

From Commission on Dental Accreditation (CODA). Accreditation standards for dental education programs. Available at: http://www.ada.org/~/media/CODA/Files/predoc.ashx; with permission. Accessed April 2, 2016.

Table 3
Predoctoral accreditation standards for pain management

2–23	Minimum Graduate Competencies In Providing General Dentistry Oral Health Care
a	Patient assessment, diagnosis, comprehensive treatment planning, prognosis, and informed consent
e	Local anesthesia, and pain and anxiety control
o	Evaluation of the outcomes of treatment, recall strategies, and prognosis
Intent	Ability to evaluate, assess, and apply current and emerging science and technology The basic knowledge, skills, and values to practice dentistry, independently, at the time of graduation The school identifies the competencies included in the curriculum based on the school's goals, resources, accepted general practitioner responsibilities, and other influencing factors The comprehensive care experiences provided for patients by students should be adequate to ensure competency in all components of general dentistry practice Programs should assess overall competency, not simply individual competencies, to measure the graduate's readiness to enter the practice of general dentistry
2–13	In-depth information on abnormal biological conditions must be provided to support a high level of understanding of the cause, epidemiology, differential diagnosis, pathogenesis, prevention, treatment, and prognosis of oral and oral related disorders
2–14	Competency in the application of biomedical science knowledge in the delivery of patient care Intent: Biological science knowledge should be of sufficient depth and scope for graduates to apply advances in modern biology to clinical practice and to integrate new medical knowledge and therapies relevant to oral health care
2–24	Competency in assessing the treatment needs of patients with special needs
Intent	Appropriate patient pool available to provide experiences that include patients with medical, physical, psychological, or social situations that make it necessary to consider a wide range of assessment and care options Assessment should emphasize the importance of nondental considerations These individuals include, but are not limited to, people with developmental disabilities, cognitive impairment, complex medical problems, significant physical limitations, and the vulnerable elderly Clinical instruction and experience with the patients with special needs should include instruction in proper communication techniques and assessing the treatment needs compatible with the special need

From Commission on Dental Accreditation (CODA): Accreditation Standards For Dental Education Programs. Available at: http://www.ada.org/~/media/CODA/Files/predoc.ashx; with permission. Accessed April 2, 2016.

Table 4
Postdoctoral accreditation standards for pain management

Endodontics

4–5	Instruction provided in:
G	Pharmacotherapeutics
H	Neurosciences

Oral and Maxillofacial Surgery

4–5	Instruction provided in basic biomedical sciences at an advanced level, including growth and development, physiology, pharmacology, microbiology, and pathologic evaluation
4–9.3	Clinical program must be supported in part by a core comprehensive didactic program on general anesthesia, deep sedation, and other methods of pain and anxiety control
4–13	Experience must include management of temporomandibular joint disease
4–13.1	Disease management includes, but is not limited to, major maxillary sinus procedures, treatment of temporomandibular joint disease, salivary gland or duct surgery, management of head and neck infections, (incision and drainage procedures), and surgical management of benign and malignant neoplasms and cysts

Periodontics

4–11	Education must provide training for the student or resident in the methods of pain control and sedation
a	In-depth knowledge in all areas of minimal, moderate, and deep sedation as prescribed by the ADA Guidelines for Teaching Pain Control and Sedation to Dentists and Dental Students
b	Clinical training to the level of competency in adult minimal enteral and moderate parenteral sedation as prescribed by the ADA Guidelines for Teaching Pain Control and Sedation to Dentists and Dental Students
Intent	Follow the ADA Guidelines for Teaching Pain Control and Sedation to Dentists and Dental Students regarding all aspects of training in minimal enteral and moderate parenteral sedation, including didactic instruction, health status assessment, monitoring, airway management, emergency care, and number of required cases The ADA Guidelines were developed and approved by the ADA Council on Dental Education and Licensure and adopted by the ADA House of Delegates
4–12	The educational program must provide instruction in interdisciplinary areas
a	The management of orofacial pain to a level of understanding

Prosthodontics

4–8	Instruction must be provided at the understanding level
f	TMDs and orofacial pain
4–14	Students or residents must be competent in the prosthodontic management of patients with TMDs and/or orofacial pain

Orthodontics

4–3.4	
g	Manage patients with functional occlusal and TMDs
4–4	Supporting curriculum: the orthodontic graduate must understand
e	Pain and anxiety control
h	Pharmacology

(continued on next page)

Table 4 (continued)	
Pediatric Dentistry	
3–3.8	Inpatient facilities to permit management of general and oral health problems for patients with special health care needs
4–10	Clinical experiences in oral facial injury and emergency care must enable students or residents to achieve competency in a and b
a	Diagnosis and management of traumatic injuries of the oral and perioral structures, including primary and permanent dentition, and in infants, children, and adolescents
b	Emergency services, including assessment and management of dental pain and infections

From Commission on Dental Accreditation (CODA). Standards for Advanced Specialty Education Programs. Available at: http://www.ada.org/en/coda/current-accreditation-standards/; with permission. Accessed April 2, 2016.

WHAT MIGHT THE FUTURE BRING FOR INTERPROFESSIONAL EDUCATION FOR PAIN MANAGEMENT AND EFFECTS ON THE COLLABORATIVE PRACTICE?

Oral health care plays a prominent role in managing a significant part of society's pain burden. Dental practitioners are or should be uniquely trained to understand and teach the diagnosis and treatment of acute dental pain, as well as chronic orofacial pain problems; that is, TMDs, trigeminal neuralgia, tension headaches, and neuropathic pain affecting oral tissues. Dental education must promote the ability for both its students and graduates to function in today's collaborative practice, with the goal that all health care providers will have confidence when treating patients who suffer from these dental pain problems.

IPE will provide a foundation for teaching the principles of pain management that will allow this goal to be reached.[15,29] The goals for pain management dental education for the collaborative practice are clear.[9,11,15,29] Members of the health care team should understand acute dental pain and its management. They should have a familiarity with the diagnosis and standards of care for chronic orofacial pain problems, such as TMDs, that affect the TMJ joint and the muscles of mastication; as well as neuropathic pain affecting oral structures, such as trigeminal neuralgia, and atypical odontalgia. Health care providers in all professions should recognize that oral health provides a window for assessing the status of chronic diseases but also that control of these chronic diseases (eg, diabetes) are necessary for optimum oral health. All members of the health team must understand the assessment of the chronic pain patient who is managed on opioids. This includes a patient's response to evidenced-based treatment, pain control methods, and functional assessments, while meeting guidelines such as those published by the Veterans Administration.[45] The most critical aspect of these policy guidelines is that the use of controlled medications follows a documented diagnosis-based plan of care and sustains the patient's quality of life and function.

The challenge is how to best insure that education at all levels is structured to teach the effective pain management necessary for the collaborative practice.[15] Accreditation standards that guide the development of pain management skills for students, and the establishment of the institutional relationships and faculty development for IPE, are required to achieve the goals of affordable health care and control of the opioid abuse crisis. Such standards will best prepare dentists, and other health care professionals, for their role in tomorrow's collaborative practice.

Table 5
Advanced graduate programs in general dentistry

Oral Medicine	
2–12–c	Establish a differential diagnosis and formulate an appropriate working diagnosis, prognosis, and management plan pertaining to but not limited to 1. Oral mucosal disorders 2. Medically complex patients 3. Salivary gland disorders 4. Acute and chronic orofacial pain 5. Orofacial neurosensory disorders
2–11	Formal instruction must be provided
A	Anatomy, physiology, microbiology, immunology, biochemistry, neuroscience and disease concepts used to assess patients with complex medical problems that affect various organ systems and/or the orofacial region
B	Pathogenesis and epidemiology of orofacial diseases and disorders
C	Concepts of molecular biology and molecular basis of genetics
D	Aspects of internal medicine and disease necessary to diagnose and treat orofacial diseases
E	Concepts of pharmacology, including the mechanisms, interactions, and effects of prescription and over-the-counter drugs in the treatment of general medical conditions and orofacial diseases
Orofacial Pain	
Goals	1. Provide education in orofacial pain at a level beyond predoctoral education relating to the basic mechanisms and the anatomic, physiologic, neurologic, vascular, behavioral, and psychosocial aspects of orofacial pain 2. Plan and provide interdisciplinary or multidisciplinary health care for a wide variety of patients with orofacial pain 3. Interact with other health care professionals in health care 4. Manage the delivery of oral health care by applying concepts of patient and practice management and quality improvement that are responsive to a dynamic health care environment 5. Function effectively and efficiently in multiple health care environments and within interdisciplinary or multidisciplinary health care teams 6. Apply scientific principles to learning and oral health care, including using critical thinking, evidence or outcomes-based clinical decision-making, and technology-based information retrieval systems 7. Enhance the dissemination of information about diagnosis and treatment or management of orofacial pain to all practitioners of the health profession 8. Encourage the development of multidisciplinary teams composed of basic scientists and clinicians from appropriate disciplines to study orofacial pain conditions, to evaluate current therapeutic modalities, and to develop new and improved procedures for diagnosis and treatment or management of such conditions, diseases, or syndromes
2–1	The orofacial pain program must be designed to provide advanced knowledge and skills beyond the DDS or DMD training
2–5	Formal instruction must be provided
C	Head and neck disease and pathophysiology with an emphasis on pain

(continued on next page)

Table 5 (continued)	
G	Epidemiology of orofacial pain disorders
H	Pharmacology and pharmacotherapeutics
2–6	The program must provide a strong foundation of basic and applied pain sciences to develop knowledge in functional neuroanatomy and neurophysiology of pain
A	The neurobiology of pain transmission and pain mechanisms in the central and peripheral nervous systems
B	Mechanisms associated with pain referral to and from the orofacial region
C	Pharmacotherapeutic principles related to sites of neuronal receptor specific action pain
D	Pain classification systems
E	Psychoneuroimmunology and its relation to chronic pain syndromes
F	Primary and secondary headache mechanisms
G	Pain of odontogenic origin and pain that mimics odontogenic pain
H	The contribution and interpretation of orofacial structural variation (occlusal and skeletal) to orofacial pain, headache, and dysfunction
2–10	Instruction and clinical training in multidisciplinary pain management for the orofacial pain patient
c	Have primary responsibility for the management of a broad spectrum of orofacial pain patients in a multidisciplinary orofacial pain clinic setting, or interdisciplinary associated services Responsibilities should include pharmacotherapeutic treatment of orofacial pain, including systemic and topical medications and diagnostic or therapeutic injections
Intent	Judicious selection of medications directed at the presumed pain mechanisms involved, as well as adjustment, monitoring, and reevaluation
Common medications	Muscle relaxants Sedative agents for chronic pain and sleep management Opioids for management of chronic pain Adjuvant analgesic tricyclics and other antidepressants for chronic pain Anticonvulsants, membrane stabilizers, and sodium channel blockers for neuropathic pain Local and systemic anesthetics for management of neuropathic pain Anxiolytics, analgesics, and anti-inflammatories Prophylactic and abortive medications for primary headache disorders Botulinum toxin injections
Common issues	Management of medication overuse headache Medication side effects that alter sleep architecture Prescription medication dependency withdrawal Referral and comanagement of pain in patients addicted to prescription, nonprescription, and recreational drugs Familiarity with the role of preemptive anesthesia in neuropathic pain

From Commission on Dental Accreditation (CODA). Accreditation Standards for Advanced General Dentistry Education Programs in Oral Medicine; and Accreditation Standards for Advanced General Dentistry Education Programs in Orofacial Pain. Available at: http://www.ada.org/en/coda/current-accreditation-standards/; with permission. Accessed April 2, 2016.

REFERENCES

1. CAIPE. Interprofessional education: a definition. London: United Kingdom Centre for the Advancement of Interprofessional Education (CAIPE); 1997.
2. World Health Organization. Framework for action on interprofessional education and collaborative practice. Geneva (Switzerland): WHO; 2010. Available at: http://apps.who.int/iris/bitstream/10665/70185/1/WHO_HRH_HPN_10.3_eng.pdf. Accessed April 3, 2016.
3. Watt-Watson J, Hunter J, Pennefather P, et al. An integrated undergraduate curriculum, based on IASP curricula, for six health science faculties. Pain 2004;110: 140–8.
4. Dowell D, Haegerich TM, Chou R. CDC guideline for prescribing opioids for chronic pain—United States, 2016. MMWR Recomm Rep 2016;65:1–49.
5. Barr H, Freeth D, Hammick M, et al. Evaluations of interprofessional education: a United Kingdom review for health and social care. London: United Kingdom Centre for the Advancement of Interprofessional Education with the British Educational Research Association; 2000. Available at: http://caipe.org.uk/silo/files/evaluations-of-interprofessional-education.pdf. Accessed March 30, 2016.
6. Washington State Agency Medical Directors' Group's Interagency Opioid Guidelines (AMDGO). Available at: http://www.agencymeddirectors.wa.gov/guidelines.asp. Accessed April 2, 2016.
7. Institute of Medicine (U.S.). Committee on advancing pain research care and education. Relieving pain in America: a blueprint for transforming prevention, Care, Education, and Research. Washington, DC: National Academies Press; 2011. p. xvii, 364.
8. International Association for the Study of Pain (IASP) [Internet]. IASP curricula; 2012. Available at: http://www.iasp-pain.org/. Accessed April 2, 2016.
9. Fishman SM, Young HM, Lucas Arwood E, et al. Core competencies for pain management: results of an interprofessional consensus summit. Pain Med 2013;14(7):971–81.
10. Interagency Pain Research Coordinating Committee (IPRCC). National Pain Strategy: A Comprehensive Population Health-Level Strategy for Pain. 2016 Draft Report. Available at: http://iprcc.nih.gov/docs/drafthhsnationalpainstrategy.pdf. Accessed April 3, 2016.
11. O'Neal M, editor. The ADA practical guide to substance use disorders and safe prescribing. Hoboken (NJ): Wiley-Blackwell; 2015.
12. Pain Management Advisory, Massachusetts Executive Office of Health and Human Services (EOHHS) Date Adopted: March 11, 2009; Amended: July 20, 2011. Available at: http://www.mass.gov/eohhs/gov/departments/dph/programs/hcq/dhpl/dentist/alerts/pain-management-advisory.html. Accessed March 22, 2016.
13. Keith DA. The prescription monitoring program in Massachusetts and its use in dentistry. J Mass Dent Soc 2015;64(3):18–21.
14. Ducharme J. Massachusetts medical schools are working together to fight the opioid crisis. The Boston Magazine: Hub Health 2016.
15. Watt-Watson J, Siddall PJ, Carr E. Interprofessional pain education: the road to successful pain management outcomes. Pain Manag 2012;2(5):417–20.
16. De Leeuw R, editor. The American Academy of Orofacial Pain. Orofacial pain: guidelines for assessment, diagnosis and management. 4th edition. Chicago: Quintessence; 2008. p. 137–8.

17. Woolf CJ. Dissecting out mechanisms responsible for peripheral neuropathic pain: implications for diagnosis and therapy. Life Sci 2004;74(21):2605–10.
18. Dinesco RC, Kenna GA, O'Neil MG, et al. Prevention of prescription opioid abuse: the role of the dentist. J Am Dent Assoc 2011;142(7):800–10.
19. Briggs EV, Carr EC, Whittaker MS. Survey of undergraduate pain curricula for healthcare professionals in the United Kingdom. Eur J Pain 2011;15(8):789–95.
20. Watt-Watson J, McGillion M, Hunter J, et al. A survey of prelicensure pain curricula in health science faculties in Canadian universities. Pain Res Manag 2009;14(6):439–44.
21. Mezei L, Murinson BB. Pain education in North American medical schools. J Pain 2011;12(12):1199–208.
22. Upshur CC, Luckmann RS, Savageau JA. Primary care provider concerns about management of chronic pain in community clinic populations. J Gen Intern Med 2006;21(6):652–5.
23. Scudds R, Scudds R, Simmonds M. Pain in the physical therapy (PT) curriculum: a faculty survey. Physiother Theory Pract 2001;17(4):239–56.
24. Voshall B, Dunn K, Shelestak D. Knowledge and attitudes of pain management among nursing faculty. Pain Manag Nurs 2012;14(4):e226–35.
25. Singh RM, Wyant SL. Pain management content in curricula of U.S. schools of pharmacy. J Am Pharm Assoc (Wash) 2003;43(1):34–40.
26. Breuer B, Cruciani R, Portenoy RK. Pain management by primary care physicians, pain physicians, chiropractors, and acupuncturists: a national survey. South Med J 2010;103(8):738–47.
27. Vadivelu N, Mitra S, Hines R, et al. Acute pain in undergraduate medical education: an unfinished chapter! Pain Pract 2012;12(8):663–71.
28. Strong J, Tooth L, Unruh A. Knowledge about pain among newly graduated occupational therapists: relevance for curriculum development. Can J Occup Ther 2000;66(5):221–8.
29. Klasser GD, Gremillion HA. Past, present, and future of predoctoral dental education in orofacial pain and TMDs: a call for interprofessional education. J Dent Educ 2013;77(4):395–400.
30. NIH Pain Consortium Centers of Excellence in Pain Education sponsored by the National Institute on Drug Abuse, NIH, Contract # HHSN271201500075C. Centers of Excellence in Pain Education (CoEPEs). Reference #: NO1DA-15-4427, 2015. Available at: http://painconsortium.nih.gov/NIH_Pain_Programs/CoEPES.html. Accessed March 22, 2016.
31. Hunter J, Watt-Watson J, McGillion M, et al. An interfaculty pain curriculum: lessons learned from six years experience. Pain 2008;140(1):74–86.
32. Johnson M, Moorhead S, Bulechek G, et al. NANDA, NOC, and NIC linkages to NANDA-I and clinical conditions. 3rd edition. St. Louis (MO): Mosby; 2012.
33. Jomar RT, de Souza Bispo VR. The most common nursing diagnosis among adults/seniors hospitalised with cancer: integrative review. Ecancermedicalscience 2014;8:462.
34. Hoben M, Chamberlain SA, Knopp-Sihota JA, et al. Impact of symptoms and care practices on nursing home residents at the end of life: a rating by front-line care providers. J Am Med Dir Assoc 2016;17(2):155–61.
35. International Association for the Study of Pain. IASP Interprofessional Curricula. Available at: http://www.iasp-pain.org/Education/CurriculaList.aspx?navItemNumber=647. Accessed April 3, 2016.

36. Abu-Saad Huijer H, Miaskowski C, Quinn R, et al. IASP curriculum outline on pain for nursing. Available at: http://www.iasp-pain.org/Education/CurriculumDetail.aspx?ItemNumber=2052. Accessed April 3, 2016.

37. Finkelman MD, Kulich RJ, Zacharoff KL, et al. Shortening the Screener and Opioid Assessment for Patients with Pain-Revised (SOAPP-R): A Proof-of-Principle Study for Customized Computer-Based Testing. Pain Med 2015; 16(12):2344–56.

38. Doorenbos AZ, Gordon DB, Tauben D, et al. A blueprint of pain curriculum across prelicensure health sciences programs: one NIH Pain Consortium Center of Excellence in Pain Education (CoEPE) experience. J Pain 2013;14(12):1533–8.

39. Herr K, Marie BS, Gordon DB, et al. An interprofessional consensus of core competencies for prelicensure education in pain management: curriculum application for nursing. J Nurs Educ 2015;54(6):317–27.

40. Committee on Measuring the Impact of Interprofessional Education on Collaborative Practice and Patient Outcomes, Board on Global Health, Institute of Medicine. Measuring the impact of interprofessional education on collaborative practice and patient outcomes. Washington, DC: National Academies Press (US); 2015.

41. Conway WA, Hawkins S, Jordan J, et al. 2011 John M. Eisenberg Patient Safety and Quality Awards. The Henry Ford Health System No Harm Campaign: a comprehensive model to reduce harm and save lives. Innovation in patient safety and quality at the local level. Jt Comm J Qual Patient Saf 2012;38(7):318–27.

42. Wawrzyniak KM, Backstrom J, Kulich RJ. Integrating behavioral care into interdisciplinary pain settings: unique ethical dilemmas. Psychol Inj L 2015;8(4):323–33.

43. Berna C, Kulich RJ, Rathmell JP. Tapering long-term opioid therapy in chronic noncancer pain: evidence and recommendations for everyday practice. Mayo Clin Proc 2015;90(6):828–42.

44. Council On Dental Accreditation (CODA). Available at: http://predoc.ashx.ashx. Accessed April 2, 2016.

45. The Management of Opioid Therapy for Chronic Pain Working Group. VA/DoD Clinical practice guideline for management of opioid therapy for chronic pain. Department of Veterans Affairs, Department of Defense, 2010. Available at http://www.healthquality.va.gov/guidelines/Pain/cot/. Accessed March 22, 2016.

Interprofessional Collaboration in Improving Oral Health for Special Populations

Paul Glassman, DDS, MA, MBA[a],*, Maureen Harrington, MPH[b],
Maysa Namakian, MPH[b], Paul Subar, DDS, EdD[c]

KEYWORDS

- Teledentistry • Virtual dental home • Health services for persons with disabilities
- Oral health • Health status • Disabilities • Patient care management
- Interprofessional relations

KEY POINTS

- People with special needs are the most underserved and have the most significant oral health disparities of any group.
- The traditional office- and clinic-based dental care delivery system does not adequately address the oral health needs of people with special needs.
- There is increasing emphasis in US general health and oral health care systems on achieving the triple aim: better experiences receiving care, better health outcomes, and lower cost per capita.
- New delivery systems are evolving that better serve people with special needs using telehealth-connected interprofessional health care teams and creating Virtual Dental Homes.
- New delivery systems, with a focus on health outcomes, require and lead to integration of oral health services with social, educational, and general health systems.

ORAL HEALTH AND PEOPLE WITH SPECIAL NEEDS

In proposing an expanded role for interprofessional collaborations to improve oral health for people with "special needs" it is useful to consider the definition of the phrase "people with special needs." There are many similar terms in use in the literature. These include "people with special needs," "children with special health care needs," "people

Disclosure: None of the authors have any conflicts to disclose.
[a] Arthur A. Dugoni School of Dentistry, University of the Pacific, 155 Fifth Street, San Francisco, CA 94103, USA; [b] Pacific Center for Special Care, Arthur A. Dugoni School of Dentistry, University of the Pacific, San Francisco, CA, USA; [c] Special Care Clinic, Arthur A. Dugoni School of Dentistry, University of the Pacific, San Francisco, CA, USA
* Corresponding author.
E-mail address: pglassman@pacific.edu

Dent Clin N Am 60 (2016) 843–855
http://dx.doi.org/10.1016/j.cden.2016.05.004
0011-8532/16/$ – see front matter © 2016 Elsevier Inc. All rights reserved.

with disabilities," "people with complex needs," among others.[1–3] Some of these terms, such as "children with special health care needs" or people with "developmental disabilities," have definitions that are found in federal laws or regulations and are used for standardized data collection and reporting or for funding purposes.[4,5] Other terms, such as "people with special needs," "people with disabilities," or "people with complex needs," do not have generally agreed on definitions, although they are widely used and useful in describing populations who experience challenges in obtaining oral health services. For the purpose of this article the term "people with special needs" is used interchangeably with the phrases listed previously. A broad definition of this terms is people who have difficulty accessing dental treatment services because of complicated medical, physical, or psychological conditions.[6]

People with complex medical, physical, and psychological conditions are among the most underserved groups in receiving dental care and consequently have the most significant oral health disparities of any group. In the 2000 US Surgeon General's report *Oral Health in America* it was noted that although there have been gains in oral health status for the population as a whole, they have not been evenly distributed across subpopulations.[1] That report noted that profound health disparities exist among populations including racial and ethnic minorities, individuals with disabilities, elderly individuals, individuals with complicated medical and social conditions and situations, low income populations, and those living in rural areas. These conclusions were reaffirmed in the 2011 report of the Institute of Medicine (IOM) *Improving Access to Oral Health Care for Vulnerable and Underserved Populations*.[7] The IOM report noted that people with disabilities are less likely to have seen a dentist in the past year than people without disabilities; that people with intellectual disabilities are more likely to have poor oral hygiene and periodontal disease and more likely to have caries than people without intellectual disabilities; that people with special needs face systematic barriers to oral health care, such as transportation barriers (especially for those with physical disabilities) and cost; that health care professionals are not trained to work with these individuals; and that dental offices are not physically suited for them to receive care. Many other reports confirm that people with chronic medical illnesses, developmental disabilities, physical and psychosocial conditions, and the aging population in America experience more oral health care problems than others who do not have these conditions.[8–15]

The Population of People with Special Needs Is Increasing Dramatically

Not only do people with special needs experience greater difficulty obtaining dental care and consequent oral health disparities, but individuals with special needs are also becoming a larger part of the population. Advances in medicine have increased the likelihood that people today live longer with comorbidities that would previously have shortened their lifespan.[16] Forty years ago, for example, the typical person with Down syndrome would have a life expectancy of roughly 12 years compared with 60 years now.[17] Because of these advances, the number of people with special needs who need oral health services is growing dramatically. According to the 2010 US Census, roughly 50 million people, or almost 20% of the US population, have a long standing health condition or disability.[18] This phenomenon is increasing as the US population ages.

Challenges in Providing Oral Health Care for People with Special Needs

There are numerous challenges in providing oral health services for people with special needs that go beyond normal considerations for other populations. These challenges often require oral health professionals to have advanced training, and personal characteristics, such as empathy, patience, and desire, to be successful.

There are several areas where providing oral health services for these populations presents unique challenges for dental professionals.

First there is a need to understand and to be prepared to work with people with a wide variety of general health conditions. Although oral health professionals do not need to have complete knowledge about every general health condition that their patients present with, it is essential that they have the knowledge and experience to know what information is needed, and the ability to gather and apply that information to provide appropriate services. This implies the need for training and ability to function in interprofessional health care teams and get consultations from and work with physicians, nurses, social workers, and other general and social service professionals.

There is also a need for oral health professionals to understand the social service systems that operate in their community and the social context in which oral health services take place. An understanding of the system and how to work with community living facilities, social service agencies, and advocacy organizations operating in their community is essential to success. The use of appropriate language when interacting with individuals with special needs and their caregivers is also important. There is a growing movement advocating for the use of "people first" language.[19] This language emphasizes that disability is a part of the human condition and all people want to be described by their abilities rather than labeled by their disabilities. An oral health professional who does not understand this language and refers to people he or she treats by saying "I treat the handicapped in my practice" risks alienating the individual, their caregiver, and those advocating for full inclusion in society.

Oral health professionals also need to understand the extraordinary vulnerability of people with special needs to abuse and neglect in society.[20,21] An essential skill is the ability to recognize abuse and neglect and their role as mandated reporters. Oral health providers are health professionals and as a part of the health care team they may find that their patients are depressed or struggling to cope with various living challenges. As critical members of the health care team, there is an obligation to intervene, provide basic diagnosis and counseling, and make appropriate referrals for follow-up in these situations. As integrated care becomes the norm, it is likely that these referral systems will become stronger and more readily accessible.

Oral health professionals also need to understand how to help people with special needs prevent oral diseases. There are special challenges presented by working with someone where communication and even procedures need to be performed by a third person, a caregiver. Some people have limited physical ability to perform oral hygiene procedures and "partial participation" programs need to be designed and carried out. This term refers to having the individual do as much as they are able to, and having a caregiver ensure that needed prevention procedures are completed either through additional physical aids, reminders, or direct procedures performed by the caregiver. There are numerous informational, physical, and behavioral obstacles to be addressed in preventing dental disease in special needs populations. These are described in detail in a caregiver training package titled "Overcoming Obstacles to Dental Health: A Training Package for Caregivers of Adults with Disabilities and Frail Elders."[22] In addition to this package, there is a large body of literature that describes the challenges and techniques for helping people with special needs prevent oral diseases.[6,23–25]

THE EVOLVING DENTAL CARE LANDSCAPE

The US oral health industry is facing tremendous pressure to change. A large and increasing segment of the population does not access the traditional oral health care system until they have advanced disease, pain and infection. As illustrated in

Table 1, Medical Expenditures Panel Survey data indicate that most (52%) dental care in the United States is purchased by those with the top family incomes, whereas those in the bottom one-third purchase only 19% of dental services.[26] Unfortunately, those groups in the bottom income strata, along with people with special needs as described previously, have most of the dental disease.[1,7] This means that dentists are increasingly treating the wealthiest and healthiest segments of the population, whereas those with the highest rates of disease go largely untreated until they have advanced disease, pain, and infection.

One result of these dramatic shifts in the dental care landscape is that visits to dental offices and dentist's incomes are decreasing.[27] Visits to general dental offices have steadily declined, by 10% starting in 2003, well before the recent recession, and continuing well into the recovery. The American Dental Association Health Policy Resources Center has cautioned the profession not to expect a return to previous periods of increasing growth and described these declines as "the new normal."[28]

Despite decreasing demand over the last several decades, the price of dental care continues to rise during that time period. As illustrated in **Fig. 1**, the Consumer Price Index for Dental Services, a marker of the average price of dental care for the average person, rose at twice the rate of the Consumer Price Index, the general rate of inflation, between 1990 and 2014.[29] This is unfortunate because dental care is far more price sensitive than general health services. As depicted in **Fig. 2**, individuals pay for dental services out-of-pocket more than they pay for any other health service except prescription drugs.[30] High out-of-pocket costs, and increasing prices in the face of falling demand, help explain why dental care is the health service most likely to be put off by people who believe that they need care but do not obtain the care because of cost as a barrier.[31] In addition to price, people with special needs face all the other barriers described previously.

NEW STRATEGIES FOR THE DENTAL CARE SYSTEM

The IOM has proposed that one of the principles that needs to be included in an oral health system that is able to address the profound and increasing health disparities

Table 1
Medical expenditures panel survey: dental expenditures by income

Family Income	Number (000,000)	% of Population	% with Expenses	Expenditures (000,000)	% of Expenditures
Poor	46.3	15	27	$6266	7
Near poor	15.0	5	28	$2321	3
Low	45.7	14	32	$8333	9
Middle	93.4	30	39	$27,073	29
High	115.2	37	54	$47,837	52

Poor, < FPL; Near poor, > FPL–125% FPL; Low, >125%–200% FPL; Middle, >200%–400% FPL; High, >400% FPL.

2010 FPL for family of 1 = $10,830, family of 4 = $22.050 (HHS Poverty Guidelines 2010, http://aspe.hhs.gov/poverty/10poverty.shtml).

Abbreviation: FPL, federal poverty line.

Data from Agency for Healthcare Research and Quality (AHRQ). Medical expenditures panel survey (MEPS). Dental services expenses general dentist visits. 2013. Available at: http://meps.ahrq.gov/mepsweb/data_stats/tables_compendia_hh_interactive.jsp?_SERVICE=MEPSSocket0&_PROGRAM=MEPSPGM.TC.SAS&File=HCFY2013&Table=HCFY2013%5FPLEXP%5FB&VAR1=AGE&VAR2=SEX&VAR3=RACETH5C&VAR4=INSURCOV&VAR5=POVCAT13&VAR6=REGION&VAR7=HEALTH&VARO1=4+17+44+64&VARO2=1&VARO3=1&VARO4=1&VARO5=1&VARO6=1&VARO7=1&_Debug=. Accessed January 15, 2016.

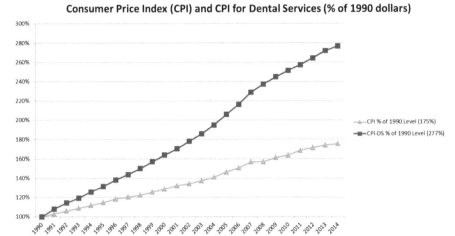

Fig. 1. Consumer price index (CPI) for dental services. (*Data from* Bureau of Labor Statistics. Consumer price index. Available at: http://www.bls.gov/cpi/cpi_dr.htm. Accessed January 15, 2016.)

described previously is the use of "collaborative and multidisciplinary teams working across the health care system."[7] This statement was based on the conclusion that "the separation of oral health care from overall health care is a factor in limiting access to oral health care for many Americans." Furthermore, the IOM indicated that "oral health is an integral part of overall health, and therefore, oral health care is an essential

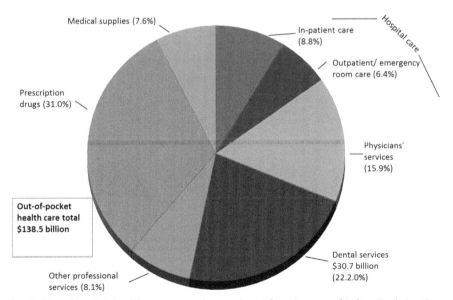

Fig. 2. Out-of-pocket health care expenditures. (*Data from* Bureau of Labor Statistics. Consumer out-of-pocket health care expenditures in 2008. Available at: http://www.bls.gov/opub/ted/2010/ted_20100325.htm. Accessed January 15, 2016.)

component of comprehensive health care."[7] These and other statements emphasize the need to increase the use of interprofessional practice as a major strategy in improving oral health. In this case, interprofessional practice refers to integrating oral health considerations and activities into educational, social, and general health systems and coordinating efforts between multiple individuals in these systems.

The IOM proposed several recommendations and potential strategies (**Fig. 3**).[7] Some of the strategies that apply to people with special needs already being considered, tested, or deployed are discussed next.

Deliver Oral Health Services in Nontraditional Settings

This is sometimes referred to as bringing oral care to "where underserved people are" be it in Head Start preschools, schools, residential facilities, nursing homes, day programs, or other community locations.

Expand the Oral Health Workforce

Strategies being tested include creating new categories of oral health professionals or expanding the scope of practice of current oral health professionals to ensure that they are able to practice to the full extent of their education and experience.

Use Nontraditional Providers

There are many significant local and national efforts underway to engage general health professionals in interprofessional practice activities to improve oral health and to integrate oral health into the systems where these professionals work.

Develop Integrated Health Homes

What began as a description of the "Medical Home" and then a "Dental Home" has now broadened to consideration of creating true integrated "Health Homes" where

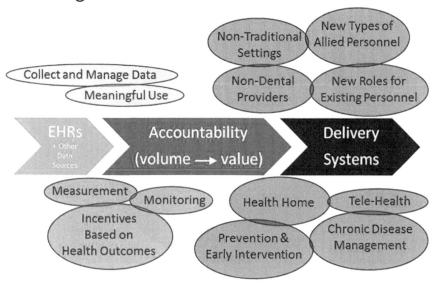

Fig. 3. Strategies for moving oral health care from volume to value. Value, health outcomes achieved per dollar spent over the lifecycle of a condition. EHRs, electronic health records.

dental health considerations and services are integrated with services delivered in general health, social service, and educational settings. Integration is supported by professionals in various disciplines and the use of interprofessional practice is emphasized.

Use Telehealth Technologies

The advent and availability of telehealth technologies is making it possible for dental practices to expand their reach to communities of people not traditionally served in dental offices and clinics. Geographically distributed telehealth-connected oral health teams are able to provide care in community locations, such as WIC sites, nursing homes, group homes, schools, and in rural communities using cloud-based electronic health records and other technology to maintain communication.

Use Tools of Chronic Disease Management

There is growing realization that the major incentives and focus in the oral health industry have been on acute surgical interventions, whereas the major dental diseases, caries and periodontal disease, are chronic diseases. There is a growing science of "chronic disease management" that emphasizes behavioral, medical, and social tools to partner with individuals and communities to manage chronic diseases. These strategies require the use of community engagement and interprofessional teams to be effective.[32]

Emphasize Prevention and Early Intervention

There is growing realization that preventing or intervening early in oral disease with minimally invasive interventions is an increasingly important tool for the oral health industry in the "era of accountability" where the emphasis is on improving oral health of the population at the lowest cost-per-capita. Again, this strategy requires the use of interprofessional teams to be effective.

INTERPROFESSIONAL PRACTICE AND VIRTUAL DENTAL HOMES

An example of emerging oral health delivery systems that incorporate the principles presented by the IOM is the Virtual Dental Home (VDH) demonstration project in California.[33] The VDH system, developed by the Pacific Center for Special Care at the University of the Pacific Arthur A. Dugoni School of Dentistry (Pacific), brings prevention and early intervention oral health services to underserved groups of children and adults. This 6-year demonstration has shown that telehealth-connected oral health teams, integrated within interprofessional teams in educational, social service, and general health systems, can reach children and adults in Early Head Start, Head Start preschools, rural communities, elementary schools, residential facilities for people disabilities, nursing homes, and community centers who are in the population groups, such as people with special needs, that might otherwise not receive any dental care until they have advanced disease, pain, or infection.[34]

The VDH system uses telehealth technology to link allied dental personnel in the community with dentists in dental offices and clinics. The system keeps people healthy in community settings by providing education, triage, case management, preventive procedures, and interim therapeutic restorations on an ongoing basis. Where more complex dental treatment is needed, the VDH connects patients with dentists in the area through "warm" referrals and case management. The system also links patients and dental providers into interdisciplinary teams. Most importantly, it brings much-needed services to individuals who might otherwise receive no care.

This system promotes collaboration between dentists in dental offices and clinics and these community-based dental hygienists and dental assistants. It promotes integration of dental care and interprofessional practice into educational, social service, and general health systems. Allied dental personnel in these community sites interact on a daily basis with administrators, family advocates in Head Start preschools, teachers, school nurses, nursing assistants and physicians in long-term care facilities and residential facilities for people with disabilities, and social services staff. All these efforts are in recognition of the reality that changing individual behavior and improved "daily mouth care" are essential components in improving the oral health of populations and this cannot be done by dental professionals in the isolation of dental offices. Interprofessional teams and community engagement are essential for success.

Pacific's VDH demonstration project in California has shown that the oral health system can increase the number of patients receiving care and better integrate dental care into overall health care without additional investment in costly infrastructure. There is a tremendous potential for expanding the reach of existing oral health care providers across the country by using this system.

PREVENTION AND EARLY INTERVENTION IN THE ORAL DISEASE PROCESS IN PEOPLE WITH SPECIAL NEEDS

Finally, the most important reason that the use of interprofessional teams is critical in improving and maintaining oral health for people with special needs is that dental professionals, working separately from educational, social, and general health systems, cannot be successful in creating the daily behaviors needed to prevent dental disease or intervene early enough to prevent the significant consequences of untreated disease.

Individual behaviors are among the most important factors leading to health.[35,36] However, influencing people to change habitual behaviors is extremely difficult. Providing information, even when it results in knowledge increase, does not necessarily lead to behavior change.[37,38] A 2000 report by the IOM on social and behavioral research stated that "To prevent disease, we increasingly ask people to do things that they have not done previously, to stop doing things they have been doing for years, and to do more of some things and less of other things. Although there certainly are examples of successful programs to change behavior, it is clear that behavior change is a difficult and complex challenge. It is unreasonable to expect that people will change their behavior easily when so many forces in the social, cultural, and physical environment conspire against such change."[39] Providing information about health-producing behaviors does not necessarily lead to behavior change. Furthermore, a 2006 study aimed at changing oral health behaviors of caregivers of people with disabilities demonstrated that caregiver knowledge about preventive procedures was improved after training, but this was only translated into behavior change and incorporation of new techniques into daily routines after a dental assistant observed the prevention session in the residential environment and provided hands-on, real time coaching for the caregiver.[25]

There are many examples of successful efforts and techniques aimed at influencing people to adopt effective oral health practices.[40] However, efforts to improve health through oral health education activities performed in a dental office are not likely to be successful in improving the oral health of many people with special needs. There are several important reasons for this conclusion. The dental office is not the best place to deliver oral health messages, oral health professionals are not the best people to deliver these messages, and the dental office is not well suited to delivering messages with the best timing. Unfortunately, the segments of the population where dental office–based education is not likely to be successful, including people with special needs, are also those segments of the population that have the highest rates of dental disease. Therefore, alternate strategies need to be used including community engagement using interprofessional teams.

Several strategies have been described to improve health communication in dental offices.[41] Unfortunately, there is evidence that these techniques are not widely used.[42] However, even if they were more widely used, dental offices would still not be the best places to deliver oral health education messages to improve the health of many segments of the population including those with special needs. A major factor is that the people with most of the dental disease in the population do not take advantage of the traditional office and clinic-based dental care system and are therefore not in dental offices.[1,7] Even for those who do visit dental offices, it is not the best place because most people are nervous, if not afraid, when they are in dental offices.[43] People are worried about what is going to happen on the way in and what has just happened, and what it will feel like later. Even though dental professionals generally perceive their offices or clinics as friendly environments, to many of their patients these office and clinics are surgical suites and not the place where they feel the most open to receiving and incorporating health information. Providing the traditional short lesson on "oral hygiene" or even a longer "anticipatory guidance" session delivered at the end of a dental appointment in a dental office may not have any impact on the subsequent behavior of the individual, or for dependent children or adults, or their caregivers.[25,44]

In many situations, oral health professionals are not the best people to delivery oral health education messages designed to change behaviors for many segments of the population. Although some communication techniques, such as motivational interviewing, have shown positive results in changing behavior, there is inadequate training in this and other behavior change techniques included in the crowded curriculum in oral health professional education programs.[43] However, even if oral health professionals had additional training and were in contact with those individuals with the greatest health disparities, there is often a cultural gap between the oral health professional and the recipient of the information.[45] Oral health professionals are generally not skilled at determining the literacy level of patients and caregivers and delivering messages at the appropriate level. In the 2010 Census, just over one-third of the US population reported their race and ethnicity as something other than non-Hispanic white alone. This group, referred to as the "minority" population, increased from 86.9 million (30.9%) to 111.9 million (36.3%) between 2000 and 2010. This represented a growth of 29% over the decade.[46] In California, for example, the "minority" population grew from 18.1 million (53.3%) in 2000 to 22.3 million (59.9%) in 2010. California is one of four states with a "majority-minority" population (ie, more than 50% of the population was minority). This distribution is markedly different than the composition of dentists in the United States. The cultural divide experienced by many groups of people results in people not fully understanding what the oral health professional is saying, people being embarrassed about talking about their personal behaviors with oral health professionals, and people concluding that oral health professionals are knowledgeable but do not understand their lives or the challenges they face in implementing the recommendations that are being given.

Finally delivering dental health messages in dental offices may not be the optimal timing for some segments of the population. Those populations of people with the greatest burden of dental diseases do not visit dental offices at all or do so infrequently.[47] Therefore messages delivered to these groups in dental offices are not delivered repeatedly and not at a time when people are the most receptive to considering changing their behavior.

The most effective messages are those delivered by people seen as trusted members of the individual's own community, delivered by multiple people on multiple occasions, and incorporating a feedback system so people who run into challenges can get additional instruction and coaching over time.[48] The ability to use these principles is enhanced by having oral health messages and coaching delivered in places where people with special needs receive educational, social, or general health services on a regular basis.[49–51] Therefore the best opportunity for oral health professionals to influence the preventive practices of people with special needs and their caregivers is to develop linkages and partnerships and work with staff in organizations delivering educational, social, and general health services.

SUMMARY

People with complex medical, physical, and psychological conditions, referred to in this article as people with special needs, are among the most underserved groups in receiving dental care and consequently have the most significant oral health disparities of any group. The traditional dental care delivery system is not able to deliver adequate services to these people with special needs for a variety of reasons. New systems of care are evolving that better serve the needs of these groups by using interprofessional teams to reach people and integrate oral health services into social, educational, and general health systems.

REFERENCES

1. U.S. Department of Health and Human Services. Oral health in America: a report of the Surgeon General. Rockville (MD): U.S. Department of Health and Human Services; National Institute of Dental and Craniofacial Research; National Institutes of Health; 2000.
2. Waldman HB, Perlman SP, Waldman HB, et al. Children with special health care needs: results of a national survey. J Dent Child 2006;73(1):57–62.
3. Glassman P, Henderson T, Helgeson M, et al. Consensus statement: oral health for people with special needs: consensus statement on implications and recommendations for the dental profession. J Calif Dent Assoc 2005;33(8):619–23.
4. Newacheck PW, Rising JP, Kim SE. Children at risk for special health care needs. Pediatrics 2007;118(1):334–42.
5. Definition of Developmental Disability. 42 USC §15002(8). 1978.
6. Glassman P, Anderson M, Jacobsen P, et al. Practical protocols for the prevention of dental disease in community settings for people with special needs: the protocols. Spec Care Dentist 2003;23(5):86–90, 160–4.
7. IOM (Institute of Medicine) and NRC (National Research Council). Improving access to oral health care for vulnerable and underserved populations. Washington, DC: The National Academies Press; 2011.
8. Oral Health America. The Disparity Cavity: Filling America's Oral Health Gap. Oral Health America, Chicago; 2000.
9. Haavio ML. Oral health care of the mentally retarded and other persons with disabilities in the Nordic countries: present situation and plans for the future. Spec Care Dentist 1995;15:65–9.
10. Feldman CA, Giniger M, Sanders M, et al. Special Olympics, special smiles: assessing the feasibility of epidemiologic data collection. J Am Dent Assoc 1997; 128:1687–96.

11. Waldman HB, Perlman SP, Swerdloff M. Use of pediatric dental services in the 1990s: some continuing difficulties. J Dent Child 2000a;67:59–63.
12. United States General Accounting Office. Oral health: factors contributing to low use of dental services by low-income populations. Report to Congressional Requesters 2000. Available at: http://www.gao.gov/new.items/he00149.pdf. Accessed June 19, 2016.
13. Horwitz S, Kerker B, Owens P, et al. The health status and needs of individuals with mental retardation. Special Olympics; 2000. Available at: http://staging.specialolympics.org/uploadedFiles/LandingPage/WhatWeDo/Research_Studies_Desciption_Pages/healthstatus_needs.pdf. Accessed June 20, 2016.
14. Oral health status and needs of Special Olympics athletes – World summer games, Raleigh, North Carolina – June 26– July 4, 1999. Special Olympics International: Unpublished report. 1999.
15. Dolan TA, Atchison K, Huynh TN. Access to dental care among older adults in the United States. J Dent Educ 2005;69(9):961–74.
16. Spencer G. US Bureau of the Census: current population reports, series P-25, no 1018, projections of the population of states by age, sex and race: 1988-2010. Washington, DC: US Government Printing Office; 1988. 29, 94, 95, 97,99, 100, 01, 03, 05.
17. Bittles AH, Bower C, Hussain R, et al. The four ages of Down syndrome. Eur J Public Health 2006;17(2):221–5.
18. Brault MW. Americans With Disabilities: 2010. U.S. Census Bureau 2012. Available at: http://www.census.gov/prod/2012pubs/p70-131.pdf.
19. CDC. Communicating with and about people with disabilities: people first language. Available at: http://www.cdc.gov/ncbddd/disabilityandhealth/pdf/disabilityposter_photos.pdf. Accessed January 15, 2016.
20. Glassman P, Chavez E, Hawks D. Abuse and neglect of elderly individuals: guidelines for oral health professionals. J Calif Dent Assoc 2004;32(4):232–5.
21. Glassman P, Miller C, Ingraham R, et al. The extraordinary vulnerability of people with disabilities: guidelines for oral health professionals. J Calif Dent Assoc 2004; 32(5):379–86.
22. Miller C, Glassman P, Wozniak T, et al. Overcoming obstacles to dental health: a training program for caregivers of adults with disabilities and frail elders. 5th edition. San Francisco (CA): University of The Pacific School of Dentistry; 2008.
23. Glassman P, Miller C. Dental disease prevention and people with special needs. J Calif Dent Assoc 2003;31(2):149–60.
24. Glassman P, Miller C. Preventing dental disease for people with special needs: the need for practical preventive protocols for use in community settings. Spec Care Dentist 2003;23(5):165–7.
25. Glassman P, Miller C. Effect of preventive dentistry training program for caregivers in community facilities on caregiver and client behavior and client oral hygiene. NY State Dent J 2006;72(2):38–46.

26. AHRQ MEPS Dental services expenses general dentist visits. 2013. Available at: http://meps.ahrq.gov/mepsweb/data_stats/tables_compendia_hh_interactive.jsp?_SERVICE=MEPSSocket0&_PROGRAM=MEPSPGM.TC.SAS&File=HCFY2013&Table=HCFY2013%5FPLEXP%5FB&VAR1=AGE&VAR2=SEX&VAR3=RACETH5C&VAR4=INSURCOV&VAR5=POVCAT13&VAR6=REGION&VAR7=HEALTH&VARO1=4+17+44+64&VARO2=1&VARO3=1&VARO4=1&VARO5=1&VARO6=1&VARO7=1&_Debug=. Accessed January 15, 2016.

27. Vujicic M, Lazar V, Wall TP, et al. An analysis of dentist's income 1996-2009. J Am Dent Assoc 2012;143(5):452–60.

28. ADA Health Policy Resources Center. A profession in transition: key forces reshaping the dental landscape. 2013.

29. Bureau of Labor Statistics: Consumer price index. Available at: http://www.bls.gov/cpi/cpi_dr.htm. Accessed January 15, 2016.

30. Bureau of Labor Statistics. Consumer out-of-pocket health care expenditures in 2008. Available at: http://www.bls.gov/opub/ted/2010/ted_20100325.htm. Accessed January 15, 2016.

31. ADA Health Services Policy Center. Research brief: financial barriers to dental care declining after a decade of steady increase. 2013. Available at: http://www.ada.org/~/media/ADA/Science%20and%20Research/Files/HPRCBrief_1013_1.pdf. Accessed June 19, 2016.

32. Glassman P, Harrington M, Namakian M. Promoting oral health through community engagement. J Calif Dent Assoc 2014;42(7):465–70.

33. Glassman P, Harrington M, Namakian M, et al. The virtual dental home: bringing oral health to vulnerable and underserved populations. J Calif Dent Assoc 2012;40(7):569–77.

34. Pacific Center for Special Care: Report of the Virtual Dental Home Demonstration: Improving the Oral Health of Vulnerable and Underserved Populations Using Geographically Distributed Telehealth-Connected Teams. Executive Summary: http://dental.pacific.edu/Documents/community/special_care/acrobat/VirtualDentalHome_Report_ExecutiveSummary_2016-0614.pdf. Available at: http://dental.pacific.edu/Documents/community/special_care/acrobat/VirtualDentalHome_Report_FullReport_2016-0614.pdf.

35. McGinnis JM, Foege WH. Actual causes of death in the United States. JAMA 1993;270(18):2207–12.

36. McGinnis JM, Williams-Russo P, Knickman JR. The case for more active policy attention to health promotion. Health Aff 2002;21(2):78–93.

37. Freeman R, Ismail A. Assessing patients' health behaviors: essential steps for motivating patients to adopt and maintain behaviors conducive to oral health. Monogr Oral Sci 2009;21:113–27.

38. Satur JG, Gussy MG, Morgan MV, et al. Review of the evidence for oral health promotion effectiveness. Health Educ J 2010;69(3):257–66.

39. The Institute of Medicine. Promoting health: intervention strategies from social and behavioral research. Washington, DC: The National Academy Press; 2000.

40. Institute of Medicine. Oral health literacy: workshop summary. Washington, DC: The National Academies Press; 2013.

41. Horowitz AM, Kleinman DV. Creating a health literacy-based practice. J Calif Dent Assoc 2012;40(4):331–40.

42. Rozier RG, Horowitz AM, Podschun G. Dentist-patient communication techniques used in the United States. J Am Dent Assoc 2011;142(5):518–50.

43. McNeil DW, Randall CL. Dental fear and anxiety associated with oral health care: conceptual and clinical issues. Chapter 12. In: Mostofsky DI, Fortune F, editors.

Behavioral dentistry. 2nd edition. Ames (IO): John Wiley & Sons, Inc; 2014. p. 165–93.

44. American Academy of Pediatric Dentistry. Guideline on periodicity of examination, preventive dental services, anticipatory guidance/counseling, and oral treatment for infants, children, and adolescents. Hoboken, NJ: John Wiley & Sons; 2009.

45. Centore L. Dental health literacy and California's clarion call. J Calif Dent Assoc 2012;40(4):352–9.

46. Humes KR. Census Briefs. Overview of race and Hispanic origin: 2010. U.S. Census 2011. Available at: http://www.census.gov/prod/cen2010/briefs/c2010br-02.pdf. Accessed June 19, 2016.

47. Wallace BB, Macentee MI. Access to dental care for low-income adults: perceptions of affordability, availability and acceptability. J Community Health 2012; 37(1):32–9.

48. Bauer S. Building pathways of trust. J Calif Dent Assoc 2012;40(4):361–3.

49. Braun B, Horowitz AM, Kleinman DV, et al. Oral health literacy: at the intersection of k–12 education and public health. J Calif Dent Assoc 2012;40(4):323–30.

50. Simmer-Beck M, Gadbury-Amyot CC, Ferris H, et al. Extending oral health care services to underserved children through a school-based collaboration. Part 1: a descriptive overview. J Dent Hyg 2011;85(3):181–92.

51. Keselyak NT, Simmer-Beck M, Gadbury-Bmyot C. Extending oral health care services to underserved children through a school-based collaboration. Part 2: the student experience. J Dent Hyg 2011;85(3):193–203.

Interprofessional Collaborative Practice

An Oral Health Paradigm for Women

Cherae Farmer-Dixon, DDS, MSPH[a],
Machelle Fleming Thompson, RDH, MSPH[b],
Daphne Young, DDS, MSPH[c], Stephanie McClure, MD[d],
Leslie R. Halpern, MD, DDS, PhD, MPH[e],*

KEYWORDS

- Interprofessional relations • Women's health • Oral health • Intimate partner violence
- Pregnancy • Medicine related osteonecrosis of the jaw
- United States Health resources and services administration

KEY POINTS

- Oral disease is among the most prevalent health problems, and discrepancies that exist regarding the health of women compared with the health of men.
- Five key concepts for women's oral health using an interprofessional collaborative framework include wellness and prevention, biologic applications, selective disease awareness, behavioral health, and interprofessional health team members' roles.
- An interprofessional collaborative team approach increases awareness among oral health care providers, along with obstetrician/gynecologists, regarding the significance of oral health during pregnancy.
- The oral health care provider is central to an interprofessional collaborative framework in identifying victims of intimate partner violence, as most injuries are facial and intimate partner violence exposure results in poor health.
- Providing interprofessional collaborative models involving both oral and overall health care professionals enable patient-centered care with patients becoming more empowered in decision making.

[a] Meharry Medical College, School of Dentistry, Nashville, TN, USA; [b] Clinical Affairs, Meharry Medical College, School of Dentistry, Nashville, TN, USA; [c] General Practice Residency, Meharry Medical College, School of Dentistry, Nashville, TN, USA; [d] Meharry Medical College, School of Medicine, Nashville, TN, USA; [e] Oral and Maxillofacial Surgery Residency, Meharry Medical College, School of Dentistry, 1005 DB Todd Jr. Boulevard, Nashville, TN 37208, USA
* Corresponding author.
E-mail address: lhalpern@mmc.edu

Dent Clin N Am 60 (2016) 857–877
http://dx.doi.org/10.1016/j.cden.2016.05.005
0011-8532/16/$ – see front matter © 2016 Elsevier Inc. All rights reserved.

INTRODUCTION

The US Surgeon General issued a report calling attention to the "silent epidemic" of dental and oral diseases suffered by millions of children and adults throughout the United States.[1] The report called for the development of a National Oral Health Plan that would "improve quality of life and eliminate health disparities by facilitating collaborations among individuals, health care providers, communities, and policymakers at all levels of society and by taking advantage of existing initiatives."[2] As a result, there is now an emphasis on examining the relationship of poor oral health and its influence on systemic disease.[3] The latter lends support for an interdisciplinary collaboration of health care professionals including the oral health care provider, in comprehensive patient care to eradicate dental health disparities and health disparities in general.[1–4]

The above collaborative effort has driven a model for innovative interprofessional collaborative (IPC) practice with respect to the oral and overall health of women. Women engage with a wide array of providers across their lifespan, often interacting more frequently with health providers compared with men; therefore, women's health can be an ideal area in which to pursue further IPC strategies.[5–9] The US Department of Health and Human Services, Health Resources and Services Administration (HRSA), Office of Women's Health in 2013, commissioned a report that provided recommendations to improve women's health education across 5 specific health professions programs: medicine, oral health/dentistry, baccalaureate nursing, pharmacy, and public health.[10] Both women's health and IPC practice are top priorities in health education, and improvements may contribute to dramatic health benefits across the population.[5–10] This article provides the reader with several examples of IPC frameworks/models designed to provide oral health care practitioners skills to enhance their role within the interprofessional team approach to the care of the female patient. The authors chose several important health disparities that have both oral and systemic manifestations that can be approached using an IPC paradigm.

Women's Overall Health Needs

The Institute Of Medicine mandated that there was a need to integrate dentistry with medicine and the health care system as a whole to provide greater research support of an oral-systemic health connection.[9] These changes in health care delivery and the reports on new health care models have helped shape the Patient Protection and Affordable Care Act, signed into law in 2010, which proposes to improve and promote "A Healthier Nation," encompasses the ideals of interprofessional collaboration.[9,11] It has recreated health care for all by addressing the quality of health care, the costs, and, most important, the advent of access to care for all.

The hypothesized "Triple Aim" as suggested by Donald Berwick, MD,[12] has the potential to remedy the significant expense of health care in the United States, improve outcomes, and increase the value of the health care dollars spent.[9,11,12] The Triple Aim model of health care can have a significant impact on women, especially with the increase in Medicaid and Medicare benefits.[12] The Centers for Medicare and Medicaid estimate that 18 million women will find insurance coverage that fits their needs in the marketplace. It is well known that women are more likely than men to require coverage, particularly during the reproductive years, and have a greater out of pocket cost; therefore, they may be unable to pay because of a concomitant wage discrepancy compared with their male cohorts.[11,12] As a result of the Affordable Care Act, women are now eligible to receive not only preventive coverage for wellness visits but also examinations for specialty needs, that is, obstetrician/gynecologist (OB/GYN) visits, without requirement of a referral from their primary care doctors.[11,12]

This concept also creates an opportunity for professions to collaborate in providing optimal comprehensive health care that is inclusive of not only medical health needs but communicative roads toward the inclusion of oral health, treatment, and prevention.

The above concept has the potential to close the gender gap between men and women with respect to awareness of health needs that are quite separate in physiology and treatment strategies based on the disease entity. Several research groups propose different health attitudes across genders and have hypothesized a gender gap in health reporting. For instance, according to Bogner and Gallo,[13] women are more likely to interpret symptoms associated with depression and low well-being as signs of emotional problems and hence get psychiatric help. This finding suggests that women perceive symptoms in different ways compared with men, so that they also seek more medical care. Hibbard and Pope[14] found that women also report higher interest and concern about health than men do. The most recent studies suggest that health matters are more salient among women that they value health more than men do and that they have more responsibility in caring for ill family members. Such findings are consistent with the idea that women pay more attention to health than men do.[7,8,10–14]

Women's Health and Oral Health

Documentation continues to list oral disease as one of the most prevalent health problems and discrepancies in the health of women compared with men.[4–6] As such, the oral health care component of the IPC model for women's health is of great interest not only to women of reproductive age but to those in midlife and the elderly. Issues such as oral health changes caused by cardiovascular disease, sexuality, domestic violence, and disease prevention are all health disparities that poor oral health can impact/exacerbate.[7] Experts in women's health define the discipline of IPC as a product of cultural, social, and psychological factors in addition to biology.[15] An IPC model for women's health and men's health can empower both the patient and their providers by identifying a comprehensive health plan that increases disease prevention and reduces health costs in the community they treat.[15]

The approach to a new paradigm of oral health as part of overall health and well-being formed the basis for a 2011 expert panel in Washington DC to design a broad curriculum that melded dentistry, medicine, pharmacy, nursing, osteopathic medicine, and public health.[16,17] A framework was crafted to develop core competencies for an interprofessional educational collaborative (IPEC) with a common goal for an interdisciplinary approach to total patient health.[17] This expert panel defines interprofessional teamwork as "the levels of cooperation, coordination and collaboration characterizing the relationships between professions in delivering patient-centered care and interprofessional team-based care … and shared responsibility for a patient or group of patients."[17] The report from this panel defines 4 broad domains of competency: values and ethics, roles and responsibilities, interprofessional communication and, most importantly, team-based care. The competencies are framed around the concept that health care should be patient/family centered, community/population oriented, relationship focused, and process oriented.

Community Models that Apply Oral Health Within an Interprofessional Collaborative Framework

The impact of IPC teamwork on the health needs of women is exemplified in the community models described below. The utilization of IPC frameworks in each model described integrates the interdisciplinary voices of both health care providers and patients to reinforce comprehensive health habits and empower better decision-making strategies for the health and well-being of women. The health issues discussed include the care of pregnant women, women who have experienced domestic violence/intimate partner violence (IPV), and women with chronic diseases in their elderly years.

Interprofessional collaborative model for oral/overall health during pregnancy

It is estimated that 6.5 million women in the United States become pregnant each year.[17] The physiologic changes that occur during pregnancy caused by hormonal changes are necessary to support and safeguard the developing fetus and prepare the mother for parturition. These systemic changes can also affect the woman's oral health.[17–23] Dental problems not only cause pain and discomfort but also can be a risk factor for preterm delivery and low birth weight babies.[18,19,21–23] Although there are standardized guidelines for health care professionals providing prenatal care, studies do not show that most health professionals providing prenatal care incorporate oral examinations as part of standard prenatal care.[17–23] As such, the IPC team approach is paramount among the OB/GYN and other health professionals (eg, dentists, dental hygienists, physicians, nurses, midwives, nurse practitioners, physician assistants) to provide pregnant women with appropriate and timely oral health care, which includes oral health education.[17–24] Based on this principle, numerous health care organizations have fostered efforts to promote oral health for pregnant women. The American Academy of Pediatric Dentistry, the American Academy of Pediatrics, the American Academy of Periodontology, the American Academy of Physician Assistants, the American College of Nurse-Midwives, the American College of Obstetricians and Gynecologists, and the American Dental Association (ADA) have issued statements and recommendations for improving oral health care during pregnancy.[24] An expert panel was convened to develop an Oral Health Care During Pregnancy Consensus Statement through a Development Expert Workgroup Meeting in 2011 convened by HRSA's Maternal and Child Health Bureau (MCHB) in collaboration with American College of Obstetricians and Gynecologists and ADA and coordinated by the National Maternal and Child Oral Health Resource Center. The implementation within this statement would bring about changes in the health care delivery service to women during pregnancy and thereby improve the overall standard of care.[24] **Box 1** describes the key points of the 2012 Consensus Statement.

Based on the above approach, a community model was developed to encourage an IPC framework that examines oral health during pregnancy.

Model A pilot study called An Interprofessional Education Approach to Increasing Access to Health Services for African American Women at Risk for Preterm-Low Birth Weight Babies (funded by the Robert Wood Johnson Foundation Center for Health Policy, Meharry Medical College, Nashville, TN) was designed to increase access to health services and improve oral health/overall health through an IPC approach. The women in the project were seen in the Meharry Dental School, Meharry Center for Women's Health Clinics (OB/GYN, Meharry Centering Pregnancy), Matthew Walker Community Health Center, Meharry 1919 Clinic, and one private OB/GYN office. The target population was African-American women at risk for preterm low birth weight babies. The participants were recruited from the centers listed above and administered a validated survey to assess their awareness, knowledge, and attitude regarding oral health as it relates to adverse pregnancy outcomes (**Tables 1** and **2**). A total of 159 surveys were collected with completed data analyzed on 146 participants (95%). The study concluded that the stronger the participant's perception

---

Box 1
Key points of 2012 consensus statement on oral healthcare during pregnancy

- Assess pregnant woman's health status and when to consult with prenatal health professional.
- Advise pregnant woman about oral health care and safety of dental treatment during pregnancy.
- Work in collaboration with oral health care professionals.
- Provide support services (social services) to pregnant women.
- Improve health services in the community.
- Assess pregnant woman's oral health status.
- Advise pregnant women about oral health care.
- Improve health services in the community.

Data from Oral Health Care During Pregnancy: A National Consensus Statement. Proceedings of Summary of an expert workgroup meeting.© 2012 by the National Maternal and Child Oral Health Resource Center, Georgetown University, Grant number H47MC00048, Health Resources and Service Administration (HRSA), US Department of Health and Human Services (DHHS).

---

that their dental health affects their overall health, the more strongly they agreed that their teeth and gums would affect whether their baby is healthy (**Fig. 1**). The results of the data analysis also suggested that insurance status, household income, and type of insurance impacted participants' perceptions of regular dental check-ups, of dental health on overall health, and the impact of their oral health on the health of their baby. The IPC team (dentist, dental hygienists, OB/GYN physicians, maternal fetal medicine physicians, nurse midwife, nurse practitioner, social worker, behaviorist, nutritionist, physician assistant, and other health care providers) participated in training workshops and seminars and shared values of delivering the message of preventive care to pregnant women to optimize birth outcomes. The goal was to instill in the pregnant patient the importance of seeking dental care as part of their prenatal care (Thompson and Farmer-Dixon, 2015).

The results of this pilot study suggest "there is a relationship between oral health during pregnancy and overall health." The IPC team, however, felt that education was lacking in familiarity with dental caries detection/gum disease and the role they could play in addressing oral health care needs within this patient population (physicians <30%; nurses ≤25%; physician assistants ≤17%, **Fig. 2**). IPC dialogue and education are still needed to build strong partnerships for patient-centered care in the management of oral health during pregnancy.

Interprofessional collaborative model for intimate partner violence identification/intervention
Violence and abuse is a serious global public health epidemic.[25,26] A multicountry study by the World Health Organization found that 25% to 50% of women interviewed reported physical assaults that resulted in injuries and, as a result, have poor health and want to commit suicide. Studies propose a strong statistical association between IPV and adverse health outcomes.[6,25–29] As such, violence and abuse have serious long-term medical consequences that last long after the initial trauma with a higher utilization of health services compared with matched cohorts who were not abused (**Fig. 3**).[30,31] Within the United States, health care invests billions of dollars yearly

Table 1
Access to dental health study

The information that you provide will help us to identify ways in which we can better take care of your oral health in an effort to reduce your chance for adverse pregnancy outcomes. Please answer questions about your feelings and experiences. There are no right or wrong answers. Your answers will be strictly confidential. Please do not write your name, or any other identifiable information on this form. Thank you for your help in this important effort to improve your overall health.

Instructions: For each of the following questions, please check the appropriate answer or circle the number that indicates your level of agreement or disagreement.

General Information

Are you pregnant?
 Yes _____ (Please complete all questions on the survey)
  If yes, how many weeks
  1–12 wk _____
  13–24 wk _____
  25 wk or greater _____
 No _____ (Please stop. Thank You.)

	Agree	Strongly Agree	Disagree	Strongly Disagree	Not applicable
About the Health of your Mouth					
1. I have regular dental check ups	5	4	3	2	1
2. I have sensitive teeth due to hot or cold foods or drinks	5	4	3	2	1
3. I have had painful aching in my mouth	5	4	3	2	1
4. I have had a toothache	5	4	3	2	1
5. I have had painful gums	5	4	3	2	1
6. I have found it uncomfortable to eat foods because of problems with my teeth, mouth, or dentures	5	4	3	2	1
7. I have been unable to brush my teeth properly because of problems with my teeth, mouth, or dentures	5	4	3	2	1
8. I have had to avoid or interrupt eating some foods because of problems with my teeth, mouth, or dentures	5	4	3	2	1
9. My diet has been unsatisfactory because of problems with my teeth, mouth or dentures	5	4	3	2	1
10. I have avoided smiling because of problems with my teeth, mouth or dentures	5	4	3	2	1
11. My dental health affects my overall health	5	4	3	2	1
12. My teeth and gums will affect whether or not my baby is healthy	5	4	3	2	1
13. I visit the dentist only when I have a toothache or In pain	5	4	3	2	1

(continued on next page)

Table 1
(continued)

Access to the Dental Clinic (Meharry Dental Clinic or Matthew Walker Dental Clinic)

	5	4	3	2	1
14. Upon arrival I usually do not have to wait long to be seen in the dental clinic	5	4	3	2	1
15. Information about the dental clinic is not easily accessible	5	4	3	2	1
16. I am involved in the decisions regarding my care	5	4	3	2	1
17. When I leave the dental clinic the instructions are clearly communicated	5	4	3	2	1
18. I can get a dental appointment within 2 wk to see my student dentist	5	4	3	2	1
19. The dental clinic hours are suitable to my schedule	5	4	3	2	1
20. I know how to reach the dental clinic if I have questions	5	4	3	2	1
21. The dental clinic has modern equipment to treat patients	5	4	3	2	1
22. Patients are treated equally regardless of their race	5	4	3	2	1
23. Patients are treated equally regardless of their age	5	4	3	2	1
24. I am satisfied with the dental care received	5	4	3	2	1
25. I would recommend the dental clinic to others	5	4	3	2	1

General Information continued

	5	4	3	2	1
26. I am comfortable talking to other health care providers about my health	5	4	3	2	1
27. I am healthier because my doctor works with other health care providers	5	4	3	2	1
28. I would like to learn more about my health from my health care provider	5	4	3	2	1

29. Do you have health insurance
    Yes _____
    No _____(Go to question 31)

29a. If yes, from which of the following do you obtain health insurance
    Employer _____ Spouse's employer_____
    Medicare_____ Medicaid_____
    Both Medicare and Medicaid_____
    Insurance you purchased_____

30. How do you normally travel to the dental clinic - Meharry/Matthew Walker
    Drive myself _____
    Have a friend or family member drive me_____
    Take public transportation

(continued on next page)

Table 1
(continued)

31. How far do you live from the dental clinic - Meharry/Matthew Walker
<1 mile _____ 1–5 miles_____ 6–10 miles _____ 11–15 miles _____
16 or more miles_____

32. How long have you been a patient here?
_____ <1 y_____ 1–3 y _____ 4–6 y_____ 7–9 y _____ 10 or more y _____

Demographic Information

33. Marital Status
_____ Married _____ Single _____ Divorce _____ Widowed_____

34. Yearly household income
Less than $20,000_____
$20,000–$29,000_____
$30,000–$39,000_____
$40,000–$49,000_____
$50,000 or more_____

Thank you for your participation.

Courtesy of Meharry Medical College, Nashville, TN (Thompson and Farmer-Dixon, Unpublished communication).

treating the consequences of abuse—too often without addressing the underlying causes.[30–32] Numerous health care bodies (AMA, Institute of Medicine, Centers for Disease Control and Prevention, ADA) recommend that all patients be asked routinely about abuse.[33,34] Early diagnosis of IPV-related injuries would significantly improve the health of victims and save billions of dollars in health care costs.[30–34]

Violence/Abuse Oral Health/Interprofessional Collaborative Paradigm

The gold standard for identifying an IPV-related injury is the patient's self-report, and, therefore, the diagnosis can be challenging.[27,33,34] The health care sector in general has identified and cared for victims of violence and abuse after the fact and are often in a quandary with respect to "igniting the process," that is, identify and intervene in IPV and domestic violence patient populations.[35,36] Within specialties, there are protocols but no commonly agreed on written guidelines for reasons such as litigation and personal experience.[33–36] With the above in mind, a solution requires that various health providers work together using an IPC approach to not only recognize the

Table 2
Linear regression model for outcome variable question 12: my teeth and gums will affect whether or not my baby is healthy

Variables in Equation	Regression Coefficients	P Value
Question 1: Perception of Regular Dental Checkups	0.064	.426, NS
Question 11: Perception That Dental Health Affects Overall Health	0.519	.000[a]
Question 30A: Insurance Status	0.009	.907, NS
Question 35: Yearly Household Income	0.028	.743, NS

Thompson and Farmer-Dixon, Unpublished communication.
Abbreviation: NS, not significant.
[a] $P<.001$.

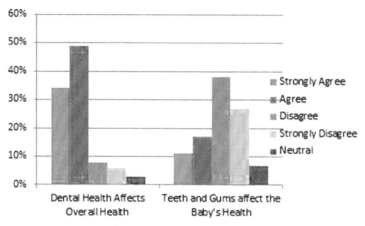

Fig. 1. Participant perception of their oral health and their baby's health.

epidemic but also integrate a common language of guidelines that can be used uniformly in all health care settings to identify victims and provide intervention.[37,38]

IPV is a frequent cause of facial injuries in victims between the ages of 18 and 64 with 75% of cases resulting in injuries to the head, neck, or mouth.[39–42] The residual effects of scars, facial asymmetries, damage to dentition, loss of masticator function, and psychological wounds persist to remind injured women the level of control by the perpetrator.[41–44] With greater than 50% of adults and children visiting the dentist, oral health care provides a pivotal point of contact for IPV victims.[42,43] Few reports, however, specify the causes or patterns of orofacial injuries in victims with IPV-related injuries using benign tools that encourage identification.[39–43] A paucity of studies have addressed health and social problems with regard to the interprofessional model and how the oral health care provider can be a significant link in this interdisciplinary chain of identifying and preventing future injuries in victims. The following are examples of community approaches using an IPC framework with oral health as a major link in the chain of identifying victims of violence and abuse for referral/intervention.

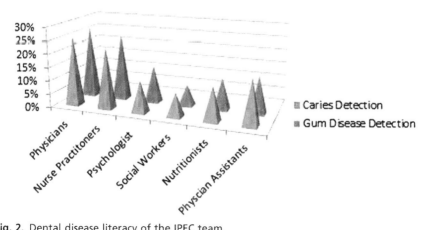

Fig. 2. Dental disease literacy of the IPEC team.

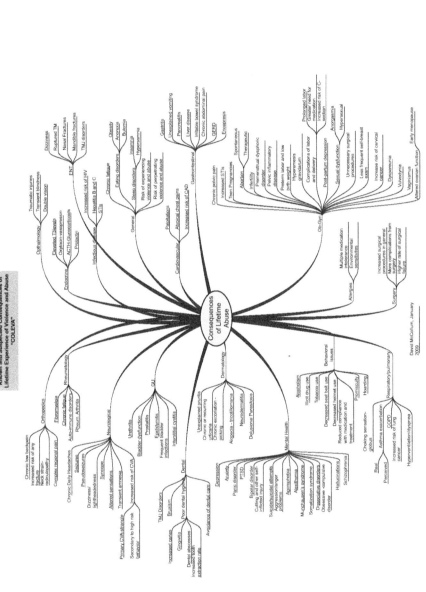

Fig. 3. COLEVA: Consequences of lifetime exposure to violence and abuse. (*From* Dolezal T, McCollum D. Hidden costs in healthcare. In: The economic impact of violence and abuse. Dolezal T, McCollum D, Callahan M, editors. Eden Prairie (MN): Academy on violence and abuse; 2009. p. 2; with permission.)

Model 1: Trauma-informed care approach

Raja and colleagues[44] suggest an oral health model to provide a framework for identification and referral of patients exposed to traumatic events. Their concept of trauma-informed care developed from experiences by oral health care providers that treat patients with a history of traumatic events at one point only but lack the tools for monitoring the survivors they identify over a longer period.[44] Dental patients with a history of traumatic experiences are more likely to engage in negative health habits and to display fear of routine dental care. Although not all patients disclose a trauma history to their dentists, some patients might. The trauma-informed care pyramid provides a framework to guide dental care providers in interactions with many types of traumatized patients using behavioral and communication skills as well as understanding the health effects of trauma and understanding how the provider's own trauma-related experiences can influence treatment strategies within an IPC framework.[38,39,44] **Fig. 4** depicts this approach, which is built on a foundation of patient communication, health effects of trauma, and the need for IPC collaboration.[44] This pyramid can be universally applied in an IPC framework across all health disciplines.[44]

Model 2: From family violence to health: an oral health approach at Dalhousie University

At Dalhousie University in Canada, dental and other health faculty crafted an IPC module that features the role of dental health professionals as central in the identification of victims of abuse.[45] The model hypothesizes the need for dental health care providers to work collaboratively with their medical, social, and legal colleagues to identify and eradicate domestic violence and IPV. This is approached from a predoctoral

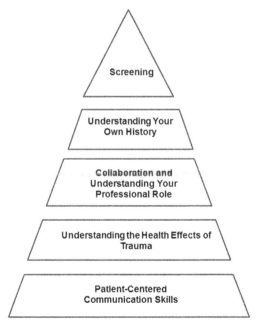

Fig. 4. Trauma-informed care pyramid. (*Adapted from* Raja S, Hoersch M, Rajagopalan CF, et al. Treating patients with traumatic life experiences. J Am Dent Assoc 2014;145(3): 241; with permission.)

perspective first followed by interdisciplinary communication via interdisciplinary focus groups. Outcomes measurements are based on qualitative parameters in which the provider becomes aware of clinical presentations of violence and abuse within the oral cavity and its effect on victims, that is, "What is the role of oral health in family violence? How might health professionals work together to allow for a better health-related quality of life in the community of victims." Quantitative risk predictors include a Likert scale approach with mean score measurements that allowed a better understanding of other health professional roles/ways to complement each other's approach to this problem and work in a health team environment that embraces cross-professional understanding for total patient care. Cross-discipline continuing education reinforces the IPC framework with regular follow-up on the outcomes measured within the interdisciplinary sphere of their health arena by feedback analyses.[45]

Model 3. Interprofessional collaborative model of violence and abuse survivors: early and long-term outcomes

Women experience more IPV than men; 4.8 million rapes and greater than 2 million injuries are enough to require multiple forms of health care (emergency room, dental care, hospital stays, and physical/psychological therapies).[25–27] The health care sector traditionally cares for victims after the fact due to the induced physical and mental health injuries. As such, the main precedence for the health care sector to address this dilemma is to develop best practice approaches that are not only team based but also aligned for rapid response to prevent further collateral damage.[35,36] Wilson and Websdale[35] crafted a paradigm "Domestic Violence Fatality Review Team" (DVFRT) the purpose of which is to provide strategies that prevent future injuries, ensure safety, and hold perpetrators and the system responsible.[35] This approach is unique because of the diversity of their team membership and more importantly because of the knowledge, experience, commitment, and goal to eradicate this chronic and sometimes fatal public health issue. The DVFRT holds the professionals, agencies, and judicial system accountable and prepares an in-depth report that is disseminated through publications, conference presentations, training, and interdisciplinary educational modules. Outcome measurements include homicide surveillance data that can examine patient demographics with respect to exposure to health care, such as, oral health and medical records, ethnicity, culture, gender, and the perpetrator's relationship to the victim.[35] Within the United states, several regions in the east and west have used the DVFRT reports as a cursory screening tool that alerted several health and social agencies to rethink their interventional strategies and compliance protocols, which were outdated and in need of interdisciplinary revision. Many states are now using DVFRT members to formulate new professional guidelines using oral health care providers as a strong link in a chain of survival for victims of violence and abuse.[35,36] Challenges, however, do remain, as the "silo" paradigm is still quite alive. Drawing on the disciplines of oral health, other health specialties, criminal justice, social services, and health policy advocates, these teams uncover basic knowledge about causation, risk, and prevention and then collectively recommend best practice patterns that offer better services and interventions to reduce future injuries and death of victims.[35,36,45]

Model 4: Facial injuries and health consequences as risk predictors for intimate partner violence exposure: Interprofessional collaborative intervention in a Tennessee community dental center

Tennessee is the fifth in the nation with respect to the number of women who are murdered each year from abuse.[46,47] Although white (non–African American [non-

AA]) victims accounted for as much as 80% of victims "who reported the incident," AA women were 3.4 times more likely to be victims compared with their non-AA cohorts.[46,47] Tennessee loses at least $10 million per year in paid work time and $33 million in health care costs because of IPV, whose identification often carried out, at least in part, in an emergency room setting.[36] Meharry Medical College (MMC) School of Dentistry in Nashville began to frame an IPC approach that uses facial injury location and questionnaires as risk predictors for identifying women with present or past exposure of IPV and uncovering those who would benefit by the health provider's awareness of exposure to this harsh life event, how it manifests itself with poor health, and how to prevent future injuries. The School of Dentistry group composed of oral health care providers and behavioral scientists are characterizing the correlation among exposure of IPV-related injuries with specific health outcomes that affect female victims (ages18–64). The group has contrasted (1) physical findings, that is, injury location (head, neck, and facial [HNF]) versus other injuries; (2) patient responses to an IPV screening questionnaire (Partner Violence Screen [PVS]); and (3) patient responses to a general health questionnaire to characterize significant health disparities secondary to exposure of IPV in women who visit the Oral Surgery Clinic at the MMC School of Dentistry.[48,49] Preliminary data support HNF injuries and positive response to the PVS screen to be statistically significant as predictors of a present or past IPV injury etiology ($P<.001$) as supported by previous studies.[48] Significant differences exist with respect to health disparities between IPV-positive/IPV-negative cohorts (**Table 3**). IPV-positive AA women, when compared with their non-AA IPV-positive cohorts, have statistically significant differences in health consequences (**Table 4**). The results of this pilot study are the first to identify the prevalence of IPV positivity in female AA versus non-AA dental patients at MMC School of Dentistry. HNF injuries and positive response to the PVS are statistically significant as predictors of a present or past IPV injury etiology ($P<.01$).

Table 3
Association between IPV and variables

Independent Variable	IPV (PVS+) Relative Frequency	Percentage	Non-IPV (PVS-) Relative Frequency	Percentage	P Value
HNF injuries	28/40	70.0	7/38	18.4	.001
Anxiety	25/40	62.5	7/38	18.4	.001
Swollen/painful joints	15/34	44.1	2/30	6.7	.001
Fatigue/tiredness	12/34	35.3	11/30	36.7	.001
Difficulty hearing	8/34	23.6	1/30	3.3	.001
Memory loss	9/34	26.5	3/30	10.0	.001
Chest pain	7/34	20.6	2/30	6.7	.001
Vaginal/pelvis pain	3/34	8.8	0/30	0.0	.001
Heart palpitation	26/34	76.5	1/30	3.3	.002
Upset stomach/heartburn	20/34	65.0	8/30	26.7	.002
Difficulty concentrating	20/34	58.8	6/30	20.0	.002
Stress/posttraumatic stress disorder	25/40	62.5	13/38	34.2	.003

This table shows association between IPV positivity and the health disparities measured. Those variables with statistical significance are bolded (Halpern et al. 2016, Violence and gender, in press).

Table 4
Association of significant variables among the races

Independent Variable	P Value	
	Non-AA (n = 21)	AA (n = 13)
Upset stomach/heartburn	.290	.001
Difficulty concentrating	.152	.002
Loss of appetite	.363	.003
Difficulty sleeping (insomnia)	.297	.003
Difficulty hearing	.094	.003
Bladder infection	.549	.037
Heart palpitation	.006	.170
Back pain	.028	.858
Memory loss	.019	.869

This table shows association of significant variables among the races. Those variables with statistical significance are bolded. (Halpern et al. 2016, Violence and gender, in press).

Significant differences exist with respect to health consequences between IPV-positive/IPV-negative. AA women when compared with non-AA cohorts have statistically significant differences in poor health. These preliminary results suggest the potential application of this protocol in screening programs to not only identify victims of IPV but also monitor their overall health and intervention to prevent future injuries in this health-poor community. We are working with our medicine and behaviorist colleagues to work out a system for communicating how well our intervention is succeeding in this patient population with respect to improvement and eradication of their health consequences (personal communication).

Interprofessional Collaborative Model for Oral Health Providers in Community Primary Care

As noted above, the World Health Organization provides a consensus statement advocating policies on oral health disease prevention and its association with chronic diseases.[1] There is a national consensus to integrate oral health into primary care.[2] However, over the last couple of decades, medical graduates are not comfortable managing older women's health with respect to oral and other disease unless they are specifically in gynecologic health care. This finding has resulted in these health workers being somewhat uncomfortable in addressing women's health, often delaying addressing these issues until discharge to outpatient practices.[50,51] Primary care providers and internists now often refer to women's health specialists, gynecologists, or to their own female nurse practitioners.[50] Women's health subsequently developed its own niche, which includes preventative care and chronic disease management, particularly in older women. This action resulted in a "silo" phenomenon, which has been a stumbling block within other specialties.[51,52]

An area of chronic disease management in older women that primary physicians are uncomfortable managing because of its atypical intraoral symptoms, is the effect of medical treatment of osteoporosis. For this reason it is important to acknowledge that IPC teams can and do play a significant role in providing comprehensive care. An excellent example of IPC collaboration occurred at Texas Tech University Health Sciences Center in Amarillo, Texas, when leaders developed a consensus statement document for the Upper Panhandle of West Texas service area.[50] The impetus to create a consensus arose when it was identified that many women on bisphosphonates were not able to access general dental care, including dental hygiene and extractions. These patients were not able to obtain general dental procedures because dentists had a fear of bisphosphonate-related osteonecrosis of the jaw now referred to as medicine-related osteonecrosis of the jaw.[53] Although the disease is rare in women receiving oral bisphosphonates for prevention and treatment of osteoporosis, access to care, nevertheless, was limited for this population, and medical providers were concerned that the risk of dying from fracture of the hip or thoracic spine was significantly higher than dying from medicine-related osteonecrosis of the jaw.[51] A debate platform was proposed in which a women's health specialist would present the pros for treatment and a dental specialist would present the cons. Fortunately, a private practice endodontist recommended that it would serve the best interest of the community to use an interdisciplinary format instead. He emphasized that providers would like to have guidance on a subject for which there is a relative deficiency of comprehensive evidence that might otherwise allow for guidelines or algorithms. In the spirit of collaboration, a half-day interprofessional forum was held, which included an audience of general dentists, dental specialists, dental hygienists, physicians, nurses, and students. A women's health specialist presented an overview of osteoporosis, an endodontist discussed bisphosphonates and osteonecrosis of the jaw, and a geriatrician served to facilitate the forum and discussions. There was a question-and-answer session after each speaker, an opportunity for patient testimony, and integrated small group breakouts to discuss local experiences and management. Feedback was collected during the forum and the evidence-based literature was reviewed and subsequently used to write a consensus document regarding management of patients considering bisphosphonate therapy for osteoporosis.[50] The document emphasized interprofessional collaboration—an IPC strategy, especially between medical and dental providers—as essential with communication being paramount. A list of providers was given for networking to provide seamless patient care. Although challenges still exist, participating in a framework of meeting annually as a regional IPEC group in a forum to share concerns and ideas regarding best approaches to manage chronic disease in geriatrics, would likely foster improved interprofessional relationships and networks, which improve patient care and outcomes (**Box 2**, SM, personal communication).

SUMMARY/FUTURE DIRECTIONS

The focus of the IPC paradigm is to treat the whole patient—mind, body, and soul by fostering critical thinking skills and engaging in a common dialogue to apply strategies

---

Box 2
Training workshop and seminar topics provided to IPC team

- Interdisciplinary approach to optimal health: An overview for health care providers
- Provider education: Identifying how health care professionals articulate and promote women's health and the importance of patient behavior and acceptance of total care
- Assessment of the oral cavity: Identification of caries, soft and hard tissue lesions unique to women
- Medical implications: the impact of medical conditions on the oral health status of the patient

that challenge the complex health care issues of the patient. This use of a team-based collaborative group will drive innovative models such as accountable-care organizations, health homes, and patient-centered specialty practices that can be used as metrics for outcome measurements of the success of an IPC strategy plan (**Box 3**). As stated in the introduction, several health services at the national level have proposed implementation of collaborative efforts to create a broader agenda for women's health curricula and application through an IPC model.

The departments of Health and Human Services, HRSA, and the Office of Women's Health in 2013, published a report to provide the background, recommendations, and implementation steps to improve women's health education across 5 specific health professions programs: medicine, oral health/dentistry, baccalaureate nursing, pharmacy, and public health.[10] The report was based on 3 expert panel meetings with the goals to:

1. Summarize the literature on women's health curricula
2. Develop key strategies or an IPEC model that would be translated across disciplines on women's health needs
3. Disseminate a plan that would create greater awareness across all disciplines as to the need to educate practitioners on the health needs of women.

Goal number 2 was especially vital, as key aspects to apply strategies include biological considerations, health and wellness, behavioral health, selected health conditions, and most importantly the role of each health practitioner in contributing to total patient care. The results of these panel proceedings were crafted as "Action Items" (**Box 4**) that provide steps for integrating educational strategies across all health disciplines and set a foundation for an IPEC collaborative framework. Active dissemination of the report, as laid out by HRSA, will improve institutional awareness of the need to improve women's health curricula, motivate the development of competencies focusing on women's health, and enhance public concern about the importance of women's health curricula in health professions education. This information will foster a legacy for better health-related quality of life not only for women but for everyone.

Oral health care is now staking its claim within this new paradigm, as the dentist may be the first line of defense not only for oral but some systemic diseases. Health care must now envision how the melding of medicine, pharmacy, nursing, psychology, other health specialties, and oral health will positively impact the paradigm already laid out to incorporate evidence-based knowledge into clinical practice. By providing models for an IPC approach to women's health both from oral and overall health care,

---

Box 3
Suggested guidelines for IPC framework in women's oral/overall health

- Analyze women's health content common across health professions.
- Create a service learning elective with ties to women's health.
- Create interdepartmental programs in women's health.
- Create interprofessional core competencies in women's health.
- Engage in interprofessional simulation exercises.
- Establish women's health clerkships and fellowships.
- Outline general and specialty women's health curriculum across disciplines.
- Secure additional funding for curricula initiatives.

Box 4
Five key content areas that experts across the health professions cited as significant for interprofessional collaboration in women's health

Role of the Health Professional

- Ethics
- Interprofessional education
- Knowledge of other health professions
- Patient-centered decision making
- Gender in provider/patient communication

Biological Considerations

- Age
- Sex
- Genetics
- Hormonal influences
- Pharmacokinetics and pharmacodynamics

Selected Conditions

- Autoimmune disorders
- Cardiovascular disease
- Endocrine disorders
- Endometriosis
- Infectious disease (especially human immunodeficiency virus)
- Pregnancy and breastfeeding (especially medications taken during pregnancy and periodontal health in pregnancy)
- Metabolic disorders
- Musculoskeletal health
- Neurologic conditions

Behavioral and Mental Health

- Anxiety/stress
- Depression/bipolar disorders
- Domestic abuse/IPV
- Eating behaviors/disorders
- Sexual behavior
- Substance abuse
- Traumatic experiences

Wellness and Prevention

- Access to care
- Environmental health
- Exercise physiology
- Hormonal transitions
- Nutrition
- Oral health

- Reproductive choice, family planning, and obstetrics
- Preventative health screening and immunizations
- Work-family balance

Experts also contributed key topics within each content area to serve as examples of shared interests across oral health, medicine, nursing, pharmacy, public health, and social work.

From U.S. Department of Health and Human Services, Health Resources and Services Administration, Office of Women's Health. Women's Health Curricula: final report on expert panel recommendations for interprofessional collaborations across the Health Professions. Rockville (MD): U.S. Department of Health and Human Services; 2013; with permission.

the patient becomes empowered in decision-making strategies for a better health-related quality of life.

REFERENCES

1. IOM (Institute of Medicine), NRC (National Research Council). Improving access to oral healthcare for vulnerable and underserved populations. Washington, DC: The National Academies Press; 2011.
2. Wilder RS, O'Donnell JA, Barry JM, et al. Is dentistry at risk? A case for interprofessional education. J Dent Educ 2008;72(11):1231–7.
3. Price SS, Funk AD, Shockey AK, et al. Promoting oral health as part of an interprofessional community based women's health event. J Dent Educ 2014;78(9): 1294–300.
4. Jackson JT, Quinonez RB, Kerns AK, et al. Implementing a prenatal oral health program through interprofessional collaboration. J Dent Educ 2015;79(3):241–8.
5. Ressler-Maerlender J, Krishna R, Robison V. Oral health during pregnancy: current research. J Womens Health 2005;14(10):880–4.
6. Scott-Storey K, Wuest J, Ford-Gilboe M. Intimate partner violence and cardiovascular risk: is there a link? J Adv Nurs 2009;65(10):2186–97.
7. Pechacek JM, Drake D, Terrell CA, et al. Interprofessional intervention to support mature women: a case study. Creat Nurs 2015;21(3):134–43.
8. WHO. Framework for action on interprofessional education and collaborative practice. Geneva (Switzerland): World Health Organization; 2010. p. 1–62.
9. Mouradian WE, Lewis CW, Berg JH. Integration of dentistry and medicine and the dentist of the future: the need for the health care team. J Calif Dent Assoc 2014; 42(10):687–95.
10. U.S. Department of Health and Human Services, Health Resources and Services Administration, Office of Women's Health. Women's Health Curricula: final report on expert panel recommendations for interprofessional collaborations across the Health Professions. Rockville (MD): U.S. Department of Health and Human Services; 2013.
11. Lee NC, Woods CM. The affordable care act: addressing the unique health needs of women. J Womens Health 2013;22(10):803–6.
12. Berwick DM, Nolan TW, Whittington J. The triple aim: care health and cost. Health Aff 2008;27(3):759–69.
13. Bogner HR, Gallo JJ. Are higher rates of depression in women accounted for by differential symptom reporting? Soc Psychiatry Psychiatr Epidemiol 2004;39(2): 126–32.
14. Hibbard JH, Pope CR. Gender roles, illness orientation and use of medical services. Soc Sci Med 1983;17(3):129–37.

15. Verdonk P, Benschop YW, de Hass HC, et al. From gender bias to gender aware-ness in medical education. Adv Health Sci Educ Theory Pract 2009;14(1):135–52.

16. Valachovic RW. Integrating oral and overall health care-on the road to interprofes-sional education and practice: building a foundation for interprofessional educa-tion and practice. J Calif Dent Assoc 2014;42(1):25–7.

17. Steinberg BJ, Hilton IV, Iada H, et al. Oral health and dental care during preg-nancy. Dent Clin North Am 2013;57(2):195–210.

18. Bobetsis YA, Barros SP, Offenbacher S. Exploring the relationship between peri-odontal disease and pregnancy complications. J Am Dent Assoc 2006;137(2):7S–13S.

19. Goldenberg RL, Culhane JF. Preterm birth and periodontal disease. N Engl J Med 2006;355:1925–7.

20. Haden NK, Catalanotto FA, Alexander CJ, et al. Improving the oral health status of all americans: roles and responsibilities of academic dental institutions. The Report of the ADEA President's Commission. J Dent Educ 2003;67(5):563–83.

21. Han YW. Oral health and adverse pregnancy outcomes – what's next? J Dent Res 2011;90(3):289–93.

22. Horton AL, Boggess KA, Moss KL, et al. Periodontal disease early in pregnancy is associated with maternal systemic inflammation among african american women. J Periodontol 2008;79:1127–32.

23. Jeffcoat MK, Geurs NC, Reddy MS, et al. Periodontal infection and preterm birth: results of a prospective study. J Am Dent Assoc 2001;132(7):875–80.

24. Oral health care during pregnancy: a national consensus statement. Summary of an expert workgroup meeting.© 2012 by the National Maternal and Child Oral Health Resource Center, Georgetown University, Grant number H47MC00048, Health Resources and Service Administration (HRSA), US Department of Health and Human Services (DHHS).

25. World Health Organization (2011). Violence. Geneva (Switzerland): Available at: http://www.who.int/topics/violence/en/, Accessed March 3, 2011.

26. World Health Organization. Violence: A public health priority. Geneva (Switzerland): WHO Global Consultation on Violence and Health; 1996. document WHO/EHA/SPI.POA.2.

27. Tjaden P, Thoennes N. Full report of the prevalence, incidence and conse-quences of intimate partner violence against women: findings from the national violence against women survey. Report for grant 93-IJ-CX-0012, funded by the National Institute of justice and the centers for disease control and prevention. Washington, DC: NIJ, 2000.

28. Campbell J, Jones AS, Dienemann J, et al. Intimate partner violence and physical health consequences. Arch Intern Med 2002;162:1157–63.

29. Campbell J. Health consequences of intimate partner violence. Lancet 2002;359:1331–6.

30. Max W, Rice DP, Finkelstein E, et al. The economic toll of intimate partner violence against women in the United States. Violence Vict 2004;19(3):259–72.

31. Dolezal T, McCollum D. Hidden costs in healthcare. In: Dolezal T, McCollum D, Callahan M, editors. The economic impact of violence and abuse. Eden Prairie (MN): Academy on Violence and Abuse; 2009. p. 1–12.

32. Tennessee Economic Council on Women (2006). The impact of domestic violence on them Tennessee economy. Available at: http://www.tn.gov/sos/ecw/domestic.violence.htm. Accessed May, 2013.

33. American College of Obstetricians and Gynecologists. Screening tools-domestic violence. Available at: www.acog.org/departments/dept_notice.cfm. Accessed March 31, 2010.

34. Black MC, Basile KC, Breiding MJ, et al. The national intimate partner and sexual violence survey (NISVS): 2010 summer report. Atlanta (GA): National Center for Injury Prevention and Control, Centers for Disease Control and Prevention; 2011.

35. Wilson JS, Websdale N. Domestic violence fatality review teams: an interprofessional model to reduce events. J Interprof Care 2006;20(5):535–44.

36. Reeves S, Sully P. Interprofessional education for practitioners working with the survivors of violence: exploring early and longer-term outcomes on practice. J Interprofess Care 2007;21(4):401–12.

37. Bell AV, Michalec B, Arenson C. The (stalled) progress of interprofessional collaboration: the role of gender. J Interprofess Care 2014;28(2):98–102.

38. Leppakoski TH, Flinck A. Paavilainen. Greater commitment to the domestic violence training is required. J Interprofess Care 2015;29(3):281–3.

39. Halpern LR. Orofacial injuries as markers for intimate partner violence. Oral Maxillofac Clin N Am 2010;22(2):239–46.

40. Huang V, Moore C, Bohrer P. Maxillofacial injuries in women. Ann Plast Surg 1998; 41:482–4.

41. Le BT, Dierks EJ, Ueeck-Homer LD, et al. Maxillofacial injuries associated with domestic violence. J Oral Maxillofac Surg 2001;59:1277–83.

42. Wilson S, Dodson TB, Halpern LR. Maxillofacial injuries as tools for diagnosis of intimate partner violence. In: Mitchell C, Anglin D, editors. Violence and abuse across the individual's lifespan. New York, NY: Oxford University Press; 2008. p. 201–16.

43. Greene PE, Chisick MC, Aaron GR. A comparison of oral health status and need for dental care between abused/neglected children and non-abused/non-neglected children. Pediatr Dent 1994;16(1):41–5.

44. Raja S, Hoersch M, Rajagopalan, et al. Treating patients with traumatic life experiences. J Am Dent Assoc 2014;145(3):238–45.

45. Johnston GM, Ryding HA, Campbell LM. Evolution of interprofessional learning: Dalhousie University's "from family violence to health" module. J Can Dent Assoc 2003;69(10). 658a-e.

46. Tennessee Domestic Violence Report, 2009-2011. Prepared by the TN Bureau of Investigation. p. 1–16.

47. Tennessee Bureau of investigation crime statistics unit (2012). TIBRS data collection: an instructional manual for the implementation of the Tennessee Incident–based Reporting *system*. 10th edition. TN Bureau of Investigation Releases "Family Violence Study". p. 1–10.

48. Halpern LR, Perciaccante VJ, Hayes C, et al. A protocol to diagnose intimate partner violence in the emergency room setting. J Trauma 2006;60(5):1101–5.

49. Ford-Gilboe M, Wuest J, Varcoe C, et al. Modeling the effect of intimate partner violence and access to resources on women's health in the early years after leaving an abusive partner. Soc Sci Med 2009;68(6):1021–9.

50. Leeper SC, Jenkins MR, Coury KA. (2008). Consensus Statement for the Panhandle and Service Region. Published and distributed to 1000 providers: Management of Patients Considering Bisphosphonate Therapy for Osteoporosis-2008 Texas Panhandle and Surrounding Service Area Consensus Statement.

51. Leibson CL, Tosteson AN, Gabriel SE, et al. Mortality, disability, and nursing home use for persons with and without hip fracture: a population-based study. J Am Geriatr Soc 2002;50:1644.
52. Hilton I. Interdisciplinary collaboration: what private practice can learn from the health center experience. J Calif Dent Assoc 2014;42(1):29–34.
53. American Association of Oral and Maxillofacial Surgeons (AAOMS) Position paper on Medication-Related Osteonecrosis of the Jaw (MRONJ). 2014. Available at: www.aaoms.org. Accessed December, 2014.

Oral Health and Interprofessional Collaborative Practice
Examples of the Team Approach to Geriatric Care

 CrossMark

Laura B. Kaufman, DMD[a,b,*], Michelle M. Henshaw, DDS, MPH[c],
Blase P. Brown, DDS, MS[d], Joseph M. Calabrese, DMD[e,f]

KEYWORDS

- Interprofessional relations • Geriatric dentistry • Patient care team • Prosthodontics
- Oral cancer • Patient care planning • Dental education • Medical education

KEY POINTS

- Most professions related to health care and their associated specialties engage in successful collaborations.
- Functional and/or cognitive impairments in older adult patients may necessitate identifying family members and caregivers to help the patient maintain optimal oral health.
- Better patient outcomes for older adults result from successful interprofessional collaboration, in conjunction with the support of the patient's family and caregivers.
- Communicating frequently with other team members helps to ensure optimal oral health outcomes over the short and long term.

INTRODUCTION

Traditionally, dental and medical education and practice take place separately, with little to no interaction between dentists and physicians during training or later in practice. There is an increased emphasis in recent years to increase interprofessional dental and medical education; the anticipated benefits include collaborative practices that lead to improved patient outcomes. Many older adults who are no longer able

[a] Department of General Dentistry, Boston University Henry M. Goldman School of Dental Medicine, 100 E. Newton Street, Boston, MA 02118, USA; [b] Section of Geriatrics, Boston University School of Medicine, MA 02118, USA; [c] Department of Health Policy and Health Services Research, Boston University Henry M. Goldman School of Dental Medicine, 560 Harrison Avenue, Boston, MA 02118, USA; [d] Department of Oral Medicine and Diagnostic Services, University of Illinois at Chicago College of Dentistry, 801 S. Paulina St, Chicago, Illinois 60612, USA; [e] Department of General Dentistry, Geriatric Dental Medicine, Boston University Henry M. Goldman School of Dental Medicine, Boston Medical Center, 100 East Newton Street, Boston, MA 02118, USA; [f] Harvard School of Dental Medicine, Boston, MA 02115, USA
* Corresponding author.
E-mail address: lbkaufma@bu.edu

Dent Clin N Am 60 (2016) 879–890
http://dx.doi.org/10.1016/j.cden.2016.05.007
0011-8532/16/$ – see front matter © 2016 Elsevier Inc. All rights reserved.

to access traditional dental office settings owing to cognitive and/or physical impairment(s) receive dental treatment in nondental settings. Meaningful patient outcomes measures, such as stabilization of weight loss and increased ability to socialize and enjoy food, is observed in some of these patients. With the rapid increase of older adults aged 65 years and over in the United States today, future directions for dental research could include validating outcome measures and assessing increased quality of life after dental treatment in frail older adults in the context of interprofessional collaborative practice.

The older adult population is expanding rapidly and life expectancy is increasing. Many dental patients are older than in the past and thanks to advances in modern dentistry and prevention,[1] the retention of natural dentition into old age is increasing. With advancing age, there may be impairment of cognitive and physical capacities, leading to less than optimal oral hygiene resulting in dental disease. According to *Healthy People 2020*, vulnerable populations, including the elderly, suffer disproportionately from dental diseases and often lack access to preventive treatments and dental care.[2] The US Department of Health and Human Services–funded training programs in geriatrics for physicians and dentists educate clinicians together to care for frail older adults' medical and dental needs (See Joskow RW: Integrating Oral Health and Primary Care: Federal Initiatives to Drive Systems Change, in this issue).

Older adult patients with complex and interrelated medical and dental conditions benefit from well-coordinated health care from a wide range of health care advocates.[3] Multiple medical comorbidities, along with cognitive and physical impairments, may have a negative impact on oral health. Coordinating care between medical and dental providers can be challenging owing to the traditional separation of medical and dental education and practice sites.

A new interprofessional education initiative model between dental and medical students at Boston University is preparing dental and medical students to communicate with each other and work together to provide comprehensive and coordinated care for their patients. Previous research has shown that students trained with an interprofessional approach to education are more likely to become collaborative team members.[4] These students are more likely to show respect and positive attitudes toward each other on future interprofessional teams and work together to improve patient outcomes. The Boston University model of interprofessional education includes a didactic module on oral and systemic health for older adults and hands on experience of intraoral screenings for medical students taught by dental students.

This article uses 2 patient case studies to help illustrate interprofessional collaborative practice. The first is an example of a successful dental–medical collaboration and a second case is one with an unsuccessful oral health outcome. In the future, more interprofessional training opportunities for students in dental and medical schools may lead to better interprofessional clinician communication and increased instances of successful patient clinical outcomes.

INTERPROFESSIONAL COLLABORATIVE PRACTICE IMPROVES PATIENT OUTCOMES IN GERIATRIC PATIENT CARE

Good oral health is vital for function, comfort, and communication, and is a critical component of overall health. Oral diseases such as dental caries (cavities/decay), periodontal disease, and oral cancer may lead to pain, functional limitations, and decreased quality of life for patients. A recent study found that many older adults, including those aged 70, 80, 90, and 100 and older are retaining their natural dentition over their lifetime, with good oral health often an indicator of good systemic health.[5] An increased understanding of the linkages between oral and systemic health, especially the association of periodontal disease with atherosclerotic vascular disease, diabetes, and stroke, heightens the need to maintain optimal oral health for older adults.[6] Collaboration with nonoral health care providers, as well as the patient's family and caregivers, are key to optimal dental treatment of older adults with multiple comorbidities.

Interprofessional team-based competencies[7] (**Table 1**) provide a framework for dentists collaborating with nondental health care providers in caring for older and frail patients. The competencies include clearly communication of the importance of integrating dental care into the patient's overall treatment plan, communication between health care providers, defining the rolls of various providers, and how to best work together for optimal patient care. Consideration of interprofessional collaboration opportunities regarding geriatric medical domains and their impacts on oral health should be made (**Table 2**).

BOSTON MEDICAL CENTER GERIATRICS: A SUCCESSFUL INTERPROFESSIONAL COLLABORATIVE PRACTICE MODEL

At Boston Medical Center, homebound older adults receive coordinated care from a team of geriatric medical, psychiatry and dental fellows and faculty, including dentists, physicians, nurses, and allied health professionals (**Fig. 1**). The important role of caregivers and family members in helping the older homebound patients is recognized, valued, and included in caregiving and treatment decision making.

Table 1
Interprofessional team core competencies, characteristics, and geriatric oral health

Interprofessional Team Core Competencies[7]	General Characteristics[7]	Geriatric Oral Health
Values and ethics for interprofessional practice	Patient and family as partners in team effort Respect and value of other members of the health care team	Patient-centered care for geriatric patients Educating medical providers on the importance of dental care for their patients at all ages and stages of life
Roles and responsibilities	Understand the skill set of the other professions Engage diverse health care professionals to improve the patient's health	Cross-referrals between dental and nondental providers Interprofessional education at all education levels
Interprofessional communication	Communicating effectively with other members of the health care team	Using communication tools such as teleconferences or Skype to facilitate effective communication
Teams and team work	Cooperating in patient centered delivery of care	Jointly develop comprehensive care plan that incorporates all disciplines Educating dental and medical providers about options to provide dental care in a nondental setting

Table 2
Geriatric medical domains impact oral health: opportunities for interprofessional practice

Geriatric Domains	Geriatric Medical	Geriatric Dental	Strategies for Medical and Dental Providers
Medications	Polypharmacy, radiation treatment or other etiologies resulting in xerostomia, and/or dysphagia	Patients often suck on sugar candies or consume high-sugar drinks to relieve symptoms of xerostomia and/or dysphagia, which may result in rampant caries	Preemptive strategies include educating the patient and other health care providers that xerostomia is a possible adverse side effect of treatment
			Proactively advise patients to treat symptoms by sipping water, using sugar-free candies and gum and/or oral lubricant; consider use of daily fluoride treatment
	Anticoagulant medication	Bleeding resulting from dental extractions	Need to consult patients' physician regarding anticoagulant therapy before a surgical procedure(s)
Mobility	Patient has a history of falling or is wheelchair bound	Patient may fall in office. Limited room for wheelchair in office	Clear hallways and operatory of potential fall hazards Design dental offices and bathrooms for wheelchair accessibility
	Patient is homebound	Limited or no access to dental care	Educate family and other caregivers to assist homebound patients in daily oral hygiene procedures Dentists can consider making a home dental visit to treat patient
Cognitive function	Short-term memory loss Dementia Depression	Poor oral hygiene Losing dentures	Frequent hygiene recall visits Extract nonsalvageable teeth Engage caregivers to help keep track of dentures
Social support	Little social support: formal (visiting nurse, home health aide, Meals on Wheels) or informal (family, neighbors, etc)	Inadequate and poor nutrition Caries and periodontal disease	Encourage and train informal and formal caregivers to provide oral hygiene assistance Use social service agencies for local resources
Physical impairment	Osteoarthritis Vision loss Hearing loss	Inability to grasp toothbrush handle or floss Difficulty seeing teeth to clean adequately Trouble hearing oral hygiene instructions	Modifying tooth brush handle with aluminum foil or tennis ball Use of children's size electric toothbrush Large print handouts of oral hygiene instructions

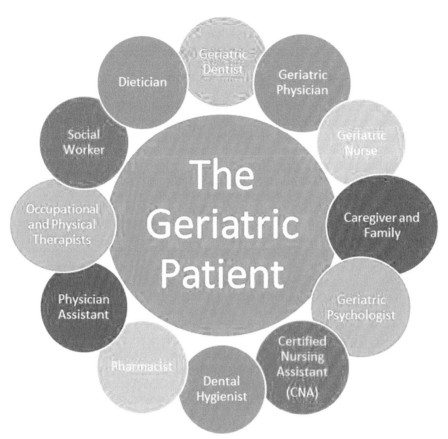

Fig. 1. Interprofessional members of an ideal geriatric patient care team. (*Courtesy of* Boston University Henry M. Goldman School of Dental Medicine, Boston, MA; with permission.)

Interprofessional components of the geriatrics training for dentists and primary care physicians (PCPs) contributing to successful collaborative practice include case discussions of patients' comorbidities with primary health care providers, complex case discussions with medical and dental components resulting in collaborative treatment planning, and interdisciplinary and evidence-based medical and dental case conferences.

CASE STUDY 1: DENTURE FABRICATION FOR A MEDICALLY COMPLEX OLDER ADULT IN A NONTRADITIONAL HEALTH CARE SETTING WITH A COLLABORATIVE TEAM

An 84-year-old homebound man with a medical history significant for chronic kidney disease, hypertension, hyperlipidemia, chronic obstructive pulmonary disease, vision impairment (legal blindness), depression, and recent weight loss was referred to geriatric dental medicine for comprehensive oral evaluation owing to a broken upper denture and weight loss. Documented in the electronic medical record notes by the PCP were periods that the patient was argumentative and depressed, as well as a diagnosis of "failure to thrive."

A discussion between the geriatric dentist, physician, and nurse case manager provided the dental team with the knowledge that the patient would likely cooperate with an oral health assessment and dental treatment and that the family was supportive of the treatment (see **Fig. 1**). The initial oral health assessment found our patient wearing ill-fitting upper and lower dentures, with a fractured acrylic flange in the maxillary buccal vestibule.

Team members included the geriatric dentist, PCP, and 2 fourth-year dental students. The entire team, including the patient and his wife, met in the same room and discussed the treatment plan. Under the direct supervision of the attending geriatric dentist, the students provided the treatment for the patient throughout the denture fabrication process, including preliminary impressions, final impressions, intermaxillary records, tooth and denture base shade selection, tooth try-in, denture insertion, and postinsertion adjustment visits as needed.

Medical concerns of note to the dental team included the patient's decreased food intake with associated weight loss and the patient's diagnosis of depression. The day of the first denture fabrication visit, the dental team stood by ready to go for a few minutes while the patient finished his breakfast. During this time the dental team took the opportunity to manage the expectations of the patient, his wife, and his son for the new dentures. Once the patient was ready, the students took the time necessary to develop a rapport with the patient, including asking him what kind of music he would like them to play on their smartphone during the visit. Upon learning that he was a retired choir director, the students promised him that they would "hold a concert" with him, that is, play piano and sing, after the last appointment.

After that seminal moment and until treatment was completed, the patient would anxiously await the arrival of the dental team. He would be on time and dressed up in a button-down shirt and tie. The patient and his family looked forward to each visit, appreciated the fact that the patient was offered the opportunity to select the music playing on the student's smartphone during each visit, and celebrated the end of the treatment with a music recital, including the patient playing the piano and singing with the students. Six months after completion of the case after a follow-up by the PCP, the patient's PCP reported that the patient had gained weight and was now actively engaging in social situations, a far cry from the man they met about 7 months earlier.

LESSONS LEARNED FROM CASE STUDY 1

Failure to thrive in older adults manifests as a state of decline resulting from chronic medical conditions and functional impairments. Patient symptoms include depression, decreased food intake, and concomitant weight loss.[8] Optimal geriatric assessment of patients with decreased food intake and concomitant weight loss should include an oral health assessment and appropriate follow-up treatment based on that (most recent) comprehensive oral health assessment. Many times, a straightforward problem such as a painful tooth or poorly functioning denture can impede the patient's ability to function or thrive in a social setting.

The time spent on building a rapport with the patient helped decrease his anxiety before beginning treatment. The dental students demonstrated excellent interpersonal skills by engaging the patient through a mutual love of music. The increase of the patient's weight after treatment is a probable successful outcome of the treatment, because it is possible that the broken and ill-fitting original dentures contributed to the patient's prior weight loss and diagnosis of failure to thrive. Additional factors contributing to the successful completion of this case included interprofessional education of all members of the geriatric dental and medical teams, exemplified by the dental referral from geriatric medicine to the geriatric dental team; the dental team collaborated with the medical team regarding best strategies for engaging the patient's cooperation; and the patient's family members, who were providing home care to the patient understood the importance of the dental treatment plan and facilitated multiple visits.

CASE STUDY 2: OROPHARYNGEAL CANCER IN AN OLDER ADULT PATIENT

Jane Doe, age 80, presented to her general dentist for an oral health evaluation and treatment following a recent diagnosis of "throat cancer." The patient's medical history included hypertension, for which she was taking an angiotensin-converting enzyme inhibitor. Her social history noted that she lives alone and has 2 adult children who live nearby. A letter from her oncologist to her dentist stated that she would be undergoing surgery, chemotherapy, and radiation therapy. Jane had read this letter and knew from conversations with her oncologist that her dentist needed to prepare her oral cavity before cancer treatment and she needed to attend follow-up appointments at the dentist during the period of oncology treatment.

The team and their anticipated roles relevant to the patient's oral health included the following:

- Patient: 80 years old; lives alone; dependent on her grown children, who live nearby, for rides to her appointments.
- Oncologist: Coordinate and provide oncology care.
- Dentist: Prepare an "oral health care plan" for patient before oncology treatment, including dental treatment to be done immediately, as well as a comprehensive prevention protocol for the patient to carry out at home during cancer treatment, along with scheduling 2-month recall visits in the dental office during cancer treatment.
- Oral surgeon: Extract teeth with poor prognosis (at risk for abscess) before cancer treatment.
- Dental office manager and dental hygienist: Coordinate preventive maintenance appointments for patient during cancer treatment.
- Nursing staff in the oncology center: Administer care as communicated from the oncologist.

Jane's oral health status has been somewhat stable for the past decade. At the time of the oropharyngeal squamous cell carcinoma (OPSCC) diagnosis, she was dentate. The 26 remaining teeth present with multiple restorations and prosthetic replacement of 2 missing teeth. Jane has been on a periodontal maintenance therapy (3-month recall visits) for a number of years.

A comprehensive oral examination including a full mouth radiographic evaluation was completed (**Fig. 2**). An oral health care plan[9,10] for preprocedure therapy and posttreatment preventative oral health management was created for Jane based on the examination findings and her high risk for developing oral complications after chemotherapy and radiation treatment (**Box 1**).

The plan was presented to Jane and shared with her adult son. Jane understood and consented to the preprocedure and posttreatment oral care treatment plan. Copies of this plan were shared electronically with Jane's oncologist and the oral surgeon who would be extracting the 3 teeth identified as having a poor long-term prognosis. The oncologist acknowledged receiving the oral health care plan from Jane's dentist and noted its comprehensiveness.

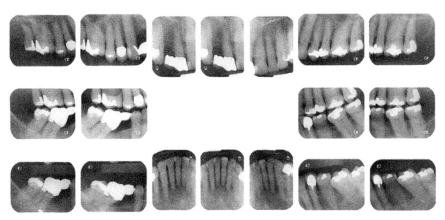

Fig. 2. Jane Doe before cancer treatment, full mouth radiographs. Shaded and light solid areas represent existing restorations with solid dark shaded areas showing carious lesions.

Box 1
Oral health care plan for Jane Doe

1. Initial scaling and prophylaxis in conjunction with oral hygiene instructions for patient and caregivers (to be repeated and reinforced at each subsequent patient encounter):
   a. Written and demonstrated use of a soft toothbrush; and
   b. Daily use of fluoride toothpaste and rinse.

2. Prescribe:
   a. Chlorohexidine mouth rinse, alcohol-free, twice daily rinse and expectorate daily, for 14 days; and
   b. Fluoride toothpaste and/or gel.

3. Referral to oral surgeon for the extraction of teeth numbers 2, 15, and 30.

4. Four quadrants of periodontal root planning and scaling.

5. Restorative treatment for teeth numbers 18 and 20.

6. Maintenance therapy in the dental office:
   a. Two-month recalls during and following cancer treatment;
   b. Alternate use of fluoride and chlorohexidine varnish; and
   c. Support patient and medical team with mucositis relief as needed.

7. Hyposalivation support:
   a. Prescription mouth rinse for the relief of mucositis and mouth sores.
   b. Continue prescription strength fluoride at home.
   c. Continue 2-month hygiene recall schedule.
   d. Use of xylitol-containing mints.
   e. Artificial saliva for daily use.
   f. Increase home and bedroom humidity.
   g. Consult with medical team concerning use of parasympathetic agonist medication.

Data from Little JW, Falace DA, Miller CS, et al. Cancer and oral care of the patient, in dental management of the medically compromised patient. Chapter 26. 7th edition. St Louis (MO): Elsevier; 2008. p. 433–61; and Jansma J, Vissink A, Spijkervet FK, et al. Protocol for the prevention and treatment of oral sequelae resulting from head and neck radiation therapy. Cancer 1992;70(8):2171–80.

After periodontal maintenance, oral surgery, and restorative procedures, custom fluoride trays were constructed for home use. Before the commencement of Jane's cancer treatment, the posttreatment portion of the oral health care plan was again presented to her, with careful explanation of each detail, stressing the importance of meticulous oral hygiene and plaque control, nutrition, hydration, and 2-month recall visits with the dental team. Jane did mention that she was now dependent on her son and daughter to bring her to all of her appointments.

An automated 2-month reminder was established using the dental offices' electronic health record and management system. Office staff meetings identified the office manager and hygienist as key individuals to coordinate the aggressive preventive schedule for Jane.

In the 12 months that have passed since the last pretreatment visit at the dental office, Jane failed to respond to any mail or telephone call/voice mail reminder to comply with the recall schedule. Contact was made with her son and daughter, but failed to get Jane to the office for recall.

Thirteen months after cancer treatment, Jane presented to the dental office with no chief complaint other than the need to get her teeth checked. During the patient interview, Jane discussed her cancer therapy complications. She had a "terrible" time with sores in the oral cavity, taste, and swallowing during and immediately after the chemotherapy and radiation treatment. She also could not get herself to come to the dentist during this time, partly owing to concern about imposing on her son and daughter, who shared time caring for her. When questioned about her oral care prevention plan and the use of fluoride, she denied ever having received the prevention plan and prescriptions. She then described the dysphagia as the most difficult complication after the cancer treatment. She found using maple syrup with every meal and snack as the only means to swallow. She stated that the oncology team nurses encouraged her to continue to use the syrup because it helped her to gain weight and receive some nutritional benefit.

A comprehensive oral evaluation and full series radiographic examination were then completed with the following results:

- No observable structural or dysmorphic alterations.
- Hyposalivation, with the absence of any observable saliva.
- Moderate plaque accumulation.
- Generalized marginal gingivitis.
- Rampant dental decay (**Fig. 3**).

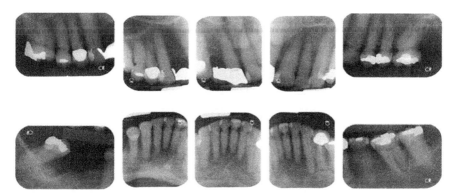

Fig. 3. After treatment: full mouth radiographs for Jane Doe with rampant caries visible as dark areas on teeth.

Treatment of the rampant postchemotherapy and radiation caries (tooth decay) became another adverse sequala of the cancer therapy and the nonimplementation of the oral health care plan. The prognosis for the patient's oral health remains guarded, with added morbidity and quality-of-life issues from the need for extensive restorative care and dental extractions, with the increased risk for osteoradionecrosis.[11]

LESSONS LEARNED FROM CASE STUDY 2

The incidence of oral cavity squamous cell carcinoma and OPSCC increases in all races with advancing age, often occurring in the geriatric population, and peaks between ages 60 and 70.[12] The diagnosis and treatment of OPSCC is commonly overseen by a medical oncologist, but typically requires the collaboration of a number of health care providers that can include the patient's PCP, an oral surgeon or head and neck surgeon, radiation oncologist, plastic surgeon, dentist, dietitian, psychologist, rehabilitation specialist, and speech therapist.[9]

From the oral health outcomes reported in this case study, missing members of the care team could be identified, whose inclusion in the care of this patient could help ameliorate potential adverse side effect of cancer therapy[10] (**Table 3**). These team members include:

- Nutritionist: Advise patient, patient's family, and medical team on proper nutritional support;
- Geriatric physician: Add medical evaluation and assessment of patient's ability to care for herself;
- Geriatric psychologist: Contribute cognitive and psychological assessment;
- Home health nurse: Provide treatment, education, and emotional support; and
- Social worker: Assess and coordinate social support.

Reaching out to the oncologist from the dental office to discuss the patient's missed visits may have helped. If the oncologist had known that the patient was not following the oral health plan, reinforcement of the importance of doing so could occur with not only the patient, but her children during one of the follow-up oncology visits.

The patient missed multiple dental appointments during cancer treatment, even though reminders were sent to the patient and her family members. Could the dental

Table 3 Cancer treatment adverse side effects: what the oncologist, dentist, and patient should know	
Potential Adverse Side Effects	Proactive Dental Treatment
Xerostomia and/or salivary gland hypofunction	Educate patient about the importance of hydrating the mouth with non–sugar-containing candies and drinks. Educate patient and caregivers about oral hygiene practices. Prescription-strength daily fluoride applications, can include rinse, toothpaste and/or custom mouth trays. Recommend follow-up dental and hygiene visits at least every 3 months during cancer treatment.
Osteoradionecrosis	Extract teeth with poor prognosis before radiation and chemotherapy.
Dysphagia	Low or no-sugar drinks to help in swallowing. Consult speech pathologist for additional strategies.

Adapted from Jansma J, Vissink A, Spijkervet FK, et al. Protocol for the prevention and treatment of oral sequelae resulting from head and neck radiation therapy. Cancer 1992;70(8):2172.

team have offered to make a home care visit to assess the oral health when they see multiple missed appointments?

Include the patient's family in the discussions regarding oral hygiene and the necessity for the patient to be monitored closely in the dental office during cancer treatment. Medical and dental team members can follow-up with patients undergoing cancer treatment. Yet, it is the caregivers who assist and reinforce the importance of maintaining oral hygiene during the months of treatment.

The medical and dental team members had the perception that their care plan and actions were adequate to meet the oral health needs of this patient. To avoid outcomes like this, dentists can use their knowledge to educate the oncology and radiation team members about the importance of daily oral hygiene, good nutrition and regular dental visits for patients during cancer treatment.

THE IDEAL GENERALIZABLE COLLABORATION OF HEALTH CARE PROVIDERS

Today people are living longer and maintaining their natural teeth into their later years. Ideally, medical and dental providers would work together as part of an interdisciplinary team to best help older adult patients maintain their oral health. Patients' ongoing oral health care can be improved through updates about the patients' cognitive, physical, and emotional status and suggestions from primary health care providers and family members. To achieve this integration of knowledge and skills, the ideal collaboration includes frequent and on-going communication between the team members. Strategies that may prove useful include:

- Recognize the need for direct communication and intentional collaborative action by the separate health care providers.[13]
- Consider implementing common electronic medical–dental records.
- Use modern communication technology, such as Skype, for team discussion about a patient's care plan, including oral health issues.
- Training health care providers to write effective referrals, discuss cases and write treatment plans that include both dental and medical care can be aided by the use of electronic health education material like Oral Health Nursing Education and Practice or the *Oral Adherence Tool Kit* and *Smiles for Life*.[14–16]

SUMMARY

The challenges for health care teams addressing oral health in patients undergoing treatment for OSCC and OPSCC are similar to those in treating geriatric patients. Creating a culture of collaboration between separate health care providers and the patient's social support systems will help ensure better patient-centered care with consistent outcomes for all patients. Oral health care providers need to forge relationships with other professions to expand their knowledge and skills to meet the needs of geriatric patients.

REFERENCES

1. Recommendations for using fluoride to prevent and control dental caries in the United States. Centers for Disease Control and Prevention. MMWR Recomm Rep 2001;50(RR-14):1–42.
2. US Department of Health and Human Services. Healthy People 2020 Oral Health Topics and Objectives. Available at: www.healthypeople.gov/2020/topics-objectives/topic/oral-health. Accessed March 11, 2016.

3. Dolce M, Aghazedeh-Sanai N, Mohammed S, et al. Integrating oral health into the interdisciplinary health sciences curriculum. Dent Clin North Am 2014;58:829–43.
4. Barker K, Oandasan I. Interprofessional care review with medical residents: lessons learned, tensions aired a pilot study. J Interprof Care 2005;19(3):207–14.
5. Kaufman LB, Setiono TK, Doros G, et al. An oral health study of centenarians and children of centenarians. J Am Geriatr Soc 2014;62(6):1168–73.
6. IOM (Institute of Medicine). Advancing oral health in America. Washington, DC: The National Academies Press; 2011.
7. Interprofessional Education Collaborative Expert Panel. Core competencies for interprofessional collaborative practice: report of an expert panel. Washington, DC: Interprofessional Education Collaborative; 2011.
8. Robertson RG, Montagnini M. Geriatric failure to thrive. Am Fam Physician 2004; 70(2):343–50.
9. Little JW, Falace DA, Miller CS, et al. Cancer and oral care of the patient, in dental management of the medically compromised patient. Chapter 26. 7th edition. St Louis (MO): Elsevier; 2008. p. 433–61.
10. Jansma J, Vissink A, Spijkervet FK, et al. Protocol for the prevention and treatment of oral sequelae resulting from head and neck radiation therapy. Cancer 1992;70(8):2171–80.
11. Reuther T, Schuster T, Mende U, et al. Osteoradionecrosis of the jaws as a side effect of radiotherapy of head and neck tumour patients: a report of a thirty year retrospective review. Int J Oral Maxillofac Surg 2003;32(3):289–95.
12. Surveillance, epidemiology, and end results (SEER) cancer statistics factsheets: oral cavity and pharynx cancer. Bethesda (MD): National Cancer Institute; 2008. Available at: http://seer.cancer.gov/statfacts/html/oralcav.html. Accessed November 18, 2015.
13. Brown BP. Meeting IPEC core competencies through a dentistry nursing partnership [Abstract]. J Dent Educ 2016;80(2):229.
14. Oral health care: begin with a class act. Oral Health Nursing Education and Practice (OHNEP) Website. Available at: http://ohnep.org/oral-health-care-begin-class-act. Accessed January 28, 2016.
15. Oncology Nursing Society. Tools for oral adherence toolkit. 2009. Available at: www.ons.org/sites/default/files/oral%20adherence%20toolkit.pdf. Accessed December 17, 2015.
16. Wells M, Swartzman S, Lang H, et al. Predictors of quality of life in head and neck cancer survivors up to 5 years after end of treatment: a cross-sectional survey. Support Care Cancer 2016;24(6):2463–72.

Addressing Health Disparities via Coordination of Care and Interprofessional Education

Lesbian, Gay, Bisexual, and Transgender Health and Oral Health Care

Stefanie Russell, DDS, MPH, PhD*, Frederick More, DDS, MS

KEYWORDS

- Interprofessional relations • Sexual behavior • Oral health • Health status disparities
- Health care disparities • Homosexuality • Transgender persons • Gender identity

KEY POINTS

- Lesbian, gay, bisexual, and transgender (LGBT) people share a common need for competent, accessible health care, dispensed without intolerance, and with an understanding of the unique but diverse health needs of the members of this group.
- Dental practitioners should recognize that, as a group, LGBT persons face greater health risks and have different health needs than heterosexual persons.
- However, data are sparse in the dental literature regarding the oral health needs of members of the LGBT community. Dental practitioners can learn much from their medical and nursing colleagues regarding the provision of culturally competent care for LGBT persons. It is likely that the best care for this group can only be achieved through interprofessional care among dental, medical, nursing, and other health care practitioners.

INTRODUCTION

LGBT stands for lesbian, gay, bisexual, and transgender. Some add the letter Q to LGBT, meaning either queer or questioning, and still others add the letters I and A for intersex and asexual, respectively. Members of this group (LGBT, LGBTQ, LGBTQIA) are also sometimes grouped together as sexual minorities. LGBT persons are a diverse group, but they share a common need for competent, accessible health

Department of Epidemiology & Health Promotion, NYU College of Dentistry, 433 First Avenue, 7th Floor, New York, NY 10010, USA
* Corresponding author.
E-mail address: stefanie.russell@nyu.edu

Dent Clin N Am 60 (2016) 891–906
http://dx.doi.org/10.1016/j.cden.2016.05.006
0011-8532/16/© 2016 Elsevier Inc. All rights reserved.

care, dispensed without intolerance, and with an understanding of the unique health needs of the members of this group. Dental practitioners, like other medical providers, need to recognize the heterogeneity of this group, and understand that, as a group, LGBT persons face greater health risks than heterosexual persons, largely because of how they are often regarded by society in general and by some health care workers.[1]

However, within the last several years, great progress in the acceptance of LGBT persons has occurred, as shown by the support of most Americans for same-sex unions, culminating in the Supreme Court's 2015 ruling that the 14th Amendment does not allow states to ban same-sex marriage[2]; however, many people argue that social gains (and the health care gains that are likely to follow) for LGBT people have not occurred equally for each LGBT subgroup. For example, bisexual men and women report worse health than gay men and lesbians, which may be partially attributable to their heightened economic, behavioral, and social disadvantages.[3] It has been also reported that lesbian and bisexual women, for example, may be less likely than gay men to adhere to some cancer-screening guidelines.[4] In addition, it should be recognized that within the LGBT group profound differences are evident with respect to race, ethnicity, and gender.[5] For example, LGBT women are more likely to experience stigma and discrimination than their male LGBT counterparts, which can make health care more costly for them because of discriminatory laws, discrimination by providers, insurance exclusions for transgender people, and inadequate reproductive health coverage.[6] In addition, LGBT persons of color are more likely to be poor than their white LGBT counterparts.[5,7]

Over the past 2 decades the medical and nursing academic communities have begun to address disparities in LGBT health by recognizing that more attention needs to be paid to understanding the health of those persons who comprise this vulnerable group.[5,8,9] An increasing number of studies investigating disparities in health and disease, and in those demographic, social, behavioral, and other factors related to these disparities, have been reported, and the literature has grown.[5] Physicians and nurses have recognized that reducing disparities also requires coordination of care and of education among providers and trainees, and have introduced curricula that respond to this need.[10–12]

Although some oral health care practitioners and academics have documented similar issues, the dental literature is less robust, and is limited to a few studies of attitudes and behaviors.[13–16] The oral health community, therefore, may learn from what medicine and nursing has already discovered; namely, that this population deserves special attention, given their increased risk for disease, and, more importantly, that through a coordinated effort of care and training, disparities in health (which are likely to extend to oral health) for this group can be minimized and/or eradicated.

The purposes of this article are:

1. To review the literature on oral health and overall health of LGBT persons in the United States and Canada, including data related to clinical findings and health care use.
2. To discuss ways in which dentists can improve the health care they provide to this vulnerable population, including how interprofessional education and collaborative practice may help to reduce oral health disparities within this group.

LESBIAN, GAY, BISEXUAL, TRANSGENDER: WHAT'S IN A NAME?

When speaking of, to, or about persons in the LGBT community there are several terms that dental practitioners should be aware of. In addition, practitioners must realize that although the acronym LGBT may be useful as an umbrella term (ie, the general and oral health needs of this community are often grouped together), each of these letters represents a specific, separate population with its own health issues. Importantly, clinicians need to recognize that this group is extremely diverse, comprising both those who identify or present as genders different from the sex assigned to them at birth (those with varying gender identities and gender expressions) and those whose sexual orientation is not solely heterosexual.

The LGBT community comprises groups defined by *sexual orientation:* including *lesbians* (women who are attracted to women), *gays* (men who are attracted to men, or persons attracted to those of the same gender, in general), *bisexual* persons (those men and women who are attracted to both men and women) and *asexual* persons (those who generally do not feeling sexual attraction) *and by gender identity*, including *transgender* (a person who crosses culturally-defined gender categories) and *intersex* (those who naturally have sex characteristics that do not fit neatly into society's definitions of male or female).[5,9,17] The term *queer* includes anyone who chooses to identify as such, while the term *questioning* refers to anyone exploring his or her own gender identity or expression, and/or sexual orientation.[17] An additional term, *gender queer*, refers to having a gender identity and/or expression that is outside of the societal norm and/or is beyond gender.[17]

Sex and Gender

In addition, clinicians should distinguish between the terms *sex* (which refers to a person's biological status including hormonal, anatomic, and physiologic characteristics; most commonly male and female) and *gender*, which is a social construct that includes the "attitudes, feelings, and behaviors that a given culture associates with a person's biological sex."[18] Clinicians should recognize that sex can be ambiguous; for example, in someone who is born with both male and female physical traits or with ambiguous genitalia (historically, these intersex children were usually assigned the sex of female because of the greater ease and effectiveness of genital surgery).[19] However, studies have shown that the historical approach to gender assignment surgery that was common in the second half of the twentieth century resulted in high rates of mental and sometimes physical health issues.[20–22]

Gender Identity

Gender identity refers to how a person identifies - as male or female, or another gender (including *transgender*, *bigender*, or *gender queer*; denunciations of the traditional classification of gender as binary).[5] *Gender identity* is linked with the term *gender expression*, which denotes how a person chooses to appear to the world and includes not only one's physical appearance, but one's personality and behavior.[5] *Gender role conformity* refers to the extent to which an individual's gender expression adheres to the cultural norms prescribed for people of his or her sex;[5] for example, a gender non-conforming woman may choose to dress and appear in clothes typically associated with men or a gender non-conforming man may choose clothing or makeup that may appear feminine though he makes no effort to hide his maleness. The term *cisgender* designates a person whose (biologic) sex, gender identity and gender expression are consistent.[5] For example, a "cis male" is a man whose biologic gender is male, he identifies as male, and he appears to the world as a male. In today's world, there are people who consider themselves *gender fluid*. That is, they resist being labeled as either "male" or "female" and may move between being male or female at different points in time.[5] *Gender dysphoria* is an uneasiness, discomfort or outright distress with one's assigned sex.[5]

Transgender

The term *transgender* is a catchall term that includes a diverse group of individuals who cross or transcend culturally defined categories of gender. Descriptive terms include *transsexual* (those who often have had, or desire, hormone therapy and/or surgery so that may live full time as a gender different from the one they were assigned to at birth); *cross-dressing* (those who present outwardly a gender different from the one they were assigned to at birth for emotional and/or sexual gratification); *transgenderists* (those who live full time in the cross-gender role, may take hormones, but do not desire surgery); *bigender* persons (who identify as both male and female); and *drag queens* and *kings* (who dress in clothes associated with the other gender usually adopting an ultra-feminine or masculine persona).[5] While the term *transgender* has received much attention lately as transgender men and women have become more visible (for example, note Bruce Jenner's very public transition to Caitlyn Jenner in 2015), this term has been around for decades, particularly in literature and film. For example, Armisted Maupin's series of popular novels,[23] which were later turned into a *Public Broadcasting System* miniseries (1993) and a theatre production, featured a transgender woman character (played by Olympia Dukakis in the television series). Hillary Swank won a "Best Actress Oscar in 1999 for her portrayal of Brandon Teena, a transgender man who was raped and murdered. Other movies, such as "Transamerica" (2006) introduced Americans to transgender people and the challenges they face. Despite their ubiquity in literature, film and in the real world, transgender persons among those who are most often the victims of the most violent hate crimes.[24] Presently, only 18 states and the District of Columbia have passed laws protecting people against discrimination based on gender expression and/or gender identity.[25] Increasingly, transgender people are finding more support in the medical and mental health professions as they "transition" to their chosen gender, which typically requires the use of hormonal therapy, plastic surgery and in some cases, gender reassignment surgery. In addition, many states and cities now support changing birth certificates and other forms of identification, although some states require medical "proof of sterilization" by sex reassignment surgery in order to warrant a gender change.

Sexual Orientation

Sexual orientation is defined by a person' preference in partners in intimate human relationship (romantic, sexual, or both; actualized or only imagined) in relation to the person's own sex/gender.[5] Persons traditionally may identify as *heterosexual* (straight or hetero), *gay*, or *bisexual*, although contemporary designations allow for divisions that are more encompassing. A self-described straight man or woman may have or have had same-sex relationships in the past or occasionally in the present but not consider himself/herself as gay. Similarly, a self-described gay person may have or have had opposite-sex relationships. Still more complicated are persons who engage in same-sex relationships without any qualifiers. More accurate assessment may include exclusively gay, mostly gay, mostly straight, or exclusively straight.

Health practitioners may be interested in knowing a patient's sexual orientation and current sexual activity to assess risk for disease, including sexually transmitted diseases. Dentists and dental hygienists specifically need to know each patient's sexual history so they can recognize any increased risk for those conditions and diseases that have oral sequelae, most notably human immunodeficiency virus (HIV) and human papilloma virus (HPV) infection, in order to assess each patient's risk for HPV-related head and neck cancer and other conditions, to assess the potential benefits of HPV vaccination, and to perform ongoing risk assessments.

What is of practical, essential importance is that health care professionals like dentists need to be both sensitive to and knowledgeable about issues of sexual orientation, gender identity, and gender expression. However, judging someone's gender using their appearance can be misleading, offensive to the person, or even dangerous for a health care provider. For example, a transgender woman may dress and appear female even though she was assigned the male sex at birth: missing this reality might lead the dentist to overlook that she is taking large doses of steroids on a daily basis. Another example is the physically fit, masculine-appearing young man with well-trimmed facial hair who may have been born female and is taking hormones to transition. In addition, for a gender-fluid person, identifying as male or female on the intake form may become a barrier to effective communication. Later in this article ways to improve the office experience for those in the LGBT community are discussed; briefly, approaches include revising the office or clinic intake form to allow persons to select from at least 3 gender options (male, female, other) is a simple way to show the intention to be inclusive. Another option is to have all restrooms in the practice or selected restrooms in the building be gender-neutral (ie, without a male/female label on the door) to increase comfort and show inclusivity. In terms of using the proper, preferred language and terminology, practitioners should realize there are some words and terms that must be avoided, because they are considered outdated, derogatory, and/or bigoted. These terms include *hermaphrodite*, *sexual preference* or *sexual identity* (as opposed to the correct terms *sexual orientation* and *gender identity*), *sex change*, *sex change operation*, *preoperative* or *post-operative* (as opposed to the correct term *transitioning*) and, of course, epithets.[26] In addition, some in the LGBT community have expressed dismay at the words *transvestite* (proper term: *cross-dressing*), *homosexual* (proper terms: *gay* or *lesbian*), *alternative* (seen as overused and non-specific) and *tolerance* (believing that LGBT persons should be more than "tolerated").

NORTH AMERICAN LESBIAN, GAY, BISEXUAL, AND TRANSGENDER POPULATION ESTIMATES

Estimating the number of people in the various categories in the population is an important, albeit difficult, undertaking that has been fraught with issues making estimates unreliable. The recent Institute of Medicine report *The Health of Lesbian, Gay, Bisexual, and Transgender People: Building a Foundation for Better Understanding*[5] reviews the US surveys that have provided population-based estimates, including (1) a 1992 survey in which about 2.8% of the men and 1.4% of the women more than 18 years of age considered themselves homosexual or bisexual; (2) a 2002 US Centers for Disease Control and Prevention survey of adults aged 18 to 44 years that found 2.3% of men identifying themselves as homosexual 1.8% as bisexual, and 1.3% of women identifying themselves as homosexual and 2.8% as bisexual; (3) a 2008 study that found that 2.2% of men identified as gay and 0.7% as bisexual, whereas 2.7% of women identified as lesbian and 1.9% as bisexual; and (4) a 2009 study that estimated that 6.8% of men and 4.5% of women self-identified as lesbian, gay, or bisexual.[5] However, there are no good, recent estimates on the proportion of transgender persons in the United States. Results of the Massachusetts Behavioral Risk Factor Surveillance Survey, one of the few population-based surveys that included a question designed to identify the transgender population, found that 0.5% of adults (aged 18–64 years) in the state identified as transgender in 2007 and 2009.[27] In Canada, 1.7% of adults aged 18 to 59 years reported being gay or lesbian and 1.3% reported being bisexual in 2014.[28]

GENERAL HEALTH AMONG LESBIAN, GAY, BISEXUAL, AND TRANSGENDER PERSONS
General Health

Although LGBT persons as a group have been shown to be disproportionally affected by several health conditions, including chronic disease, sexually transmitted infections, mental disorders, and injury/violence (including intimate partner violence),[27] disease rates and related conditions vary by subgroup. Although in some cases these health disparities are related to an increased tendency among some within this group for high-risk activities (eg, HIV infection among gay men), in other cases these conditions are related to the long-standing discrimination and social stigma that LGBT persons continue to face. Discrimination may affect a person's income and employment, and is therefore related to whether the person can obtain and keep health insurance. In addition, social stigma is related to poor mental health and poor coping skills, including risky sexual behaviors and substance abuse.[9] Not being able to be open about sexual orientation and/or gender identity likely increases stress and limits social support; both of these negatively affect health.[29] Understandably, health-related risky behaviors and poorer health are more common among those LGBT people who have experienced the most discrimination; one study of young adults rejected by their own families showed that this group was 8.4 times more likely to have made attempts at suicide, 5.9 times more likely to report high levels of depression, 3.4 times more likely to use illegal drugs, and 3.4 times more likely to have risky sex.[30] Importantly, sexual orientation and gender identity have been shown to interact with other recognized risk factors for poor health, including socioeconomic status, race, and ethnicity.[6,31] In addition, in these rapidly changing times, groups that might have been at a disadvantage in the past may now no longer be subjected to the same level of discrimination because public attitudes have changed.[32] For example, a recent study showed that self-reported poor health was no worse (and possibly better) among gay men and lesbians compared with heterosexual men and women.[6] Because of the heterogeneity of the LGBT group, we will separately discuss the general health of each of the major sexual minority groups: gay men, lesbians, bisexual persons, and transgender persons separately.

Gay Men

Gay men, as a group, are at higher risk of sexually transmitted diseases compared with heterosexual men. HIV infection continues to be a major issue affecting gay and bisexual men. Between 2009 and 2013, the HIV infection rate increased by 12% in this group; most alarmingly increasing by 22% among those aged 13 to 24 years.[33] Black and Hispanic gay and bisexual men were disproportionally represented in this group: in 2010, black men accounted for 10,600 (36%) and Hispanic/Latino men accounted for 6700 (22%) of all estimated new HIV infections. In addition, HPV[34,35] and hepatitis infections are also more common in gay men compared with heterosexual men.[36] Gay men also seem to be at increased risk for some cancers. Although most research has focused on the increased incidence of those cancers associated with sexually transmitted viruses, recent studies have shown that gay men have increased risk for skin cancer[37] because of a disparity in sun and tanning bed use between gay and heterosexual men; and for lung cancer, because gay men have higher rates of tobacco use.[38] Gay men, as well as bisexual men, have higher rates of anal cancer (which is associated with HPV infection),[39] Kaposi sarcoma (which is associated with herpes virus type 8 and HIV infections),[39] and non-Hodgkin lymphoma and hepatocellular carcinomas (which are associated with hepatitis B and C infections)[38] compared with heterosexual men. Studies have shown that gay men have higher rates of depression and anxiety compared with heterosexual men.[40] Some studies have shown that gay men are more likely to smoke and use illicit drugs compared with heterosexual men.[27]

Lesbians

As a group, lesbians are more likely to be overweight or obese compared with heterosexual women, and are therefore at higher risk for obesity-associated conditions, including diabetes, cardiovascular disease and stroke, and breast and colon cancer.[41] Lesbians are less likely than heterosexual women to have had a full-term pregnancy, placing them at higher risk for those cancers that are reduced in women who have been pregnant and have breastfed, including breast, endometrial, and ovarian cancers. It has also been reported that lesbians have higher rates of arthritis compared with heterosexual women.[36] Lesbians are more likely to smoke than heterosexual women,[27] increasing their risk for lung cancer and other smoking-related diseases. Although recent data suggest that alcohol use among lesbians has decreased, heavy drinking and drug abuse (eg, moderate marijuana use) have been reported to be more common among lesbians than heterosexual women,[27] especially among younger women. Regarding mental health, lesbians report higher rates of depression and anxiety compared to heterosexual women. Lesbians may use preventive health care services less frequently than heterosexual women, and are less likely to receive routine screenings, such as a Pap tests, clinical breast examinations, and mammograms.[6]

Bisexuals

Several population-based studies have shown that bisexual persons have overall worse health than heterosexuals, gays, and lesbians.[27] Bisexuals are more likely to be poor and are more likely to be unemployed.[27] Bisexual persons have some of the highest rates of disease-related risk behaviors, including smoking and substance abuse disorders.[42,43] However, within the bisexual population, risks tend to vary by sex/gender and, as is the case for gay men, lesbians, and transgender persons, by other demographic characteristics, including race/ethnicity and socioeconomic status. Like gay men, bisexual men are at increased risk for HIV and HPV infection,[34] and for other sexually transmitted diseases. Bisexual men have been found to have higher hepatitis rates compared with heterosexual men.[36] Bisexual women are more likely to report higher-risk sexual behaviors, smoking, substance abuse, and binge drinking than other groups.[27,42] Like lesbians, bisexual women are at increased risk for those cancers related to being nulliparous. Studies have shown that mental health issues, including increased worry and anxiety, depression, suicide ideation, and emotional stress, are more prevalent in the bisexual population compared with either the gay/lesbian or heterosexual communities.[27,44]

Transgender Persons

Information regarding transgender health is limited, and the data that are available come from small studies of convenience samples; for example, those persons attending clinics, rather than population-based samples.[44,45] In general, the specific health concerns of female-to-male transgender persons are less well understood than those for male-to-female persons.[9] Transgender persons have unique health needs; some of these needs depend on whether they choose to take hormones and/or undergo surgery. Estrogen-progestin hormones are associated with thrombo-embolic disease, and testosterone has been associated with an increase in liver enzyme levels, loss of bone mineral density, and increased risk for ovarian cancer. However, although the risk for these diseases is likely increased in transgender persons taking these hormones, few studies have evaluated the long-term effects of these hormones in transgender persons. One unique health issue among transgender persons is the problems that are related to a sex/gender identity mismatch.[4] For example, a woman who identifies as male but retains female reproductive organs may avoid having cervical cancer screenings and pelvic examinations. Information regarding the prevalence of mental disorders in transgender persons is also lacking, because no population-based data are available. However, studies have shown that suicide ideation and suicide attempts are common within the transgender population.[44] It has been estimated that between 16% and 60% of transgender persons have experienced physical violence and that 13% to 66% have experienced sexual assault; racial and ethnic minority transgender women are at the highest risk. Although the exact prevalence of HIV infection among transgender persons is not known, one study found that HIV prevalence among a group of transgender women in 12 cities varied between 5% and 68%, and was higher among black and Hispanic transgender women. Studies estimate that between 45% and 74% of transgender persons smoke; alcohol use is also high. In addition, drug use, including marijuana, crack cocaine, methamphetamines, and injection drug use, seems to be common among transgender persons.

Health Care Access and Use

LGBT persons are less likely to have access to appropriate and necessary medical care,[46] including preventive care; are less likely to have health insurance; and are less likely to use some medical care. Many within the LGBT community struggle to access health care because they are uninsured.[9] In the United States, same-sex marriage was not universally recognized before 2015; therefore, access to a partner's health benefits was limited to those (few, but increasing) states that recognized same-sex marriage.[47] Lesbians and bisexuals are less likely to have health insurance compared with both heterosexuals and gay men and lesbians.[9,27] Transgender persons are least likely to have insurance, and health insurance that covers appropriate care for transgender patients is lacking.[9] Lesbians and bisexuals are less likely to have a regular health care provider compared with both heterosexuals and gay men and lesbians.[27] Transgender persons report barriers to their use of preventive services[48] and are most likely to report having trouble finding health care providers who are knowledgeable about their unique health issues.[4] Finding a provider who is competent in LGBT health has also been a problem for lesbians, gays, and bisexuals.[46] A recent study found that heterosexual providers implicitly and explicitly favor heterosexual patients rather than LGBT patients.[1]

MEDICAL AND NURSING APPROACHES TO ADDRESSING DISPARITIES

A dilemma that is common to all health disciplines is a lack of data. Demographic surveys, collected for years in health education programs, by faculty, and by practitioners, do not generally include data on sexuality, or provide options for gender identity beyond male/female. Electronic health records do not include expanded designations for gender, ask for preferred pronouns, or include opportunities for patients to define alternative family patterns. In addition, curricula in the health professions do not include meaningful information about LGBT and LGBT health. A 2011 survey of medical deans[10] showed a wide variation of time and curriculum topic areas that included information about LGBT/LGBT health. Of the 132 medical schools surveyed, the average amount of time in the curriculum was 5 clock hours. Fifty-five percent of schools used written examinations to evaluate knowledge, 35% included standardized patients, 31% used faculty-observations and patient interactions, and 29% did not evaluate teaching of LGBT topics. To our knowledge, no such survey concerning coverage of LGBT issues has been performed or published in dentistry.

In 2013, the Health Resources Services Administration published *LGBT Training Curricula for Behavioral Health and Primary Care Practitioners*.[49] Nursing seems to have recognized the need for nursing education to address LGBT health. Recommendations for nursing education include the creation of culturally sensitive nursing care plans for LGBT patients, clinical placements of students in diverse settings, and increasing access to LGBT interest groups.[11] In addition, the Association of American Medical Colleges (AAMC) released a comprehensive document: *Implementing Curricular and institutional Climate Changes to Improve Health Care for Individuals Who Are LGBT, Gender Nonconforming, or Born with DSD*.[50] The AAMC document provides an excellent bridge to knowledge, curriculum opportunity, and steps toward institutional climate change. The result is to provide insights and make progress toward meeting the unmet needs of LGBT persons.

The Gay Lesbian Medical Association (GLMA) has been a visible force in medicine. The American Medical Association included GLMA as a component in 2000. Over its 30 years of existence, the GLMA has been a strong advocate for LGBT health with efforts such as white papers, companion paper on LGBT health for Healthy People 2020, and support for LGBT advocacy in other professions such as nursing, physician's assistants, and pharmacy. Along with the Institute of Medicine report,[5] the resources provided by the GLMA are likely to be useful to dental practitioners and educators seeking information.

RECOMMENDATIONS FOR DENTISTRY

The first article in the dental literature that addressed LGBT issues appeared in 2004.[13] Since then, the few articles that have explored this area reinforce the observation that dental school diversity programs are not inclusive of LGBT[14] persons and that students are unprepared to meet the needs of LGBT patients.[15] However, dentistry lags behind medicine and nursing regarding recognition of this area, and has not yet worked to gather data, does not have a profile of LGBT persons with regard to clinical practice or dental education, and does not offer guidelines for curricula for US dental education institutions.

In an effort to provide guidance on these issues, we have compiled a list of recommendations is presented in **Box 1** and resources that are available are listed in **Table 1**, largely from organizations that advocate for LGBT health but also from the medical and nursing fields. We recognize that there are some local clinics designed to meet the oral health care needs of those in the LGBT community and have provided information on those organizations, believing that these clinics might serve as a model for the appropriate delivery of care for LGBT persons. We urge oral health researchers, educators, and practitioners to recognize the unique needs of this population and to recognize the diversity within this group, and appeal to those in the dental community to follow the lead of our medical and nursing colleagues.

Box 1
Suggestions for oral health clinicians, educators, and researchers to improve LGBT oral health care

Suggestions for clinicians[51]

- Become educated about the specific health issues facing LGBT people, and be knowledgeable about the recommended standards of practice for LGBT patients, such as those found at http://www.glbthealth.org/CommunityStandardsofPractice.htm.
- List your practice in the GLMA directory as an LGBT-friendly office.
- Be sensitive: make sure you and your office staff know which pronouns to use when referring to a transgender patient or same-sex couple.
- Displaying an LGBT-friendly sign (Human Rights Campaign equal sign or rainbow flag) that shows your office is a welcoming, safe space for everyone.
- Make sure your medical history and other data forms allow for male/female/transgender and use neutral terms like "partner" or "spouse" rather than "single," "married," or "divorced." Use "parent 1" and "parent 2" to include same-sex couples raising children. See the sample form in **Table 1**: Resources.
- Avoid making assumptions about patients based on their appearance.
- When taking a sexual history, ask, "Are your current or past sexual partner's men, women, or both?"
- Listen attentively. Be sensitive to the fact that this disclosure may be difficult for your patients.

Suggestions for educators[52]

- Recognize the role of dental education in eliminating LGBT oral health disparities.
- Educate students and faculty regarding the specific health issues facing LGBT people.
- Provide education about the health needs of individuals who are LGBT, gender nonconforming, and/or born with DSD, and the role of academic dentistry and the oral health care system in supporting these populations.
- Create and integrate professional competencies to improve oral health care for LGBT persons.
- Make oral health clinics LGBT friendly (see suggestions for clinicians).
- Use existing frameworks and materials available to the medical and nursing academic communities in order to facilitate teaching and learning.
- Highlight national resources and curricular innovations within academic medicine and nursing.
- Use clinical scenarios and discussion points, including clinical teaching cases and questions for learning.
- Using the AAMC's MedEdPORTAL to Advance Curricular Change introduces MedEdPORTAL as a venue for accessing and sharing curricular materials to enhance teaching about individuals who are or may be LGBT, gender nonconforming, and/or born with DSD.

Suggestions for oral health researchers[53]

- Move toward building a more solid evidence base for LGBT oral health.
- Consider adapting the current research agenda to include collection of data on LGBT populations.
- Design studies to specifically collect data on sexual and gender minorities and document the prevalence of, incidence of, and risk factors for oral disease by subgroup.
- Because it is well known that LGBT individuals face barriers to equitable medical care because of lack of health insurance, fear of discrimination from providers, lack of providers who are

well trained in the health needs of LGBT individuals, and dissatisfaction with services, oral health researchers should investigate whether or not the same is true for oral health care.

- Designing studies that seek to understand the experiences of LGBT individuals seeking oral health care, disparities, provider attitudes and education, and ways in which the care environment could be improved would provide a solid base from which to address these inequities.

- Recognize that the body of evidence assembled to date for LGBT health is sparse, and that most areas have no research or require considerable additional work. Therefore, there are important opportunities to answer many research questions.

Table 1
Resources available for health care providers, educators, and researchers

Title	Description	Location of Resource
General		
Lesbian, Gay, Bisexual, and Transgender Health. Healthy People 2020	Healthy People 2020 site provides information regarding issues and health care goals for LGBT persons	https://www.healthypeople.gov/2020/topics-objectives/topic/lesbian-gay-bisexual-and-transgender-health?topicid=25
The Williams Institute	Dedicated to conducting rigorous, independent research on sexual orientation and gender identity law and public policy, including health care policy	http://williamsinstitute.law.ucla.edu/
Planned Parenthood Out for Health	Provides outreach, education, and information to LGBT persons and their health care providers about the importance of inclusive and respectful care	http://www.outforhealth.org/
Center of Excellence for Transgender Health	Mission is to increase access to comprehensive, effective, and affirming health care services for trans communities	http://transhealth.ucsf.edu/
Practice		
Guidelines for Care of Lesbian, Gay, Bisexual and Transgender Patients. Gay and Lesbian Medical Association	Comprehensive, 60-page document on how to provide sensitive care to the LGBT community	http://www.glma.org/_data/n_0001/resources/live/Welcoming%20Environment.pdf
Sample medical/dental forms. The Fenway Institute	Sample forms for intake, medical history, dental information	http://fenwayhealth.org/documents/patientservices/FenwayClient_Registration_v11.pdf http://fenwayhealth.org/documents/patient-services/Dental_Medical_History_December_2011.pdf

(continued on next page)

Table 1
(continued)

Title	Description	Location of Resource
Coleman E, et al. Standards of care for the health of transsexual, transgender, and gender-nonconforming people, version 7. World Professional Association for Transgender Health. Int J Transgend 2011;13: 165–232	Comprehensive document provides clinical guidelines for health professionals working with transsexual, transgender, and gender-nonconforming people. Best practices for improving physical and mental health	http://www.wpath.org/uploaded_files/140/files/IJT%20SOC,%20V7.pdf
The Fenway Institute	An interdisciplinary center for research, training, education, and policy development, focusing on ensuring access to quality, culturally competent health care for traditionally underserved communities, including LGBT people	http://fenwayhealth.org/the-fenway-institute/
Finding an LGBT-friendly Healthcare Provider. GLMA	Online directory of LGBT-friendly healthcare providers. Allows practitioners to self-identify as LGBT friendly and create a listing	http://www.glma.org/
Transgender Health Resources. GLMA	Resources for health care providers regarding the provision of culturally competent and compassionate health care, education about transgender health issues	http://www.glma.org/index.cfm?fuseaction=Page.viewPage&pageId=948&grandparentID=534&parentID=938&nodeID=1
Ten Things Transgender Persons Should discuss with Their Healthcare Care Provider. GLMA	Provides information on important issues in transgender health	http://www.glma.org/index.cfm?fuseaction=Page.viewPage&pageID=692
Education		
Implementing Curricular and Institutional Climate Changes to Improve Health Care for Individuals Who Are LGBT, Gender Nonconforming, or Born with DSD: A Resource for Medical Educators	Comprehensive report for medical providers and educators to better serve LGBT and gender-nonconforming people and those with differences in sex development	aamc.org

(continued on next page)

Table 1
(continued)

Title	Description	Location of Resource
ADEA Gay-Straight Alliance	A resource for information, advocacy and support for schools, students, faculty, administrators, and staff with a commitment to create more inclusive environments	http://www.adea.org/about_adea/governance/Pages/Gay-StraightAlliance.aspx
Research		
The Health of Lesbian, Gay, Bisexual, and Transgender People Building a Foundation for Better Understanding. Institute of Medicine. March, 2011	At the request of the NIH, the Institute of Medicine evaluated current knowledge of the health status of lesbian, gay, bisexual, and transgender populations; identified research gaps and opportunities; and outlined a research agenda to help NIH focus its research in this area	http://www.nationalacademies.org/hmd/Reports/2011/The-Health-of-Lesbian-Gay-Bisexual-and-Transgender-People.aspx
The Center for Population Research in LGBT Health, the Fenway Institute	Center that supports and stimulates research to fill critical knowledge gaps related to the health of sexual and gender minorities	http://fenwayhealth.org/the-fenway-institute/education/the-center-for-population-research-in-lgbt-health/ http://lgbtpopulationcenter.org/web-resources/#funding
NIH	NIH funding opportunities in LGBT health	http://grants.nih.gov/funding/searchGuide

Abbreviation: NIH, National Institutes of Health.

SUMMARY

It is apparent that LGBT persons have unique but diverse health needs, and that these needs are best addressed only when competent, accessible health care is available. Dental practitioners should recognize that, as a group, LGBT persons face greater health risks and have different health needs than heterosexual persons. Although specific data regarding oral health care and dental needs are sparse, dental practitioners can and need to learn about this vulnerable group in order to address any disparities in oral health that likely mirror those in general health. Working with medical and nursing colleagues to understand the unique needs of this group is an efficient and reasonable way that dentists can provide culturally competent care for LGBT persons.

REFERENCES

1. Sabin JA, Riskind RG, Nosek BA. Health care provider's implicit and explicit attitudes toward lesbian women and gay men. Am J Public Health 2015;105(9): 1831–41.

2. Obergefell et al. v Hodges, Director Ohio Department of Health, et al., 14-556 (2014) Supreme Court of the United States. Available at: https://www.supremecourt.gov/opinions/14pdf/14-556_3204.pdf. Accessed February 25, 2016.

3. Bisexual community. In, Re: searching for LGBTQ Health. Available at: http://lgbtqhealth.ca/community/bisexual.php. Accessed February 25, 2016.

4. Quinn GP, Sanchez JA, Sutton SK, et al. Cancer and lesbian, gay, bisexual, transgender/transsexual, and queer/questioning (LGBTQ) populations. CA Cancer J Clin 2015;65(5):384–400.

5. Institute of Medicine (US) Committee on Lesbian, Gay, Bisexual, and Transgender Health Issues and Research Gaps and Opportunities. The health of lesbian, gay, bisexual, and transgender people: building a foundation for better understanding. Washington (DC): National Academies Press (US); 2011. Available at. http://www.ncbi.nlm.nih.gov/books/NBK64810/.

6. Gorman BK, Denney JT, Dowdy H, et al. A new piece of the puzzle: sexual orientation, gender, and physical health status. Demography 2015;52(4):1357–82.

7. Lesbian, gay, bisexual and transgender persons and socioeconomic status. American Psychological Association. Available at: http://www.apa.org/pi/ses/resources/publications/factsheet-lgbt.pdf. Accessed March 28, 2016.

8. Krehely J. How to close the LGBT health disparities gap. Washington DC: Center for American Progress; 2009. Available at: http://cancer-network.org/media/pdf/lgbt_health_disparities_gap_race.pdf. Accessed March 20, 2016.

9. Johnson CV, Mimiaga MJ, Bradford J. Health care issues among lesbian, gay, bisexual, transgender and intersex populations in the United States: introduction. J Homosex 2008;54(3):213–24.

10. Obedin-Maliver J, Goldsmith ES, Stewart L, et al. Lesbian, gay, bisexual, and transgender–related content in undergraduate medical education. JAMA 2011;306(9):971–7.

11. Lim FA, Brown DV Jr, Jones H. Lesbian, gay, bisexual, and transgender health: fundamentals for nursing education. J Nurs Educ 2013;52(4):198–203.

12. Carabez R, Pellegrini M, Mankovitz A, et al. "Never in all my years... ": nurses' education about LGBT health. J Prof Nurs 2015;31(4):323–9.

13. More FG, Whitehead AW, Gonthier M. Strategies for student services for lesbian, gay, bisexual, and transgender students in dental schools. J Dent Educ 2004;68:623–32.

14. Behar-Horenstein LS, Morris DR. Dental school administrators' attitudes toward providing support services for LGBT-identified students. J Dent Educ 2015;79: 965–70.

15. Anderson JI, Patterson AN, Temple HJ, et al. Lesbian, gay, bisexual, and transgender (LGBT) issues in dental school environments: dental student leaders' perceptions. J Dent Educ 2009;73:105–18.

16. Madhan B, Gayathri H, Garhnayak L, et al. Dental students' regard for patients from often-stigmatized populations: findings from an Indian dental school. J Dent Educ 2012;76(2):210–7.

17. Green ER, Peterson EN. LGBTQI terminology. Riverside (CA): LGBT Resource Center at University of California; 2004. Available at: http://www.lgbt.ucla.edu/documents/LGBTTerminology.pdf. Accessed March 2, 2016.

18. The guidelines for psychological practice with lesbian, gay, and bisexual clients, adopted by the APA Council of Representatives, February 18-20, 2011. Available at: http://www.apa.org/pi/lgbt/resources/guidelines.aspx. Accessed February 8, 2016.

19. Intersex Society of North America. What's the history behind the intersex rights movement? Available at: http://www.isna.org/faq/history. Accessed February 10, 2016.

20. Wherrett DK. Approach to the infant with a suspected disorder of sex development. Pediatr Clin North Am 2015;62(4):983–99.

21. Hiort O, Birnbaum W, Marshall L, et al. Management of disorders of sex development. Nat Rev Endocrinol 2014;10:520–9.

22. Dreger AD. 'Ambiguous sex'–or ambivalent medicine? Ethical issues in the treatment of intersexuality. Hastings Cent Rep 1998;28(3):24–36.

23. Maupin A. Tales of the city. New York, NY: Harper & Row; 1978.

24. US Department of Justice, Federal Bureau of Investigation. Hate crime statistics, 2014. 2015. Available at: https://www.fbi.gov/about-us/cjis/ucr/hate-crime/2014/resource-pages. Accessed February 10, 2016.

25. American Civil Liberties Union. Know your rights: transgender people and the law. Available at: https://www.aclu.org/know-your-rights/transgender-people-and-law. Accessed February 10, 2016.

26. GLAAD media reference guide - terms to avoid. Available at: http://www.glaad.org/reference/offensive. Accessed March 27, 2016.

27. Conron KJ, Mimiaga MJ, Landers SJ. A population-based study of sexual orientation identity and gender differences in adult health. Am J Public Health 2010;100(10):1953–60.

28. Statistics Canada. Same-sex couples and sexual orientation by the numbers. 2015. Available at: http://www.statcan.gc.ca/eng/dai/smr08/2015/smr08_203_2015#a3. Accessed March 2, 2016.

29. Centers for Disease Control and Prevention. Gay and bisexual men's health: stigma and discrimination. Available at: http://www.cdc.gov/msmhealth/stigma-and-discrimination.htm. Accessed March 28, 2016.

30. Ryan C, Huebner D, Diaz RM, et al. Family rejection as a predictor of negative health outcomes in white and Latino lesbian, gay, and bisexual young adults. Pediatrics 2009;123(1):346–52.

31. Hsieh N, Ruther M. Sexual minority health and health risk factors: intersection effects of gender, race, and sexual identity. Am J Prev Med 2016;50(6):746–55.

32. Saad L. U.S. acceptance of gay/lesbian relations is the new normal. Available at: http://www.gallup.com/poll/154634/acceptance-gay-lesbian-relations-new-normal.aspx. Accessed March 1, 2016.

33. Centers for Disease Control and Prevention. HIV/AIDS: HIV among gay and bisexual men. Available at: http://www.cdc.gov/hiv/group/msm/index.html. Accessed March 28, 2016.

34. Reiter PL, McRee AL, Katz ML, et al. Human papillomavirus vaccination among young adult gay and bisexual men in the United States. Am J Public Health 2015;105(1):96–102.

35. Chin-Hong PV, Vittinghoff E, Cranston RD, et al. Age-specific prevalence of anal human papillomavirus infection in HIV-negative sexually active men who have sex with men: the EXPLORE study. J Infect Dis 2004;190(12):2070–6.

36. Ward BW, Joestl SS, Galinsky AM, et al. Selected diagnosed chronic conditions by sexual orientation: a national study of US adults, 2013. Prev Chronic Dis 2015;12:E192.

37. Mansh M, Katz KA, Linos E, et al. Association of skin cancer and indoor tanning in sexual minority men and women. JAMA Dermatol 2015;151(12):1308–16.

38. Boehmer U, Miao X, Linkletter C, et al. Adult health behaviors over the life course by sexual orientation. Am J Public Health 2012;102(2):292–300.

39. Machalek DA, Poynten M, Jin F, et al. Anal human papillomavirus infection and associated neoplastic lesions in men who have sex with men: a systematic review and meta-analysis. Lancet Oncol 2012;13(5):487–500.

40. Boehmer U, Miao X, Linkletter C, et al. Health conditions in younger, middle, and older ages: are there differences by sexual orientation? LGBT Health 2014;1(3): 168–76.

41. Eliason MJ, Ingraham N, Fogel SC, et al. A systematic review of the literature on weight in sexual minority women. Womens Health Issues 2015;25(2):162–75.

42. Meyer IH, Dietrich J, Schwartz S. Lifetime prevalence of mental disorders and suicide attempts in diverse lesbian, gay, and bisexual populations. Am J Public Health 2008;98(6):1004–6.

43. Operario D, Gamarel KE, Grin BM, et al. Sexual minority health disparities in adult men and women in the United States: National Health and Nutrition Examination Survey, 2001-2010. Am J Public Health 2015;105(10):e27–34.

44. MacCarthy S, Reisner SL, Nunn A, et al. The time is now: attention increases to transgender health in the United States but scientific knowledge gaps remain. LGBT Health 2015;2(4):287–91.

45. Feldman J, Brown GR, Deutsch MB, et al. Priorities for transgender medical and healthcare research. Curr Opin Endocrinol Diabetes Obes 2016;23(2):180–7.

46. Khalili J, Leung LB, Diamant AL. Finding the perfect doctor: identifying lesbian, gay, bisexual, and transgender-competent physicians. Am J Public Health 2015;105(6):1114–9.

47. Landers S. Civil rights and health–beyond same-sex marriage. N Engl J Med 2015;373(12):1092–3.

48. Radix AE, Lelutiu-Weinberger C, Gamarel KE. Satisfaction and healthcare utilization of transgender and gender non-conforming individuals in NYC: a community-based participatory study. LGBT Health 2014;1(4):302–8.

49. Health Resources Services Administration. LGBT training curricula for behavioral health and primary care practitioners. Available at: http://www.hrsa.gov/LGBT/lgbtcurrcicula.pdf. Accessed March 16, 2016.

50. Hollenback AD, Eckstrand KL, Dreger A. Implementing curricular and institutional climate changes to improve health care for individuals who are LGBT, gender non-conforming, or born with DSD: a resource for medical educators. Washington DC: Association of American Medical Colleges; 2014. Available at: www.aamc.org/lgbtdsd.

51. Human Rights Campaign. Available at: http://www.hrc.org/resources/coming-out-to-your-doctor. Accessed April 1, 2016.

52. American Association of Medical Colleges. Implementing curricular and institutional climate changes to improve health care for individuals who are LGBT, gender nonconforming, or born with DSD. 2014. Available at: https://www.aamc.org/download/414172/data/lgbt.pdf?__hssc=109962074.1.1459521211613&__hstc=109962074.30def43bc428b7473d398456ef0ea60f.1459521211613.1459521211613.1459521211613.1&__hsfp=1149225117&hsCtaTracking=bd4a6b49-1c77-4054-8711-b55bde24e45b%7C090ff0e5-8d01-493d-8527-9fc74327757d. Accessed April 1, 2016.

53. National Institutes of Health. Recommendations. 2011. Available at: http://www.ncbi.nlm.nih.gov/books/NBK64812/. Accessed April 1, 2016.

The Evolving Role of Dental Responders on Interprofessional Emergency Response Teams

Michael D. Colvard, DDS, PhD, MTS, MS[a],*,
Benjamin J. Vesper, PhD, MBA[a], Linda M. Kaste, DDS, MS, PhD[b],
Jeremy L. Hirst, MS, MBA[c], David E. Peters, JD[d],
James James, MD, DrPH, MHA[e], Rodrigo Villalobos, DDS, MSc, MS[f],
E. John Wipfler III, MD[g,h,i]

KEYWORDS

- Disaster response • Disaster medicine • Interprofessional relations • Pandemics
- Dentist emergency responders • Mass vaccination
- Pandemic and All Hazards Preparedness Reauthorization Act • Emergency medicine

KEY POINTS

- Oral health care professionals can serve as responders and should be actively involved in all stages of disaster and pandemic planning within their local communities.
- Through emerging state and federal laws, dental responders can legally provide triage, immunization/vaccination, and infrastructure support during declared pandemics and disasters.
- Dentists can serve a critical role as triage coordinators and "medic" members of tactical emergency medical support and forensic investigative teams.

Continued

[a] Department of Oral Medicine and Diagnostic Sciences, Dental Medicine Responder Training Office, College of Dentistry, University of Illinois at Chicago, 801 South Paulina Street (MC 838), Chicago, IL 60612-7213, USA; [b] Department of Pediatric Dentistry, College of Dentistry, University of Illinois at Chicago, 801 South Paulina Street (MC 850), Chicago, IL 60612, USA; [c] DuPage County Office of Homeland Security and Emergency Management, 418 North County Farm Road, Wheaton, IL 60187, USA; [d] UIC Police Department, University of Illinois at Chicago, 943 West Maxwell Street, Chicago, IL 60608, USA; [e] Society for Disaster Medicine & Public Health, 11300 Rockville Pike, Rockville, MD 20852, USA; [f] Dental School, Universidad Latina de Costa Rica (ULATINA), San Jose, Montes de Oca, San Pedro, 11501 Costa Rica; [g] Department of Emergency Medicine, University of Illinois College of Medicine at Peoria, 1 Illini Drive, Peoria, IL 61605, USA; [h] Emergency Department, OSF Saint Francis Medical Center, 530 Northeast Glen Oak Avenue, Peoria, IL 61637, USA; [i] Peoria County Sheriff's Office, 301 North Maxwell Road, Peoria, IL 61604, USA
* Corresponding author.
E-mail address: colvard@uic.edu

Dent Clin N Am 60 (2016) 907–920
http://dx.doi.org/10.1016/j.cden.2016.05.008
0011-8532/16/$ – see front matter © 2016 Elsevier Inc. All rights reserved.

Continued

- The dental profession needs to continue to advocate for dentists and hygienists to be included as key members of the response team.
- Oral health care providers must be paramount in educating their medical colleagues on the importance of dental skills in catastrophic events and pandemic response.

INTRODUCTION

The number of natural, pandemic, man-made (anthropogenic), and terrorism-related events are increasing worldwide. These events are multifactorial, but are heavily influenced by increased population growth, increasing urbanization of populations, and global climate disruptions and their influence on societal well-being.[1,2] Because economic and health consequences impact climate-related events, deleterious events to humanity are only expected to increase in the future,[3] and significant international health concerns can arise from these events. Examples of recent events include Hurricane Katrina (2005), the Joplin, Missouri, tornado (2011), Hurricane Sandy (2012), the Ebola virus outbreak (2014), and the Zika virus outbreak (2015).

During Hurricane Katrina, 11 hospitals and numerous dental offices in New Orleans, LA, were flooded.[4] In Mississippi, the storm damaged another 14 hospitals and 3 federal medical facilities and caused partial or complete damage to more than 60% of dental practices in the affected counties.[4] The storm affected dentists on a personal level as well; a reported 44 dentists in Mississippi lost their homes as a result of the hurricane.[5] As such, these problems can be magnified when dental and medical personnel and facilities are situated in the area of the disaster.

Although disasters and pandemics are becoming more prominent in recent years, the concept of using medics and disaster response teams to respond to military and large-scale disaster events can be traced back to the early Greeks and the Roman legions.[6] This is not surprising; first responder duties have always had a strong association with military conflicts and disasters. During the Middle Ages, the Order of St. John of Jerusalem (later known as the Order of Malta International) was created and charged with providing military defense of the sick and security of medical centers and main roads,[7] and later filled a crucial medical role during the Crusades in Europe.[8] This set the foundation for modern traumatology and a military system of prehospital emergency medical services based on the triage and transport of casualties; the creation of this modern system is widely credited to Baron Dominique Jean Larrey (1766–1842).[6] This example of military medic duties from the 18th century, along with the continuous efforts of the various Catholic Orders providing medical and first responder care, continues to this day and serves as a model for the emergence of modern first responder entities such as the American Red Cross[9] and the worldwide civilian emergency medical technician and paramedic response systems.[10] This article reviews the history of first responders, their roles and important legislation as it relates to dental responders—specifically the role of dentists on an interprofessional response team, and with a particular focus on dentists providing immunizations.

ETYMOLOGY OF "RESPONDERS" AND EVOLUTION OF INTERPROFESSIONAL RESPONSE TEAMS

Today the term "emergency response providers" is legally defined in Section 2 of the US Homeland Security Act of 2002.[11] This act defines the term as inclusive of

"Federal, State, and local emergency public safety, law enforcement, emergency response, emergency medical (including hospital emergency facilities), and related personnel, agencies, and authorities." This definition makes no distinction between responders arriving immediately upon the onset of a disaster and those arriving many hours or days after the initial "surge" period (eg, responders who aid in identification and recovery efforts), even though the skills and personnel needed at different time intervals after the onset of an emergency event may be vastly different.

The initial response to an event is particularly critical to effectively contain and mitigate a disaster or pandemic; as such, it is necessary to identify and define "first responders" separately from other responders. President George W. Bush provided a definition for first responder in the 2003 Homeland Security Presidential Directive HSPD-8 as follows[12]: "individuals who in the early stages of an incident are responsible for the protection and preservation of life, property, evidence, and the environment." According to HSPD-8, these individuals include the emergency response providers defined in the US Homeland Security Act of 2002 and "emergency management, public health, clinical care, public works, and other skilled support personnel (such as equipment operators) that provide immediate support services during prevention, response, and recovery operations."

The US Department of Health and Human Services released the first National Health Security Strategy in 2009, which was designed to lay out a baseline strategy to minimize the health consequences of large-scale disasters.[13] The subsequent National Health Security Review 2010 to 2014[14] and the National Health Security Strategy and Implementation Plan 2015 to 2018[15] describe the progress made toward this goal and updated strategies to improve response. These and other comprehensive response plans incorporate a broad array of interdisciplinary health professionals from different professional backgrounds and organizations, including all levels of government (local, regional, state, and federal), corporations, community organizations, the nonprofit sector, academia, and the scientific community (**Fig. 1**). The dentist, serving as a dental responder, and as a participating member in the interprofessional first responder team, is included in all of these plans.[13] As these response plans become more collaborative in nature in the future, the further interprofessional development of oral health professionals on a disaster response team will be critical (**Fig. 2**).

Traditional first responder activities have typically been performed by public health professionals such as physicians, nurses, physician assistants, and emergency medical technicians. Dental professionals, however, have long served in civilian and military first responder capacities during natural disasters, anthropogenic disasters, and pandemic events, assisting various investigative and law enforcement agencies when processing missing people and identifying anthropological remains.[16] The nature of this work is typically conducted during the recovery efforts in the day(s) after a disaster; therefore, dentists have not traditionally been included as part of the interdisciplinary first responder teams initially called to a disaster scene.

In addition to being trained in forensic identification and biometric informatics,[17–20] oral health providers have the capacity to respond to disasters, provide immunizations, and provide triage care.[21] Over the past decade, selected states and the US Congress have passed legislation that has defined the dental responder and has expanded the legal authority of oral health care providers to serve in such first responder activities.

DENTAL RESPONDER LEGISLATION

Commissioned dentists in the US National Guard services, all branches of the Active Duty and Reserved Armed Forces of the United States, and the majority of

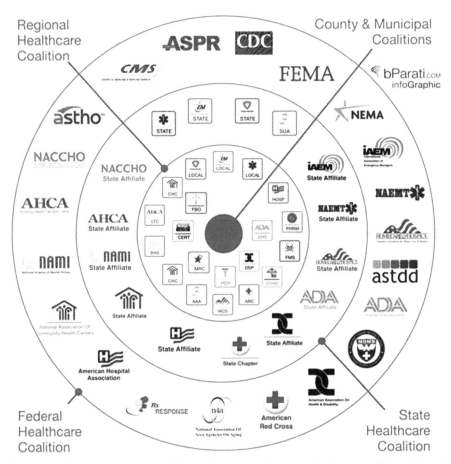

Fig. 1. Local, regional, state, and federal organizations contributing to all-hazards and pandemic preparedness and response. (*Courtesy of* bParati Consulting, Chatham (IL); with permission.)

international military forces, have a long history of providing military mass casualty and triage support as part of military medical and humanitarian response teams.[2,22,23] These dentists provide anesthesia care and management, triage care and management, immunization care and management, and attend to the oral and maxillofacial care and trauma of military forces in battlefield and home station conditions. Military dentists also have a long tradition of providing forensic identification support after battlefield events and military accidents.[16] In the United States and international civilian communities, dentists have traditionally provided first responder care for the forensic identification of casualties from mass disasters, as integral members on disaster mortuary operational teams. However, the idea of a civilian dentist acting as a full-spectrum first responder (ie, practicing care as a military dentist or disaster mortuary operational team dentist) within civilian first response teams—in concert with traditional health care professionals such as physicians, nurses, and emergency medical technicians—was not introduced into the scientific literature until 1996 by Morlang.[23]

2002 – 2012
where we were...

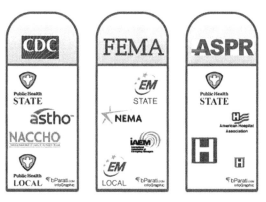

2014
where we are...

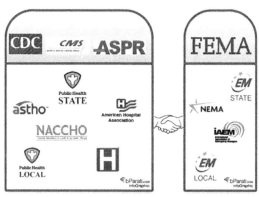

2017
where we are going...

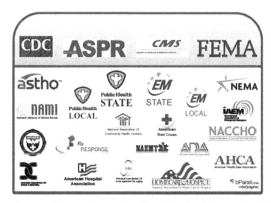

Fig. 2. Interprofessional and collaborative evolution of organizations involved in pandemic and all-hazard planning and response. (*Courtesy of* bParati Consulting, Chatham (IL); with permission.)

The September 11, 2001, terrorist attacks in the United States further served to increase awareness of the potential benefit of dental first responders. After those attacks, numerous medical and dental strategy, theory, and policy experts and clinicians, at the federal and state levels, suggested that the American dental profession needed to define and describe a cohesive vision to establish membership protocols and outline clinical duties for civilian dentists to become members of medical disaster response teams. This vision had to be synergistic with the current standard operation procedures used by the emergency response community and one that could be translated into actual changes in the state dental practice acts for each state in the United States.[24–27]

State Legislation

Illinois has been at the forefront to advance legislation incorporating dental professionals as first responders on disaster response and immunization teams.[16] This effort to define a cohesive vision and policy for the dentist to serve as a civilian first responder was reported by Colvard and coworkers in 2006.[16] Policy and strategy work by the authors leading up to the release of this paper, in concert with state and national professional support (including the Illinois State Dental Society, American Dental Association, and numerous other organizations),[28–39] resulted in Illinois Public Act 49 to 409, which was signed into law in 2005. Through this legislation Illinois defined the "dental emergency responder" and became the first state to amend their state dental practice act to introduce the concept of the civilian dental responder providing emergency medical care, triage, and immunizations during a disaster event. The Illinois Dental Practice Act defined a dental emergency responder as a licensed dentist or dental hygienist "who is appropriately certified in emergency medical response, as defined by the Department of Public Health." Dentists and dental hygienists are described as "acting within the bounds of his or her license when providing care during a declared local, state or national emergency."[18]

In 2015, the Illinois Dental Practice Act was amended via Public Act 99-0025 to change "dental emergency responder" to "dental responder."[40] The "dental responder" is defined as "a dentist or dental hygienist who is appropriately certified in disaster preparedness, immunizations, and dental humanitarian medical response consistent with the Society of Disaster Medicine and Public Health and training certified by the National Incident Management System or the National Disaster Life Support Foundation."

California has also made notable strides to support the dental responder. In contrast with Illinois, California did not directly alter its dental practice act, but rather introduced additional legislation that was designed to reduce the barriers confronting dentists who wished to participate as first responders. The California Dental Association sponsored AB 2210 in 2008. This bill, which was signed into law in 2008 and became effective January 1, 2009, "allows the California Dental Board to suspend compliance with any provision of the Dental Practice Act that would adversely affect a licensee's ability to provide emergency medical care that is consistent with his/her training."[41] Through this law, California dental professionals who provide emergency care voluntarily and without compensation during declared disasters are provided indemnity. Several other states have expanded their public health and "good Samaritan" laws to include dentists among potential responders supporting a state or national declared disaster response.[18]

Although Illinois and California have addressed the inclusion of the dental responders through changes in legislation, other states continue to advocate on the behalf of the dental responder through nonlegislative actions. For example, a number of academics, physicians, and state organizations in New York have provided support over the past decade to include and properly train dentists for first responder activities.[25,42–48] In Texas, the Texas Military Forces annually conducts Operation Lone Star, a training event for state and local partners to train for disaster response; this event includes dentists, dental assistants, and dental students.[49]

A number of civilian and military health care professionals and response organizations (such as the American Red Cross) operating at state and local levels continue to support dentists to become first responders and to be actively involved in responder research and training exercises. Notably, the United States Assistant Secretary for Preparedness and Response, responsible for overseeing the US Medical Reserve Corps (MRC), has specifically named dentists and dental assistants as possible "front line" health providers capable of providing "surge" capacity during the first 12 to 72 hours of an emergency.[50] The MRC network currently consists of nearly 1000 community-based response units throughout the United States and US territories.[51]

Federal Legislation

While individual states debate legislative actions to incorporate dental responder activities into each state's dental scope of practice, important federal legislation was recently passed to support disaster response activities of oral health care providers. The 2013 reauthorization of the Pandemic and All-Hazards Preparedness Act (PAHPA) gives dentists and dental hygienists the legal authority to support national emergency, disaster, and forensic needs by providing clinical care and infrastructure for "walking well" care, pandemic vaccination support, biometric information, and forensic dentistry.[52]

Three key changes were introduced in the PAHPA, which defined the inclusion of oral health care providers in public health emergency planning and response[52]:

1. Dental health care facilities are incorporated under ambulatory care facilities during public health emergencies;
2. Dental health assets (including dentists and dental hygienists) are incorporated after medical assets in medical triage activities during a disaster; and
3. Training efforts for dental professionals responding to public health emergencies are supported.

The PAHPA serves as a critical starting point for legally introducing dental responders into pandemic and disaster planning and response activities within the United States, but it does not describe the implementation of oral health care providers into these activities. Dentists and hygienists who wish to serve as dental responders will need to become integrated into interprofessional local, state, and federal disaster response teams.

IMMUNIZATION CAPACITY OF DENTISTS

Initial response to a public health emergency occurs at the local level and, as such, is typically coordinated by local/county response teams. Given that the disasters typically faced by a local health department depend on their geographic location, it is critical that disaster response team training occurs at the local level so that all health responder team members are best prepared for potential location-specific emergencies that may arise. As such, the greatest need for dental responders will likely be as members of local disaster response teams. Many communities already have MRC units, Civilian Emergency Response Teams, and similar teams in place to help coordinate the local health care response during emergency situations.

Only a very limited number of publications defining local-level emergency response planning and training activities designed specifically for dental responders have been reported to date in the scientific literature.[16,18,21,24–26,53] This is likely owing to a number of factors, including (1) the federal legislation supporting the inclusion of dental responders was only passed recently, and local organizations may not be aware of the change in legislation; (2) the 2013 reauthorization of the PAHPA does not provide guidance for implementing oral health care professionals onto pandemic and disaster response teams, and local health organizations may not know how to begin this process; and (3) resources to provide training may be limited and are likely to first be allocated to the traditional physician and nurse responders. Although the PAHPA states that training activities for dental responders are supported, it does not say in what capacity this support will occur.

One such immunization training activity has been reported. In late 2013, the Operation Sustained Adaptive Prophylaxis influenza mass vaccination drill was developed and conducted by the DuPage County Health Department in Wheaton, Illinois.[21] The exercise was designed to train potential dental responders in a simulated pandemic immunization response scenario, using just-in-time (JIT) training. The protocol was modified from an H1N1 influenza mass vaccination clinical protocol previously used by certified public health nurses, as provided by the local health department. The main goals of the exercise included validating the use of dentists as an emergency response resource; testing the vaccination throughput using the current plans, protocols, and procedures of the health department; validating that the correct vaccination dispensing protocol were used (drug selection, amount, technique); and validating the use and effectiveness of the JIT training.

Fifteen dental professionals (8 hygienists and 7 dentists) from the local MRC served as dental responders in the 1-hour exercise. JIT training consisted of an approximately 15-minute-long video describing inoculation techniques (watched as a group), a 10-minute group discussion reviewing the specific protocol to be used, and 15 minutes at his or her individual station to review independently the protocol and practice techniques. Community volunteers served as the "patients" for the drill. To replicate realistic operational conditions of a mass vaccination, patients were given simulated vaccine administration records. Patients presented the vaccine records to the dental responder, who was then responsible for the appropriate selection and administration of the vaccine. A porcine model was used to simulate the vaccination injection of patients. Trained nurses and emergency response personnel oversaw the exercise and evaluated the dental responders for medical history documentation, vaccination procedures, and patient throughput and error rates. **Fig. 3** shows pictures from the exercise.

Overall, the results of the dental responders were found to be similar to those documented by the DuPage County Health Department in mass influenza clinics previously conducted by certified public health nurses. A total of 335 patients were treated during the hour-long exercise, corresponding to an average throughput rate of 22.3 patients per dentists per hour. Among the 335 patients, 7 medical errors (incorrect vaccine dosage administered and/or incorrectly documented vaccine administration records) were documented, corresponding with a medical error rate of 2.1%. These results were found despite noting the 15 dental responders had vastly different backgrounds and professional experiences. This suggests validation of the use of the JIT training methodology and validation of the dental profession in general as a valuable immunization resource. It was further noted that 3 of the vaccinators did not possess the necessary vaccine administration skills to competently conduct the drill, thereby emphasizing the importance of local responder teams to regularly conduct training exercises such as this to ensure their team members are adequately prepared to respond to a pandemic or disaster.

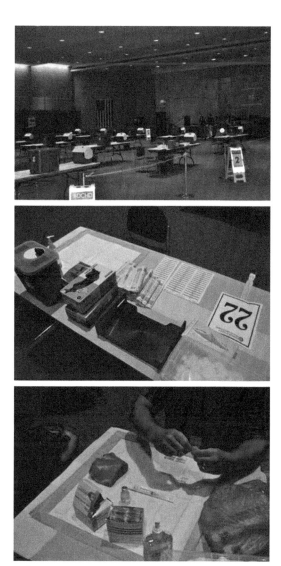

Fig. 3. The setup of a mass vaccination pandemic immunization response exercise completed by dentists. (*From* Colvard MD, Hirst JL, Vesper BJ, et al. Just-in-time training of dental responders in a simulated pandemic immunization response exercise. Disaster Med Public Health Prep 2014;8:249; with permission.)

SUMMARY

Although dentists have traditionally served on civilian interprofessional disaster response teams, their role has typically been limited to the forensic identification of remains. Oral health care professionals diagnose and treat medical conditions in their daily activities, just like their colleagues from other health care disciplines. Such activities include surgical care, anesthesia care, administering immunizations, providing appropriate (triage and tactical) support care during emergency response and triage interventions, following up with patients, and referring patients to other medical experts. These same skills and infrastructure assets are used during pandemic and disaster response activities. Dentists also possess a unique diagnostic skill set for forensic dental, oral, and facial data gathering and analysis—additional skills that are important during first responder activities. As such, dental professionals are uniquely positioned at the forefront of emerging biometric and forensic standards and technologies, and therefore can play a critical role in first responder and health security efforts.

Recent work has sought to drastically expand the purview of dentists and hygienists in disaster and pandemic planning and response. Toward this goal, work over the past decade has focused primarily on:

1. Policy advancements to legally expand the role of the civilian dental responder, and
2. Educating other health care professionals and the public to better understand the dentists' and hygienists' skill sets, and how these unique skills can be incorporated into interprofessional disaster response teams to enhance the overall quality and efficacy of emergency response efforts.

Policy advancements during the past decade, on both the state and federal levels, have resulted in significant progress in expanding the role of the dental responder beyond traditional forensic identification activities. Illinois has made the most legislative progress on the state level, through amendments made to the Illinois Dental Practice Act that define and include dental responder activities in the dentist's regular scope of practice. The 2013 reauthorization of the Pandemic and All-Hazard Preparation Act introduced dental professionals into federal legislation overseeing public health emergency response. This was a crucial achievement for the dental profession, but significant work remains to further implement the changes outlined in the act.

To this end, efforts to educate other disaster responders, other health care professionals, and the public as to the value of including dental responders are on-going. Training exercises such as the immunization drill conducted by the DuPage County Health Department (Wheaton, IL) provide documented evidence of the capacity and capability of dental professionals to participate in pandemic and disaster planning and response.[21] As dentists become more involved in first responder activities in the future, it is critical that similar training drills continue to be developed and executed.

Although advocacy efforts have increased in recent years, to date, only a relatively small number of local, state, and federal response teams actively recruit and incorporate dentists in their first responder efforts. As such, the dental community needs to continue educating other health care professionals and the public. Disaster response requires the integrated response of health professionals, and interprofessional communication is critical among members of a response team.[54] As such, all stakeholders, regardless of their health care profession, need to work together in the strategic planning, hands-on preparation drills, and active response situations to ensure the health consequences of such hazards are minimized and the response efforts can be completed as quickly and efficiently as possible. Oral health care professionals should be actively involved in all stages of disaster and pandemic planning and response within their local communities.

Now that federal legislation is in place recognizing the dental profession as responders, work must focus on solidifying collaborations among the health professions. The dental community as a whole needs to continue to advocate for dentists and hygienists to be included as key members of the response team and must educate other health professions and the public as to the critical role oral health professionals can play in disaster and pandemic response. Likewise, consensus building among various government agencies, professional organizations, and the public must continue,[18] and fundamental changes to the dental curriculum that require oral health professionals to receive disaster and pandemic response training should be implemented. Strategy sessions and hands-on training drills can serve as important interprofessional educational tools, allowing dentists and dental students to learn pandemic and disaster response techniques alongside other health care providers, while also enabling current and future dental professionals to provide valuable input into response activities. One suggested method to provide real-world interprofessional relations training to oral health care providers is to include dentists and hygienists as vaccinators during seasonal flu vaccination clinics commonly hosted by county health departments, hospitals, and universities.

Dentists and hygienists interested in training to become dental responders are urged to actively participate in their local communities through units such as the MRCs and Civilian Emergency Response Teams. Additionally, appropriately qualified dentists could serve as members on local tactical emergency medical support teams.[55] There are also several nongovernmental organizations and religious organizations that sponsor responder teams and seek dentists for the unique skill sets oral health care professionals can provide during all-hazard and pandemic events. Additionally, interested individuals should contact their local county health departments, county coroner's offices, and/or the various federal responder teams (such as disaster medical assistance teams and disaster mortuary operational teams) for participation opportunities. All teams listed require active licensure, advanced training and education, and experience for participation. Finally, the various levels of National Guard, Reserves Armed Forces, and Active Duty military train and staff responder teams able to respond to the full spectrum of chemical, biological, radiologic, nuclear, and explosive events that could potentially occur around the world. The dentist and oral health care community can make significant contributions to the intraprofessional and interprofessional collaborations among health care providers by serving on response teams within their communities.

REFERENCES

1. Aitsi-Selmi A, Murray V. Protecting the health and well-being of populations from disasters: health and health care in the Sendai framework for disaster risk reduction 2015-2030. Prehosp Disaster Med 2016;31:74–8.
2. Siri JG, Newell B, Proust K, et al. Urbanization, extreme events, and health: the case for systems approaches in mitigation, management, and response. Asia Pac J Public Health 2015;28(2 Suppl):15S–27S.
3. Core Writing Team, Pachauri RK, Meye LA. Climate Change 2014: Synthesis Report. Contribution of Working Groups I, II and III to the Fifth Assessment Report of the Intergovernmental Panel on Climate Change. Geneva (Switzerland): IPCC; 2014. p. 151.
4. Mosca NG, Finn E, Joskow R. Dental care as a vital service response for disaster victims. J Health Care Poor Underserved 2007;18:262–70.
5. Hurricane Katrina: Medical support/demobilization/transition plan for the state of Mississippi. Washington, DC: US Department of Health and Human Services; Mississippi Department of Health; 2006.
6. Goniewicz M. Effect of military conflicts on the formation of emergency medical services systems worldwide. Acad Emerg Med 2013;20:507–13.
7. 1048 to the Present Day. In: Sovereign Order of Malta. 2016. Available at: www. orderofmalta.int/history/. Accessed February 24, 2016.

8. Moeller C. Hospitallers of St. John of Jerusalem. In: The catholic encyclopedia. New York: Robert Appleton Company; 1910. Available at: http://www. newadvent.org/cathen/07477a.htm. Accessed January 19, 2016.

9. American Red Cross. 2016. Available at: www.redcross.org/. Accessed January 25, 2016.

10. What is EMS? In: National Registry of Emergency Medical Technicians. 2016. Available at: www.nremt.org/nremt/about/What_is_EMS.asp. Accessed January 25, 2016.

11. Homeland security act of 2002. Washington, DC: US Congress; 2002.

12. Bush GW. Homeland Security Presidential Directive HSPD-8. Washington, DC: US Department of Homeland Security, 2003.

13. National health security strategy of the United States of America. Washington, DC: US Department of Health and Human Services; 2009.

14. National health security review of the United States of America 2010-2014. Washington, DC: US Health and Human Services; 2014.

15. National health security strategy and implementation plan 2015-2018. Washington, DC: US Health and Human Services; 2015.

16. Colvard MD, Lampiris LN, Cordell GA, et al. The dental emergency responder: Expanding the scope of dental practice. J Am Dent Assoc 2006;137:468–73.

17. ANSI/NIST-ITL 1-2011 Update:2013. Data format for the interchange of fingerprint, facial & other biometric information. Washington, DC: American National Standards Institute; 2013.

18. Colvard MD, Naiman MI, Mata D, et al. Disaster medicine training survey results for dental health care providers in Illinois. J Am Dent Assoc 2007;138:519–24 [quiz: 536–7].

19. Glick M. Why don't dentists provide immunizations? A missed opportunity. J Am Dent Assoc 2013;144:1098–100.

20. Zohn HK, Dashkow S, Aschheim KW, et al. The odontology victim identification skill assessment system. J Forensic Sci 2010;55:788–91.

21. Colvard MD, Hirst JL, Vesper BJ, et al. Just-in-time training of dental responders in a simulated pandemic immunization response exercise. Disaster Med Public Health Prep 2014;8:247–51.

22. Flores S, Mills SE, Shackelford L. Dentistry and bioterrorism. Dent Clin North Am 2003;47:733–44.

23. Morlang WM. Dentistry's vital role in disaster preparedness. J Calif Dent Assoc 1996;24:63–6.

24. Chmar JE, Ranney RR, Guay AH, et al. Incorporating bioterrorism training into dental education: report of ADA-ADEA terrorism and mass casualty curriculum development workshop. J Dent Educ 2004;68:1196–9.

25. More FG, Phelan J, Boylan R, et al. Predoctoral dental school curriculum for catastrophe preparedness. J Dent Educ 2004;68:851–8.

26. Pretty IA, Webb DA, Sweet D. Dental participants in mass disasters–a retrospective study with future implications. J Forensic Sci 2002;47:117–20.

27. Weber CR. Dentistry's role in biodefense. Pa Dent J (Harrisb) 2003;70:32–4.

28. Colvard MD. Handbook of dental practice. Preface. Dent Clin North Am 2007;51: xv–xvii.

29. Shackelford LS, Halliday CG. Foreword. Dent Clin North Am 2007;51:xi–xiii.

30. Guay AH. The role dentists can play in mass casualty and disaster events. Dent Clin North Am 2007;51:767–78.

31. Coule PL, Horner JA. National disaster life support programs: a platform for multidisciplinary disaster response. Dent Clin North Am 2007;51:819–25.

32. Glotzer DL, Rekow ED, More FG, et al. All hazards training: incorporating a catastrophe preparedness mindset into the dental school curriculum and professional practice. Dent Clin North Am 2007;51:805–18.

33. Hagen JC, Parota B, Tsagalis M. TOPOFF 2 and the inclusion of dental professionals into federal exercise design and execution. Dent Clin North Am 2007; 51:827–35.

34. Janssen JA, Lampiris LN. Disaster response in Illinois: the role for dentists and dental hygienists. Dent Clin North Am 2007;51:779–84.

35. Lee MS, Heilicser B. Oral health professionals within state-sponsored medical response teams: the IMERT perspective. Dent Clin North Am 2007;51:879–94.

36. Mosca NG. Engaging the dental workforce in disaster mitigation to improve recovery and response. Dent Clin North Am 2007;51:871–8.

37. Naiman M, Larsen AK Jr, Valentin PR. The role of the dentist at crime scenes. Dent Clin North Am 2007;51:837–56.

38. Stewart A, Cordell GA. Pharmaceuticals and the strategic national stockpile program. Dent Clin North Am 2007;51:857–69.

39. Watson-Alvan S, Alves-Dunkerson J. The importance of a shared vision in emergency preparedness: engaging partners in a home-rule state. Dent Clin North Am 2007;51:785–803.

40. Public act 099-0025. Springfield (IL): Illinois General Assembly; 2015.

41. Emergency response policy statement. Sacramento (CA): California Dental Association; 2011.

42. Glotzer DL, Psoter WJ, Rekow ED. Preparing for a terrorist event: a scenario-driven approach. N Y State Dent J 2004;70:26–9.

43. Han SZ, Alfano MC, Psoter WJ, et al. Bioterrorism and catastrophe response: a quick-reference guide to resources. J Am Dent Assoc 2003;134:745–52.

44. Fernandez JB, Glotzer DL, Triola MM, et al. A unique role for dental school faculty: telephone triage training and integration into a health departments' emergency response planning. Am J Disaster Med 2008;3:141–6.

45. Glotzer DL, More FG, Phelan J, et al. Introducing a senior course on catastrophe preparedness into the dental school curriculum. J Dent Educ 2006;70: 225–30.

46. Glotzer DL, Psoter WJ, Rekow ED. Emergency preparedness in the dental office. J Am Dent Assoc 2004;135:1565–70.

47. Glotzer DL, Rinchiuso A, Rekow ED, et al. The Medical Reserve Corps.: an opportunity for dentists to serve. N Y State Dent J 2006;72:60–1.

48. Psoter WJ, Park PJ, Boylan RJ, et al. National emergency response programs for dental health care professionals. J Am Dent Assoc 2008;139:1067–73.

49. Operation Lone Star. In: Texas Military. 2015. Available at: https://tmd.texas.gov/operation-lone-star-2015-dental-care. Accessed January 15, 2016.

50. Volunteering with the MRC. In: Medical Reserve Corp. 2015. Available at: www.medicalreservecorps.gov/leaderFldr/QuestionsAnswers/Volunteering. Accessed January 19, 2016.

51. About the Medical Reserve Corps. In: Medical Reserve Corp. 2016. Available at: www.medicalreservecorps.gov/pageviewfldr/About. Accessed January 25, 2016.

52. H.R. 307-Pandemic and all-hazards preparedness reauthorization act of 2013. Washington, DC: US Congress; 2013.

53. Dixon K. My experience at the 2015 MI-MORT disaster exercise. J Mich Dent Assoc 2015;97:36–8.

54. Newell BJ, Pittman JC, Pagano HP, et al. Responding to the 2014 Ebola outbreak: the value of effective interprofessional communication during emergency response. Disaster Med Public Health Prep 2015;1–2.
55. TEMS Overview. In: National Tactical Officers Association. 2016. Available at: https://ntoa.org/sections/tems/. Accessed January 25, 2016.

Policy Development Fosters Collaborative Practice

The Example of the Minamata Convention on Mercury

Daniel M. Meyer, DDS[a], Linda M. Kaste, DDS, MS, PhD[b],*,
Kathy M. Lituri, RDH, MPH[c], Scott Tomar, DMD, MPH, DrPH[d],
Christopher H. Fox, DMD, DMSc[e], Poul Erik Petersen, DDS, Dr Odont, MSc (Sociology)[f]

KEYWORDS

- Dentistry • Oral health • Public policy • Environmental policy
- Interprofessional relations • Dental amalgam • Mercury • Global health

KEY POINTS

- The oral health community has responsibilities in interprofessional policy development that affect the general and oral health of the public.
- Dentistry must assure involvement in science-based responses, with recognized expertise and advocacy, albeit without governmental standing.
- Professional dental organizations can work to optimally respond, find common ground, and cooperate regarding complicated interprofessional health issues.
- Establishing interprofessional partnerships enables collaboration on health issues and ensures that those outside of dentistry understand the importance of oral health.
- The development of the Minamata Convention on Mercury showed the significance of the commitment by oral health stakeholders, sustained longevity of effort, science-based evidence, understanding of policy development ranging from local to global levels, and the dental profession working effectively in interprofessional collaborations.

[a] American Dental Association, 211 E. Chicago Avenue, Chicago, IL 60611, USA; [b] University of Illinois at Chicago College of Dentistry, 801 South Paulina Street, Room 563A, MC 850, Chicago, IL 60612, USA; [c] Boston University Henry M. Goldman School of Dental Medicine, 560 Harrison Avenue, #340, Boston, MA 02118, USA; [d] University of Florida College of Dentistry, 1329 SW 16th Street, Suite 5180, PO Box 103628, Gainesville, FL 32610, USA; [e] International Association for Dental Research, 1619 Duke Street, Alexandria, VA 22314, USA; [f] University of Copenhagen Faculty of Health Sciences School of Dentistry, Oester Farimagsgade 5, PO Box 2099, DK-1014 Copenhangen K, Denmark
* Corresponding author.
E-mail address: kaste@uic.edu

Dent Clin N Am 60 (2016) 921–942
http://dx.doi.org/10.1016/j.cden.2016.05.009
0011-8532/16/$ – see front matter © 2016 Elsevier Inc. All rights reserved.

dental.theclinics.com

INTRODUCTION

This article provides an example of interprofessional collaboration concerning policy development based on the impact of a global public health problem resulting from environmental accumulation of mercury. Contained are an overview of mercury and the environmental health issues related to mercury, a brief primer of policy and policy stakeholders, and a description of the collaborations including dentistry specifically concerning the Minamata Convention to create global policy to restrict environmental contamination with mercury.

INTRODUCTION TO THE MERCURY ISSUES WARRANTING GLOBAL ENVIRONMENTAL POLICY DEVELOPMENT
Mercury in the Environment

Mercury is a chemical element known by the symbol Hg from its former name, hydrargyrum, or liquid silver.[1,2] It is ubiquitous and found naturally in the environment throughout the world in 3 forms: elemental (or metallic), as part of an inorganic compound (eg, mercuric chloride), or as part of an organic compound (eg, methylmercury and ethylmercury). In its pure, elemental form, mercury is the only metal that is a liquid at room temperature. Mercury has been used to create alloys or amalgams with other metals, produce dental fillings, extract gold from its ores, and help extend the life of dry cell batteries. It can be released as the result of production or improper disposal of several mercury-containing products, including electrical applications (eg, switches and fluorescent lamps), paints, batteries, chlor-alkali, seed grain fungicides, scientific instruments (eg, thermometers and barometers), dental amalgam, topical antiseptics, antibacterial salves, and skin-lightening creams.[3]

Global mercury assessment is intended as a basis for decision making, with an emphasis on anthropogenic emissions (mercury going into the atmosphere) and releases (mercury going into water and land); that is, those associated with human activities.[2,4] An estimated 5500 to 8900 tonnes (1 tonne = 1000 kilograms) are emitted and reemitted to the atmosphere from 3 sources:

1. Naturally (10%) from geological weathering and geothermal activity
2. Anthropogenic (30%), mostly from artisanal and small-scale gold mining and coal burning
3. Reemissions (60%) of previously released mercury that has built up over decades and centuries in surface soils and oceans without a determinable original source

A comparison of percentage of sector contributions to total anthropogenic emissions is shown in **Table 1**,[2] including cremation attributable to dental amalgams. North American emissions are notable at roughly 3% of total global emissions.[2,4] Local and regional mercury depositions throughout the world have gradually increased contamination levels in the environment to the point that countermeasures have been enacted in recent decades to reduce anthropogenic mercury emissions. Because of long-range distribution and transport of mercury globally, nations with minimal mercury releases and other areas remote from industrial activity may be adversely affected. For example, increased mercury levels are observed in the Arctic, far from the sources of any significant releases.[2]

Although natural emissions of mercury into the environment continue, human activities have exceeded natural emissions over the last 200 years and need to be controlled.[5] Mercury can be repeatedly mobilized, deposited, and remobilized between air, water, and soil indefinitely. Although many countries have shown reductions

Table 1
Global emission inventory, 2010, by-product/unintentional (B/U) and intentional (I) assessed sectors by percentage of total anthropogenic emissions

Sector	Percentage
(I) Artisanal and small-scale gold mining	37
(B/U) Coal burning	24
(B/U) Primary production of nonferrous metals	10
(B/U) Cement production	9
(B/U) Large-scale gold production	5
(I) Consumer product waste	5
(B/U) Contaminated sites	4
(B/U) Primary production of ferrous metals	2
(I) Chlor-alkali industry	1
(B/U) Oil refining	1
(B/U) Mine production of mercury	1
(B/U) Oil and natural gas burning	1
(I) Cremation (dental amalgam)[a]	<1

[a] Does not include preparation of dental amalgam fillings and disposal of removed fillings containing mercury.

Adapted from UNEP. Global mercury assessment 2013: sources, emissions, releases and environmental transport. Geneva (Switzerland): UNEP DTIE Chemicals Branch; 2013. Available at: http://www.unep.org/PDF/PressReleases/GlobalMercuryAssessment2013.pdf; with permission.

of use and release of mercury, mercury can be transported by wind and ocean currents so it can only be controlled effectively by coordinated global programs.

Furthermore, mercury is very noxious to human health, particularly to fetal and childhood development. Each form has its own toxicologic profile, affecting the nervous, digestive, and immune systems, and specific organs such as lungs, kidneys, skin, and eyes. In adults, exposure to excessive levels of mercury has been linked to reduced fertility, brain and nerve damage, and heart disease. Hence, mercury is a global threat to human and environmental health, with organic mercury generally considered the most toxic, followed by elemental mercury, and then inorganic mercury.[6]

Mercury Use in Dental Amalgam

Dental amalgam has been used widely as a restorative dental material since the early 1800s.[7] The clinical properties of amalgam, including its ease of placement, high compressive strength, low cost, and long-term survival rates, remain largely unrivaled. During the past decades, a decrease in the use of dental amalgam and a corresponding increase in the use of tooth-colored restorative materials such as dental composites has occurred, primarily driven by esthetics.[8]

Since the inception of dental amalgam, claims have been made about the possibility of detrimental health effects caused by the mercury in its mix.[7] The health concerns and debates over the use of mercury in amalgam restorations are not new.[9,10] For more than a hundred years, numerous assertions have implicated dental amalgam for causing or contributing to neurologic diseases, adverse health conditions, and toxic illnesses. No evidence for these assertions has been found by well-designed clinical studies.[11,12] Two clinical trials sponsored by US National Institutes of Health National Institute of Dental and Craniofacial Research (NIH-NIDCR) involving more than 1000 children in Portugal and the US New England region, evaluating the potential effects of mercury from amalgam, provide sound data supporting the continued use of dental amalgam.[11,12] These two children's amalgam trials found no adverse effects in the 5 years following the placement of dental amalgam. Nonetheless, increasing concern over mercury in the environment has led to a worldwide movement against dental amalgam.[13,14]

Dental Mercury in the Environment

Dental amalgam mercury release from cremated bodies is measurable at the global level[2] (see **Table 1**). Although the amount emitted contributes to less than 1% of the global burden (as measured from cremation), the amount is estimated to be about 3.6 tonnes.[2] Mercury may also be emitted during the preparation and disposal of fillings. In 2005, ENVIRON International Corporation, with funding from the American Dental Association (ADA), prepared a scientific assessment that calculated the amount of mercury attributable to amalgam wastewater that is discharged in effluent from US sewage treatment plants into surface water.[15] This scientific assessment found that a total of approximately 0.4 tons of mercury enters surface water each year.[15] The US Environmental Protection Agency (EPA) oversaw the validation of this approach and principally agreed with ENVIRON's conclusions.[16] Therefore, dental amalgam represents a small but quantifiable part of the overall mercury burden worldwide.[15]

The EPA, among other efforts to limit human-related environmental contamination with mercury, seeks reduction of mercury release into the environment from dental offices.[17] The Clean Water Act (CWA) was established in 1948 to give federal and state EPA, and even local municipal sewerage authorities, direct legal authority to protect waterways by limiting the discharge of mercury in all its forms, including the mercury in amalgam.[18] The EPA sets broad minimum requirements in which states can elect to be more stringent. Typically, states regulate waste by granting permits to a municipal sewerage treatment plant, often referred to as the publicly owned treatment works (POTW). The permit limits the total amount of chemicals, such as mercury, the plant may discharge. POTW can either remove pollutants that enter the plant or limit their discharge into its sewerage system.

The EPA and the ADA are long-time collaborators on seeking means to reduce dental mercury environmental release. The ADA included amalgam separators as part of the ADA best management practices in October 2007. The EPA, the National Association of Clean Water Agencies, and the ADA have common commitments to reduce mercury levels in the environment through voluntary dental amalgam wastewater reduction measures.[19] A key component of the ADA best management practices is recycling. Working with the EPA and recyclers, the ADA has been leading efforts to develop a national consensus standard for the use of amalgam separators to recycle waste amalgam in the dental office. The ADA has tested, according to ISO standards, amalgam separators that are available in the United States and have published peer-reviewed articles in its journal on the qualities of alternative brands and how dentists should choose a separator.[20,21]

Estimates of mercury consumption include dental applications and are shown in **Table 2**.[22] Total consumption seems to be highest in the east/southeast Asia region, where it approaches twice that of the next highest region. The relative contributions to consumption via dental application is around one-third of total consumption for several regions. The North American region, although it has the third highest total, is has a low percentage from dental applications.[22]

Table 2
Percentage of average selected dental applications (estimated from cremation and dental use) of total mercury consumption by world region, 2010, ordered by total mercury consumption

World Region	Total	Estimated as Dental Application (%)
East and southeast Asia	504	13.3
European Union (27 countries)	253	35.6
North America	213	16.0
South Asia	129	18.6
South America	100	33.0
CIS and other European countries	63	15.9
Middle-eastern states	53	30.2
Central America and the Caribbean	47	36.2
Sub-Saharan Africa	34	17.6
North Africa	20	25.0
Australia, New Zealand, and Oceania	17	23.5
Total	1433	21.4

Adapted from AMAP/UNEP, 2013. Technical background report for the global mercury assessment. Geneva (Switzerland): Arctic Monitoring and Assessment Programme, Oslo, Norway/UNEP Chemicals Branch; 2013. p. vi. 263; with permission.

Patient Care and Economic Considerations

Dental caries, although largely preventable, is the most common chronic disease, reaching across the human lifespan, not only in the United States but also worldwide.[4] For restoration of dental caries, to date, tooth-colored materials are inferior to amalgam as fillings, especially for posterior teeth: they are far more technique sensitive, have lower clinical survival rates, are more expensive, and are far more difficult to adapt to proper tooth form under restricted clinical conditions such as in developing countries.[4,23,24] In addition, economically, no adequate alternative for dental amalgam exists. Amalgam's combination of durability and low cost is unmatched by any other dental restorative material. Chadwick and colleagues,[25] found that, "When the initial cost and the longevity are considered together, resin composite turns out to be from 1.7 to 3.5 times more expensive than amalgam." Multiple economic evaluations comparing the use of dental materials, including dental amalgam, have shown that dental amalgam is more cost-effective and cost-beneficial than tooth-colored alternatives, and it has a longer functional time and lower theoretic cost per year of function.[26,27]

Banning the use of dental amalgam globally would have a strong economic impact from a dental perspective, particularly for practice in resource-poor locations. The impact would be most pronounced in low-income countries with limited access to dental materials, underfunded health care delivery systems, and/or inadequate numbers of practitioners trained to provide safe and effective alternatives. Studies have estimated the macroeconomic impact of regulating or banning the use of amalgam restorations in the United States.[28] Beazoglou and colleagues[28] estimated the direct costs of a ban on the use of amalgam restorations: a ban on their use in children and young people aged 0 to 19 years would increase dental expenditures by about $1.1 billion per year (totaling $13 billion from 2005 through 2020). Banning amalgam in the United States is estimated to increase dental expenditures by about $8.2 billion in the first year and lead to an increase of $98.1 billion from 2015 through 2020, based on an estimate of an average increase of $52 per restoration.[28]

INTRODUCTION TO POLICY DEVELOPMENT IN ORAL HEALTH

The environmental laws that regulate the disposal of mercury from dental amalgam rely on a conservative approach to effluent limits because it is not known what happens to substances in the environment hundreds or thousands of years in the future. Experts do know a lot about the clinical safety of dental amalgam and mercury in patients because of the volume of peer-reviewed scientific studies that have been published over the past several decades. For providers who are not familiar with environmental laws, the use of environmental modeling assumptions of questionable scientific validity, uncertainty factors, safety factors, and the shifting burden of proof to the provider or alleged polluter can be bewildering and seem patently unfair. A review of policy and public policy is presented here before moving to the specifics of the Minamata Convention. It should be noted that the Minamata Convention applies at the global level, pending adoption at the country level, and having implications at local and professional levels.

Overarching Definition and Context of Policy Development for Oral Health

There is no universally agreed-on definition of the word policy. The term is used in different ways in different contexts. The Merriam-Webster dictionary (http://www.merriam-webster.com/) provides several definitions of policy, including:

- "A definite course or method of action selected from among alternatives and in light of given conditions to guide and determine present and future decisions"
- "A high-level overall plan embracing the general goals and acceptable procedures especially of a governmental body"

Those related definitions capture some of the key attributes of policy making: it involves general agreement on goals and a broad roadmap on the actions that would help achieve those goals. In many ways, policy making can be thought of as a type of decision making. Governments, institutions, and organizations vary in the policy-making processes, but in general policy making comes down to a decision by a governing body. In most situations, policy development involves receiving input from key stakeholders, negotiation, and compromise. Policy making in oral health is no exception to that general rule. The diversity of opinion among stakeholders requires that various constituents within and outside of the oral health community come together to reach mutually agreed-on goals and chart the broad pathway to achieve them.

Public Policy Processes

Governments enact public policies in many domains that directly or indirectly affect population oral health, including but not limited to health care, education, food, water, licensure, and environment. Governmental policy is frequently reflected in legislative and regulatory action (ie, laws and regulations), and the actions supporting a set of agreed-on goals therefore enter the political realm. In the United States, policies that affect oral health are enacted at every level of government. For example, federal policy governs the mechanism of federal funding for dental research, national surveillance of oral diseases, safety of oral health workers, and mandated coverage of children's dental services under Medicaid. State policies affect domains such licensure and scope of practice of oral health personnel and facilities, support for public universities and oral health training programs, and level and mechanism of reimbursement for Medicaid services. Both federal and state environmental policies affect factors such as the manufacture, use, and disposal of dental materials. Local government policy affects factors such as community water fluoridation, zoning for health care facilities, and school health programs. It is worth mentioning that there are influences on policies in North America from global ministries such as the World Health Organization (WHO) with the Pan American Health Organization as the regional component for the Americas, and the United Nations Environment Programme (UNEP). For oral health issues the organizations involved include the Oral Health Programme at WHO (Headquarters in Geneva, Switzerland; http://www.who.int/oral_health/en/) and the Environment Program at UNEP (Headquarters in Nairobi, Kenya; http://www.unep.org/About/). Both have regional offices as well, in the Americas, Africa, eastern Mediterranean, Europe, southeast Asia, and western Pacific.

The development of a global health treaty, and hence global public policy, requires a detailed process and involvement from the members of the United Nations (UN) and WHO. For example, in this article, the UNEP initiated the policy development because the issue is based on environmental contamination that caused public health concerns from the global production, transport, and release of mercury in the environment. Numerous reports were generated to collect the scientifically valid evidence and a process to develop a legally binding instrument (LBI) with an intergovernmental negotiating committee (INC) established to prepare it (**Fig. 1**)[5]. The meetings of the INC are numbered to help follow the process; for example, the first meeting is INC1. When the LBI is generated it is reviewed by the global governmental representatives. A convention is held for the signing of the LBI, which is named after the convention, by the representatives. On agreement the representatives take the convention to their countries (parties) for approval, called ratification. On reaching 50 ratifications, the convention becomes a treaty to be enacted by the ratifying parties. The process is enhanced by regional and other subgroup meetings outside of the INC meetings. The LBI can be further modified during the process of ratification. Research archives on treaties can be found at http://research.un.org/en/docs/law/treaties. Details on the process

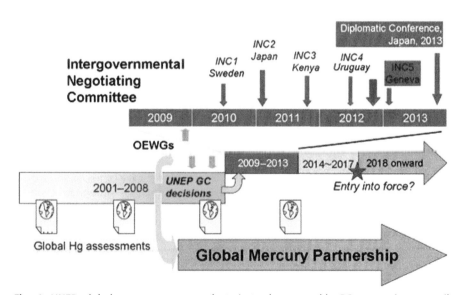

Fig. 1. UNEP global mercury program (a twin-track approach). GC, governing council; OEWG, open-ended working group. (*From* Bayne SC, Petersen PE, Piper D, et al. The challenge for innovation in direct restorative materials. Adv Dent Res 2013;25:12; with permission.)

(eg, of the Convention on the Rights of Persons with Disabilities) can be seen in the *Handbook for Parliamentarians on the Convention on the Rights of Persons with Disabilities* at http://www.un.org/disabilities/default.asp?id=212.

Regardless of the level of government, policy development is often the result of advocacy, input, analysis, and negotiation. Examples in the United States of resources on policy making and the importance of information to congress include a 2009 review by Stine,[29] and a focus in academic research is a 2015 thesis by Schneiderman.[30] UNEP has developed the Toolkit for Identification and Quantification of Mercury Releases to assist countries in undertaking such work. The toolkit is available at the UNEP Web address (www.chem.unep.ch/mercury/Toolkit/default.htm).

Policy Among Several Nongovernmental Stakeholders

Many organizations and institutions enact their own specific policies that reflect their goals, often with a set of supporting recommendations or actions on how to achieve them. Most major dental and public health organizations have a formal policy-making mechanism. Overviews of the major policy-making oral health organizations in the United States involved with the Minamata Convention are presented here.

The American Association for Dental Research (AADR) is a nonprofit organization with more than 3700 members in the United States. AADR's mission is to advance research and increase knowledge for the improvement of oral health, support and represent the oral health research community, and facilitate the communication and application of research findings (http://aadr.org/i4a/pages/index.cfm?pageid=3452#. Vp2I-fkrJdg). AADR currently has policy statements in effect and is heavily involved in advocacy at the federal level in support of its mission.

The ADA, the largest and oldest member organization representing dentists in the United States, with more than 158,000 members, enacts policy through the input of multiple levels of the organization. ADA's 11 councils serve as policy-recommending bodies within their specific areas of expertise. The House of Delegates (the 480-member governing and legislative body of the ADA representing the constituent [state] dental societies, the federal dental services, and dental students) has sole authority to formally enact policy for the association (ADA Constitution and Bylaws 2015; https://www.ada.org/~/media/ADA/Member%20Center/FIles/ADA_2015_Bylaws.ashx). The ADA currently has several hundred policies in effect, reflecting the organization's position on a wide range of topics relevant to oral health and safe practice of dentistry (http://www.ada.org/en/member-center/leadership-governance/~/media/1156718AF2E042D08AA6C3677A604C35.ashx). The ADA also seeks to influence public policy through advocacy and lobbying.

The American Public Health Association (APHA) champions the health of all people and communities (http://www.apha.org/about-apha). Health policy is a major focus of this organization, which is more than 140 years old and brings together more than 25,000 members from all fields of public health. Through its policy statement proposal process, the various components within APHA work together to establish formal evidence-based position statements on public health issues, which helps guide the organization's advocacy efforts and enables each community within the larger organization to leverage the capability and visibility of APHA to help achieve its goals. Policy statement proposals are voted on by the APHA Governing Council, the representative legislative body of the association. Successful policy statement proposals generally come about through collaboration and compromise because they must satisfy the goals and perspectives of the general public health community. APHA currently has approximately 1400 policy statements in effect (http://www.apha.org/policies-and-advocacy/public-health-policy-statements/policy-database). The APHA Oral Health

Section, with nearly 500 members, is one of 31 member sections within APHA, and, as part of a large, diverse public health organization, has unique opportunities to ensure an oral health perspective, as well as challenges when the perspectives within and among various sections and interest groups are not completely aligned, thus making collaboration, negotiation, and compromise key to advancing a dental public health agenda.

All 3 of these US-based organizations are major components in their respective international networks. The AADR is the largest division of the International Association for Dental Research (IADR), whose primary mission is to advance research and increase knowledge for the improvement of oral health worldwide (http://www.iadr.org/i4a/pages/index.cfm?pageid=3283#.Vp5QlvkrJdg). The ADA is the US National Dental Association member of the World Dental Federation (FDI), which represents the global dental profession to international, intergovernmental, governmental, voluntary, and other organizations (http://www.fdiworldental.org/about-fdi/mission/the-voice-of-dentistry.aspx#sthash.j8H5lgi7.dpuf). The APHA is a member of the World Federation of Public Health Associations (WFPHA), whose mission is to promote and protect global public health. The WFPHA is accredited as a nongovernmental organization (NGO) in official relations with the WHO (http://www.wfpha.org/about-wfpha).

Governmental Policy Development Specific to the Minamata Convention on Mercury

In parallel with other activities concerning environmental mercury, in 1997, the WHO held a consultation meeting on the use of dental amalgam.[4] The objective of this consultation was to provide more information to the member states. WHO Oral Health was requested to review again the WHO/FDI consensus statement and if necessary draft a relevant document on dental amalgam use, taking into account the benefits but also the risks for individual, occupational, and environmental health of restorative materials. The project was thoroughly scrutinized by the WHO Programmes on Environmental Health and Occupational Health.[4] The consensus statement on restorative dental care also emphasized the need for further research on alternatives to dental amalgam. These actions show that global attention to amalgam predates the Minamata Convention process.

In 2001, UNEP agreed to conduct a global assessment of mercury and its compounds, including information on the health effects, sources, long-range transport, prevention strategies, and control technologies, hence starting the process that led to the Minamata Convention. In 2003, significant evidence was published of large-scale global harm from mercury and its compounds, warranting further international action to reduce the risks to human health and the environment.

In 2009, the UNEP Governing Council mandated the development of a global LBI on mercury because it was determined that voluntary actions to control mercury waste were insufficient and that there was a need for an LBI. An INC was established to prepare an LBI on mercury (http://www.unep.org/chemicalsandwaste/Mercury/Reportsand Publications/GlobalMercuryAssessment/tabid/1060889/Default.aspx).

Also in 2009, the WHO Global Oral Health Program organized a meeting in Geneva, Switzerland, in cooperation with UNEP. From this meeting, a report on dental restorative materials concluded that dental amalgam is an effective restorative material. Consequently, the report *Future Use of Materials for Dental Restoration*[4] highlights the current scientific evidence on dental materials, including amalgam and nonamalgam restorative materials, and gathered information for future recommendations on the use of dental restorative materials, paying key attention to avoiding environmental pollution. The comprehensive review pointed out that existing alternative materials to dental amalgam are not ideal because of limitations in their durability, fracture resistance, and wear. The report also notes the widespread public health threat from any proposed or impending ban of dental amalgam. Long term, it was critically important for WHO, FDI, IADR, and national dental associations to increase global awareness about the importance of the relationship of oral health to general health and well-being by emphasizing the value of risk assessment, prevention, disease management, and minimal intervention care. Preventing and managing oral diseases diminishes the need to use amalgam and other restorative material alternatives.

During this 2009 WHO meeting, consideration was given to the importance of strengthening oral health promotion and disease prevention as the strategy to reduce the use of restorative dental materials. In the case of tooth decay, the best care possible should be provided to meet patients' needs. The meeting recognized the variation in dental practice among countries and the challenges faced by middle-income and low-income countries providing dental care, hence likely resulting in different approaches to dental caries management in different countries that need to be considered in oral health policy, training personnel, and development and planning of specific public health programs. It was noted that only a few countries, of high income, had initiatives to phase out the use of amalgam.

Among countries using amalgam, additional costs, especially if not part of their current systems, would be added by requiring systems for waste management to prevent environmental release of mercury to the environment. Following a review of existing evidence and much deliberation, the meeting recognized the huge challenges faced in dental restoration, disease prevention, and oral health promotion globally. As a result, the meeting considered that all currently existing methods and materials to manage dental caries need to remain available to dental professions in the short and medium terms.

Furthermore, the meeting noted that although alternative dental restorative materials may be desirable from an environmental health perspective, a progressive move away from dental amalgam would depend on adequate quality of these materials. Existing alternative dental materials are not ideal because of limitations in durability, fracture resistance, and wear resistance. Therefore, the meeting recognized the need for strengthening of research into the long-term performance, possible adverse effects, and viability of such materials.

Consideration of phasing down instead of targeting to phasing out dental amalgam arose at this 2009 WHO meeting. A multipronged approach with short-term, medium-term, and long-term strategies should be considered. Alternatives to dental amalgam exist but the quality of such materials needs to be further improved for use in public health care. The meeting suggested important strategies that can be put in place while waiting for new materials to be developed. The roles of WHO, UNEP, and NGOs such as the IADR and the FDI, user groups, and industry were seen as critical and it was decided that further meetings must be convened to discuss the way forward and to develop strategies to address issues in both developed and developing countries.

THE MINAMATA CONVENTION ON MERCURY

In January 2013, at the conclusion of INC5, the INC agreed on the text of what is now The Minamata Convention on Mercury. More than 750 participants attended that session, representing 137 governments, as well as 57 nongovernmental and 14 intergovernmental organizations. Hence, wording was agreed on by 147 nations.[31] Following a round of regional group meetings, delegates to the convention addressed several complex policy and technical issues, including mercury air emissions and releases to water and land, health aspects, and the phase-out (ban) and phase-down (limits and control) dates for specified products and processes.[32]

The Minamata Convention text[33] was formally adopted in Japan on the 10 October 2013 and was made available to countries for signature. The main objective of the Minamata Convention was to protect human health and the environment from anthropogenic emissions and releases of mercury and mercury compounds (www. mercuryconvention.org). The convention establishes a range of measures to control the supply and trade of mercury. It sets limitations on mercury sources, such as primary mining, small-scale gold mining, manufacturing processes, and mercury-added products.

The convention title of Minamata has historic and health significance. Minamata disease was first seen in Japan in 1956 at Minamata.[34] The illness is a form of severe methylmercury poisoning. Between 1932 and 1968, an industrial acetaldehyde plant released massive amounts of effluents containing methylmercury compounds into Minamata Bay and subsequently, into the Minamata River and the Shiranui Sea. The methylmercury bioaccumulated in the fish, shellfish, and the large marine life, which constituted much of the local diet. The mass exposure led to severe, chronic poisoning to more than 200,000 residents of the coastal areas.[34] Since the Minamata disaster, there has been a growing international awareness and need to control the anthropogenic sources of mercury.

Some of the key elements of the Minamata Convention were to control mercury by banning new mercury mines, phasing out of existing mines, controlling measures on air emissions and surface water releases, regulating artisanal and small-scale gold mining, and banning, phasing out, or limiting (phasing down) specified mercury-added products.[33] At the end of 2015 there were 128 nation signatures and 20 ratifications, and as this article goes to press at the end of March 2016 there are 25 ratifications (http://www.mercuryconvention.org/Countries/tabid/3428/Default.aspx). The convention shall enter on the ninetieth day after the date of deposit of the fiftieth instrument of ratification, acceptance, approval, or accession (article 31, item 1), which means that the convention will come into force as a treaty, once it has been ratified by 50 signatory countries. It becomes law in the ratifying countries only.

Coverage of Dental Amalgam in the Minamata Convention Process

Because dental amalgam contains mercury, its environmental impact was considered, debated, and addressed in the convention/treaty negotiations. In the initial draft, dental amalgam was included in the list of industrial mercury-added products to be phased out or banned. WHO Oral Health took the lead to create text to phase down the use of dental amalgam. With this input and collaborative efforts, it was agreed that dental amalgam use would be included as a phase-down, without a specific time frame. The statement is shown in **Box 1**.[33]

Coordinated efforts by parties described later led to the separation of dental amalgam for phase-down considerations rather than the general phase-out. Although there are 9 provisions in the Minamata Convention for phasing down dental amalgam,[33] to be compliant with the convention wording, governments do not need to adopt all of the provisions but must implement at least 2 of these provisions. The wording was designed to allow significant flexibility to account for local circumstances. This flexibility means that each country has options to comply with it as a treaty in its own unique way.

Throughout the process the FDI/ADA and IADR representatives conducted multiple meetings with the US and other national delegations. FDI and IADR representatives presented formal, scientifically based interventions throughout the negotiations. The

---

Box 1
Provisions from the Minamata Convention on Mercury for dental amalgam

Measures to be taken by a party to phase down the use of dental amalgam shall take into account the party's domestic circumstances and relevant international guidance and shall include 2 or more of the measures from the following list:

1. Setting national objectives for dental caries prevention and health promotion, thereby minimizing the need for dental restoration

2. Setting national objectives for minimizing its use

3. Promoting the use of cost-effective and clinically effective mercury-free alternatives for dental restoration

4. Promoting research and development of quality, mercury-free materials for dental restoration

5. Encouraging representative professional organizations and dental schools to educate and train dental professionals and students on the use of mercury-free dental restoration alternatives and on promoting best management practices

6. Discouraging insurance policies and programs that favor dental amalgam use rather than mercury-free dental restoration

7. Encouraging insurance policies and programs that favor the use of quality alternatives to dental amalgam for dental restoration

8. Restricting the use of dental amalgam to its encapsulated form

9. Promoting the use of best environmental practices in dental facilities to reduce releases of mercury and mercury compounds to water and land

From Minamata Convention on Mercury: texts and annexes. 2013. Available at: http://www.mercuryconvention.org/Portals/11/documents/Booklets/Minamata%20Convention%20on%20Mercury_booklet_English.pdf. Accessed April 7, 2016; with permission.

---

verbal and written statements were designed to protect the environment and to safeguard oral health care, eliminating the risk that an amalgam ban would slip through the treaty negotiations without a thorough vetting.[35] WHO emphasized the importance of strengthening dental caries prevention, which would contribute to reducing the need for any restorative dental care. The WHO Oral Health, FDI/ADA, IADR, International Dental Manufacturers (IDM), and other respected health care organizations were aligned in principle on supporting prevention efforts and advocating for research to develop safe and effective alternative treatment options. Dentistry collectively argued against a ban and in favor of a public health (prevention) approach to the issue. A concerted effort to focus on preventing dental disease, combined with responsible handling of amalgam waste and funding for research for alternative materials would reduce the use of amalgam (and limit its environmental impact) and promote public health.

American Dental Association Involvement with Expertise and Advocacy

The ADA actively participated in the UNEP INC process since its launch in 2009. Although the ADA did not have a formalized, NGO relationship with UNEP, the ADA was involved in providing its scientific acumen as representative members of the FDI and the IADR delegations. In addition, the ADA worked closely with the US State Department, the EPA, and the US Food and Drug Administration (FDA) to inform those who did not fully understand the negative public health impact that would result from banning a safe and cost-effective dental restorative material.

The ADA helped to inform the US delegation during those meetings about the positions that were advocated for by the WHO, ADA, FDI, IADR, organized dentistry, and its stakeholders.[35,36]

From the beginning of the UNEP INC process, the ADA responded to the possibility that the INC political process would interfere with the doctor-patient relationship. Issues were immediately raised by national dental associations throughout the world about government representatives who did not understand the oral health consequences that would result from banning or limiting the use of safe and effective dental restorative materials. In response to those concerns, the ADA worked with the FDI and IADR to advocate on behalf of the public and the profession about the potentially negative public health impact that could result from a ban on dental amalgam, both in the United States and throughout the world. ADA representatives to the FDI and the IADR delegations provided professional expertise and regulatory guidance to work in tandem with the WHO to help make clear to government delegations participating in the INC meetings that dental amalgam should not be equated or confused with elemental mercury, inorganic mercury, or organic mercury compounds.

The ADA provided extensive scientific evidence on its Web site, ADA.org, from well-designed laboratory and clinical studies from numerous health care organizations, including the US Centers for Disease Control and Prevention, FDA, WHO, and FDI. The professional organizations were in agreement that dental amalgam is a safe and effective cavity-filling material. Other science-based professional organizations, such as the Alzheimer's Association, American Academy of Pediatrics, Autism Society of America, and National Multiple Sclerosis Society, also made clear that dental amalgam does not create adverse health conditions or cause identifiable diseases (http://www.ada.org/en/press-room/press-kits/dental-fillings-press-kit/dental-amalgam-what-others-say).

As clearly stated by the FDA, although high levels of exposure to elemental mercury have been associated with adverse health effects, the levels released by dental amalgam fillings are not high enough to cause harm in patients (http://www.fda.gov/MedicalDevices/ProductsandMedicalProcedures/DentalProducts/DentalAmalgam/ucm171094.htm). Consistent with the EPA's position, the Scientific Committee of the European Commission also addressed safety concerns for patients, professionals, and the use of alternative restorative materials. The committee independently concluded that dental amalgams are effective and safe, both for patients and dental personnel, and also noted that alternative materials have clinical limitations and toxicologic hazards (http://ec.europa.eu/health/scientific_committees/consultations/public_consultations/scenihr_consultation_24_en.htm).

The ADA followed through with letters to the US State Department, reiterating its evidence-based scientific rationale[37] to promote health and address environmental concerns. In addition to the ADA, several US professional organizations sent letters to the State Department expressing their respective evidence-based views on dental amalgam in support of protecting the public's health. The Academy of General Dentistry, American Academy of Pediatric Dentistry, American Academy of Periodontology, American Association of Oral and Maxillofacial Surgeons, American Association of Orthodontists, and the Hispanic Dental Association all expressed their concerns. The US Association of State and Territorial Dental Directors also supported the unique opportunity to implement an oral health care model, based on disease prevention, health promotion, and materials science research. These congruent measures have helped to ensure optimal oral health, particularly for the most disadvantaged patients in need of dental care in the United States and throughout the world.

International Association for Dental Research Involvement as Facilitator and Science Advocate

In addition to partnering with the FDI, ADA, IDM, and the WHO Oral Health Programme, IADR made substantive contributions to the 2009 WHO and UNEP meeting on *Future Use of Materials for Dental Restoration.*[4] In 2010, the IADR was accepted into the UNEP Global Mercury Partnership. IADR shared the overall goal of the UNEP partnership, which was "to protect human health and the global environment from the release of mercury and its compounds by minimizing and, where feasible, ultimately eliminating global, anthropogenic mercury releases to air, water and land.[4]"

IADR hosted and published the proceedings of the Dental Materials Innovation Workshop (DMIW), which took place December 10 to 11, 2012, at King's College London. The meeting was sponsored by IADR, WHO, UNEP, FDI, and King's College London Dental Institute. The proceedings are published in the November 2013 issue of the IADR/AADR *Advances in Dental Research,*[38] an E-supplement to the *Journal of Dental Research.* The DMIW was timed as part of IADR's commitment to the UNEP Global Mercury Partnership and as an NGO participant in the UNEP negotiations to develop the Minamata Convention on Mercury.

The IADR participated in the UNEP negotiations along with the FDI, the ADA, and the IDM. Working as a team, the dental NGOs advocated that a phase-down of dental amalgam was only possible with enhancement of dental prevention, further research on suitable alternatives, and the use of best management practices for dental amalgam waste. Those provisions are largely intact in the signed convention.

World Federation of Public Health Associations/American Public Health Association

As an accredited NGO in official relations with the WHO, the WFPHA collaborates with the WHO to advance public health through the promotion of prohealth policies, strategies, and best practices around the world. The federation also holds consultation status with the UN Economic and Social Council (http://www.wfpha.org/about-wfpha). In April 2012, the WFPHA general assembly and council approved the establishment of the WFPHA Oral Health Working Group (OHWG; http://www.wfpha.org/oral-health-wg#the-working-group). Around this same time, the OHWG and the Oral Health (OH) Section of APHA became aware of a WFPHA letter signed by the Environmental Workgroup calling for the deliberate phase-out and ban of dental amalgam. The letter was aligned with the release of a June 2012 report authored by nondental professionals involving the Chair of the WFPHA Environmental Workgroup and member of the Occupational Health and Safety (OHS) Section of APHA. The WFPHA letter and report supported language in early drafts of the Minamata Convention for dental amalgam to be included on the list of industrial mercury-added products to be phased out or banned.

The OH Section of APHA immediately mobilized and strategically prepared a policy proposal statement for the preservation and phase-down of dental amalgam, which was submitted as a late-breaker policy statement at the APHA annual meeting in October, 2012. *Dental Amalgam—Preserving a Proven Dental Material* was thus passed, but with challenges from members of the OHS Section and the Environment (ENV) Section. The writers of the OH Section policy reached out to the Policy Committee Chairs of both the OHS Section and ENV Section in an effort to address their concerns and find common ground. When the language of the Minamata Convention was accepted (January 2013), including language for the phase-down of amalgam, further discussions occurred, including a face-to-face meeting at the 2013 APHA annual session that led to an agreement to work together. In January 2014, via conference call, it was decided that because all sections were in agreement with the language of the Minamata Convention, that the sections would accept that language. Subsequently, the OH Section of APHA arranged for there to be an OHS speaker at an April 2014 dental public health conference, where there was also a roundtable presentation on the Minamata Convention and its meaning to dentistry. In addition, an interprofessional invited speaker panel session, The Minamata Convention on Mercury: Implications for the Environment, Occupational Health and Dental Public Health, was held at the November 2014 APHA annual meeting.

SUBSEQUENT DENTAL ACTIVITIES

Government authorities and dental stakeholders will need to continue to work together to address the complexity of barriers that must be overcome to develop a new cost-effective material that replaces dental amalgam. Researchers and clinicians need to work in harmony to sort through the complexities of regulatory approval, intellectual property rights, distribution challenges, educational models, creating state-of-the-art information, and transferring skills to the workforce. Inconsistent national and international regulatory systems often create seemingly insurmountable demands on dental manufacturers.[39] Translating novel research products into clinical practice creates educational challenges for dental students, providers, and the dental workforce, which are ongoing concerns.

In April 2015, a European review by the Scientific Committee on Health and Environmental Risks of the environmental impact of dental amalgam confirmed that, when suitable precautions are provided, dental amalgam does not pose a significant risk.[6] Precautions include using amalgam separators and appropriate waste disposal.

The ADA and national dental associations working through the FDI have passed resolutions and policies, affirming that the signing of a globally binding treaty on the use of mercury is a sensible outcome that recognizes the practicalities of improving oral health globally. For many years, numerous recognized health care organizations have stressed the importance of avoiding a complete phase-out of the use of mercury in dentistry, particularly in a short time frame, without an adequate substitute for dental amalgam. The FDI's General Assembly approved policies to ensure that flexible approaches are available to take into account each country's domestic circumstances. The FDI encourages national policies by member associations to phase down dental amalgam, as well as devoting more resources to promote prevention; appropriately funded health care systems; materials science research; and the production of accurate, peer-reviewed information on the efficacy of all dental materials. The ADA, FDI, and IADR continue to seek a balance between being good stewards to sustain a safe environment and the use of amalgam or advanced non–mercury-based materials to promote oral health and well-being.

World Dental Federation: Implementation Plan

The FDI, with the support of the IADR, IDM, national dental associations, and dental stakeholders, created a series of education and advocacy initiatives to protect and maintain public health gains, improve oral health worldwide, and strengthen environmental stewardship through sound lifecycle management approaches.[40] National dental associations, including the ADA and the AADR, took roles in providing critical expertise to inform governments on the opportunities to improve health and protect the environment, consistent with objectives of the Minamata Convention, without compromising the professional roles of providers being able to deliver safe, effective, and affordable oral health care.

Publications and guidance for understanding and achieving the goals of the Minamata Convention from the FDI are listed in **Box 2**.[40–44] The FDI documents are intended to supply information to national dental associations, providers, patients, government officials, and media on the provisions, responsibilities, and commitments of the Minamata Convention on Mercury.

Role of Dentists and Dental Teams Regarding Implementation

In support of the Minamata Convention, providers are reminded to integrate the following into their clinical practices.[43,45–48] As members of the dental and medical professions, there are shared responsibilities to meet the objectives of the convention in order to protect human health and the environment from anthropogenic emissions and releases of mercury. These issues are not new to dental practitioners, with Hiltz's[49] discussion in 2007 providing an example. The impact of the convention is not limited to amalgam, but includes other health care equipment, such as thermometers and sphygmomanometers, that are to be phased out. WHO has provided guidance on national strategies for compliance.[50]

Given that amalgam may sometimes be the best choice, or the only option, for effectively restoring carious posterior teeth, the WHO, FDI, IADR, IDM, ADA, APHA, and EPA fully support the proper handling of dental amalgam, amalgam separation technologies, and the recycling of mercury waste. It is anticipated that coordinated implementation of the obligations of the convention will lead to an overall reduction in mercury levels in the environment over time.

Dentists should discuss all dental restorative options with their patients. There is no universal alternative or one-size-fits-all restorative material that matches amalgam's characteristics. The chemical, biological, and environmental effects of any restorative material need to be considered by both dentists and patients. Dentists and patients must also consider involvement in support of dental research for optimal dental materials and disease prevention. Although this current focus is on the fate of amalgam waste, it is likely that the impact of waste from all dental materials will be evaluated

---

Box 2
Publications and guidance for understanding and achieving the goals of the Minamata Convention available from the FDI

- FDI policy statement: dental amalgam and the Minamata Convention on Mercury[40]: http://www.fdiworldental.org/media/55201/6-fdi_ps-dental_amalgam_and_minamata_adopted_gab_2014.pdf

- Use and future use of materials for dental restoration – FDI advocacy toolkit[41]: http://www.fdiworldental.org/media/9450/use_of_materials_english.pdf

- Dental restorative materials and the Minamata Convention on Mercury – guidelines for successful implementation[42]: http://www.fdiworldental.org/media/54670/minamata-convention_fdi-guidelines-for-successful-implementation.pdf

- Understanding the Minamata Convention and its effect upon oral health care – practical advice for dentists[43]: http://www.fdiworldental.org/media/67938/minamata-convention_practical-advice-for-dentists.pdf

- FDI vision 2020 – shaping the future of oral health[44]: http://www.fdiworldental.org/media/12308/idj_vision_2020_editorial.pdf and http://www.fdiworldental.org/media/12303/idj_vision_2020_final.pdf

in more detail in the future.[51] Amalgam separators significantly reduce particulate mercury in wastewater effluent. However, separators are unlikely to capture nanoparticles or chemicals, such as bisphenol A, from resin composites or other dental materials.[20,21,52] There is only limited information available on the ultimate fate and environmental impact of these particles and chemicals.[5] The identified waste products from dental amalgam need to be kept in the proper context in consideration of the unknown and potentially adverse consequences from other dental restorative materials.[53,54]

Dental caries remains a global burden that extends far beyond the destruction of hard tooth structure. The Minamata Convention clearly highlights the important role of disease management within any oral health care strategy, but it was not designed to reverse the progression of past dental diseases. There will always be a public health need for dental materials to restore dentitions and maintain public health. Dental caries causes pain, suffering, and compromised health, and results in economic burdens to individuals, governments, and third parties. The costs for providing definitive treatment far exceed the resources to prevent disease.

Recent global trends have generally shown a decline in caries in many developed countries, whereas, in the same time frame, there has been a dramatic increase in some developing countries. These trends largely reflect changes in dietary patterns, including increased and more frequent consumption of sugar.[1] Dental teams have an important role to help their patients and communities understand that adopting healthier behaviors leads to improved health and well-being. Each member of the dental team has an opportunity to participate in programs designed to increase oral health literacy in their communities. Public health education programs for the community should be tailored in consideration of individual risk factors and needs.

SUMMARY

The Minamata Convention is the first major international treaty-level effort to identify dentistry and its global public health leadership role advocating for preventive programs, clinical care, and dental research, albeit from the context of environmental mercury release. Crucial roles were played by the dental stakeholders during the negotiations to balance the need to protect the environment and best management practices, together with the responsibility to support quality oral health care. The convention includes a full range of forward-thinking provisions to advance oral health care as well as to help protect the environment. These provisions include oral health promotion through risk assessment and disease prevention, dental materials research, and guidelines for best management practices to limit amalgam waste. The profession of dentistry has responsibilities and roles that could not bo ropro sented by others in the process of this policy development designed for overall health.

Protecting the environment while reducing the need for dental restorations will lead to improved access to care and, ultimately, significant improvements in health and well-being for all populations. As new dental restorative materials are developed, it will be necessary for policy makers to realize that no restorative material is entirely free of risk. Meeting the challenges to develop a cost-effective alternative to replace dental amalgam provides the dental profession with a unique opportunity to work collaboratively to drive global innovation for the development of advanced research, preventive techniques, and advanced restorative materials.

The Minamata Convention is an example of the requisite levels of expertise, communications, collaboration, cooperation, and commitment that are necessary to develop relevant and meaningful interprofessional policies that can have a significant impact on dentistry. It is hoped that the Minamata Convention helps to show that, although such issues may seem to arise rapidly and without warning, dentistry must be poised as an informed, understanding, knowledgeable, organized, and effective advocate to ensure that expert oral health professionals are able to provide an optimal, positive impact from the onset.

The dental profession must be prepared to fully participate in interprofessional collaborations with all stakeholders and build on such experiences to effectively address current and future public health demands and needs. Examples of several other existing areas undergoing policy development and implementation policy are discussed in this issue and include at the institutional and accreditation levels for interprofessional education[55]; emergency response[56]; genetics[57]; and affordable, appropriate, and accessible health care, including oral health care.[58–64] Appropriate use of antibiotics, although not included in this issue, is another important topic warranting interprofessional collaboration on policy.[65–67]

The oral health community has responsibilities in interprofessional policy development that affect the general and oral health of the public. Dentistry must ensure that it is involved in scientifically based responses, with recognized expertise and advocacy, albeit without governmental standing. Professional dental organizations can work to optimally respond, find common ground, and cooperate regarding complicated interprofessional health issues. Establishing interprofessional partnerships enables collaboration on health issues and helps ensure that those outside of dentistry understand the importance of oral health. The development of the Minamata Convention on Mercury showed the significance of the commitment by oral health stakeholders, sustained longevity of effort, science-based evidence, understanding of policy development ranging from local to global levels, and the dental profession working effectively in interprofessional collaborations.

ACKNOWLEDGMENTS

The authors with to thank the AADR, ADA, APHA, FDI, IADR, WFPHA, and their constituencies for the work they do towards optimal oral and general health for all.

REFERENCES

1. Petersen PE. The World Health Report 2003: Continuous improvement of oral health in the 21st century – the approach of the WHO Global Oral Health Programme. Community Dent Oral Epidemiol 2003;31(Supp 1):3–24.
2. UNEP. Global mercury assessment 2013: sources, emissions, releases and environmental transport. Geneva (Switzerland): UNEP DTIE Chemicals Branch; 2013. Available at: http://www.unep.org/PDF/PressReleases/GlobalMercury Assessment2013.pdf.
3. UNEP. List of alternatives to mercury-added products. 2008. Available at: http://www.unep.org/chemicalsandwaste/Portals/9/Mercury/Products/flyer%20final1% 20%20mercury-free%20alternatives.pdf. Accessed January 4, 2016.
4. Petersen PE. (2010) Future use of materials for dental restoration: report of the meeting convened at WHO HA. Geneva, Switzerland, November 16–17, 2009.
5. Bayne SC, Petersen PE, Piper D, et al. The challenge for innovation in direct restorative materials. Adv Dent Res 2013;25:8–17.
6. SCENIHR (Scientific Committee on Health and Environmental Risks). Opinion on the safety of dental amalgam and alternative dental restoration materials for patients and users. Opinion adopted April 29, 2015. Available

at: http://ec.europa.eu/health/scientific_committees/emerging/docs/scenihr_o_046.pdf. Accessed March 20, 2016.

7. Hyson JM Jr. Amalgam: its history and perils. J Calif Dent Assoc 2006;34:215–29.
8. Mackert JR, Wahl MJ. Are there acceptable alternatives to amalgam? J Calif Dent Assoc 2004;32:601–10.
9. Jones DW. A Scandinavian tragedy. Br Dent J 2008;204:233–4.
10. Hancocks SA. Quick silver problem; slower reactions. Br Dent J 2008;204:593.
11. DeRouen TA, Martin MD, Leroux BG, et al. Neurobehavioral effects of dental amalgam in children: a randomized clinical trial. JAMA 2006;295(15):1784–92.
12. Bellinger DC, Trachenberg F, Barregard L, et al. Neuropsychological and renal effects of dental amalgam in children: a randomized clinical trial. JAMA 2006; 295(15):1775–83.
13. BIO Intelligence Service. Study on the potential for reducing mercury pollution from dental amalgam and batteries. Final report prepared for the European Commission – DG ENV. 2012. Available at: http://ec.europa.eu/environment/chemicals/mercury/pdf/final_report_110712.pdf. Accessed March 20, 2016.
14. Parliamentary Assembly of the Council of Europe. Resolution 1816: health hazards of heavy metals and other metals – (Rapporteur: Jean Huss, Doc. 12613, text adopted by the Standing Committee, acting on behalf of the assembly, on 27 May 2011). Available at: http://assembly.coe.int/nw/xml/XRef/Xref-XML2HTML-en.asp?fileid=12818&lang=en. Accessed February 28, 2016.
15. Vandeven JA, McGinnis SL. An assessment of mercury in the form of amalgam in dental wastewater in the United States. Water Air Soil Pollut 2005;164:349–66.
16. American Dental Association. Summary of Recent study of dental amalgam in wastewater, August 5, 2005. Available at: http://www.ada.org/~/media/ADA/Member%20Center/FIles/topics_amalgamwaste_summary.pdf?la=en. Accessed April 6, 2016.
17. US Environmental Protection Agency. Effluent guidelines. Available at: https://www.epa.gov/eg and dental amalgam effluent guideline. Available at: http://www.epa.gov/eg/dental-effluent-guidelines. Accessed April 6, 2016.
18. US Environmental Protection Agency. Summary of the Clean Water Act. Available at: http://www.epa.gov/laws-regulations/summary-clean-water-act. Accessed April 6, 2016.
19. American Dental Association. Amalgam waste best management. Available at: http://www.ada.org/en/member-center/oral-health-topics/amalgam-waste-best-management. Accessed April 6, 2016.
20. Fan PL, Batchu H, Chou HN, et al. Laboratory evaluation of amalgam separators. J Am Dent Assoc 2002;133:577–84.
21. Chou HN, Anglen J. An evaluation of amalgam separators. J Am Dent Assoc 2012;143:920–1.
22. AMAP/UNEP, 2013. Technical Background Report for the Global Mercury Assessment 2013. Arctic Monitoring and Assessment Programme, Oslo, Norway/UNEP Chemicals Branch, Geneva, Switzerland. vi+ 263 pp. Available at: http://www.amap.no/documents/doc/Technical-Background-Report-for-the-Global-Mercury-Assessment-2013/848. Accessed July 11, 2016.
23. Soncini JA, Maserejian NN, Trachtenberg F, et al. The longevity of amalgam versus compomer/composite restorations in posterior primary and permanent teeth: findings from the New England Children's Amalgam Trial. J Am Dent Assoc 2007;138(6):763–72.
24. Kovarik RE. Restoration of posterior teeth in clinical practice: Evidence base for choosing amalgam versus composite. Dent Clin North Am 2009;53:71–6.

25. Chadwick BL, Dummer PM, Dunstan FD, et al. What type of filling? Best practice in dental restorations. Qual Health Care 1999;8:202–7.
26. Roulet JF. Benefits and disadvantages of tooth-coloured alternatives to amalgam. J Dent 1997;25:459–73.
27. Tobi H, Kreulen CM, Vondeling H, et al. Cost-effectiveness of composite resins and amalgam in the replacement of amalgam class II restorations. Community Dent Oral Epidemiol 1999;27:137–43.
28. Beazoglou T, Eklund S, Heffley D, et al. Economic impact of regulating the use of amalgam restorations. Public Health Rep 2007;122(5):657–63.
29. Stine DD. Science and technology policymaking: a primer. Congressional Research Service; 2009. Available at: http://www.fas.org/sgp/crs/misc/RL34454.pdf. Accessed July 11, 2016.
30. Schneiderman G. Determinants of science policy change and the need for reform in congressional decision-making and political science research. 2015. Undergraduate Honors Theses. Paper 987. Available at: http://scholar.colorado.edu/honr_theses/987. Accessed February 28, 2016.
31. Fifth session of the intergovernmental negotiating committee to prepare a global legally binding instrument on mercury (INC 5). Available at: http://www.mercuryconvention.org/Negotiations/INC5/tabid/3439/Default.aspx. Accessed April 7, 2016.
32. Intergovernmental negotiating committee to prepare a global legally binding instrument on mercury. Report of the intergovernmental negotiating committee to prepare a global legally binding instrument on mercury on the work of its fifth session. Geneva/UNEP. Distributed March 14, 2013. Available at: http://www.unep.org/hazardoussubstances/Portals/9/Mercury/Documents/INC5/5_7_REPORT_ADVANCE.pdf. Accessed April 7, 2016.
33. Minamata Convention on Mercury: texts and annexes. October 10, 2013. Available at: http://www.mercuryconvention.org/Portals/11/documents/Booklets/Minamata%20Convention%20on%20Mercury_booklet_English.pdf. Accessed April 7, 2016.
34. Hachiya N. The history and the present of Minamata Disease – Entering the second half of a century. Japan Med Assoc J 2006;49(3):112–8.
35. Hancocks SA. A sense of place. Br Dent J 2013;214(3):91 [Reprinted: A sense of place. J Am Dent Assoc 144:349-350].
36. Meyer DM. ADA advocates for public health in UN discussion. J Am Dent Assoc 2013;144(4):350–1.
37. US Environmental Protection Agency (2008). Memorandum of understanding on reducing dental amalgam discharges. Available at: http://www.epa.gov/sites/production/files/2015-06/documents/reducing-dental-amalgam-discharges-mou-dec-2008.pdf. Accessed April 7, 2016.
38. Rekow ED. IADR Dental Materials Innovation Workshop. Adv Dent Res 2013;25:1–48.
39. Rekow ED, Bayne SC, Carvalho RM, et al. What constitutes an ideal dental restorative material? Adv Dent Res 2013;25:18–23.
40. FDI policy statement: Dental amalgam and the Minamata Convention on Mercury. Available at: http://www.fdiworldental.org/media/55201/6-fdi_ps-dental_amalgam_and_minamata_adopted_gab_2014.pdf. Accessed January 4, 2016.
41. Use and future use of materials for dental restoration – FDI advocacy toolkit. Available at: http://www.fdiworldental.org/media/9450/use_of_materials_english.pdf. Accessed January 4, 2016.

42. Dental restorative materials and the Minamata Convention on Mercury – guidelines for successful implementation. Available at: http://www.fdiworldental.org/media/54670/minamata-convention_fdi-guidelines-for-successful-implementation.pdf. Accessed January 4, 2016.

43. Understanding the Minamata Convention and its effect upon oral health care – practical advice for dentists. Available at: http://www.fdiworldental.org/media/67938/minamata-convention_practical-advice-for-dentists.pdf. Accessed January 4, 2016.

44. FDI vision 2020 – shaping the future of oral health. Available at: http://www.fdiworldental.org/media/12308/idj_vision_2020_editorial.pdf and Available at: http://www.fdiworldental.org/media/12303/idj_vision_2020_final.pdf. Accessed January 4, 2016.

45. American Dental Association. Best management practices. 2007. Available at: http://www.ada.org/~/media/ADA/Member%20Center/FIles/topics_amalgamwaste_brochure.ashx. Accessed January 4, 2016.

46. UNEP module 4 mercury use in healthcare settings and dentistry. 2008. Available at: http://www.unep.org/hazardoussubstances/Portals/9/Mercury/AwarenessPack/English/UNEP_Mod4_UK_Web.pdf. Accessed January 4, 2016.

47. American Dental Association. Best management practices. 2016. Available at: http://www.ada.org/1540.aspx. Accessed January 4, 2016.

48. ADA. Best practices in waste management. 2007. Available at: http://www.ada.org/~/media/ADA/Member%20Center/FIles/topics_amalgamwaste_brochure.ashx. Accessed April 7, 2016.

49. Hiltz M. The environmental impact of dentistry. J Can Dent Assoc 2007;73(1):59–62. Available at: http://www.cda-adc.ca/jcda/vol-73/issue-1/59.html. Accessed April 6, 2016.

50. WHO. Developing national strategies for phasing out mercury-containing thermometers and sphygmomanometers in health care, including in the context of the Minamata Convention on Mercury: key considerations and step-by-step guidance. Geneva (Switzerland): World Health Organization; 2015.

51. Schmalz G, Arenholt-Bindslev D. Biocompatibility of dental materials. Berlin; Heidelberg: Springer; 2009.

52. The International Organization for Standardization. Dentistry — Amalgam separators. ISO 11143:2008. Geneva, Switzerland. Available at: http://www.iso.org/iso/iso_catalogue/catalogue_tc/catalogue_detail.htm?csnumber=42288. Accessed July 11, 2016

53. Joskow R, Barr JR, Calafat AM, et al. Exposure to bisphenol A from bis-glycidyl dimethacrylate-based dental sealants. J Am Dent Assoc 2006;137:353–62.

54. Van Landuyt KL, Yoshihara K, Geebelen B, et al. Should we be concerned about composite (nano-) dust? Dent Mater 2012;28:1162–70.

55. Gordon SC, Donoff RB. Problems and Solutions for Interprofessional Education in North American Dental Schools. Dent Clin North Am 2016;60(4):811–24.

56. Colvard MD. Dentistry's role in disaster response: preface. Dent Clin North Am 2007;52(4):xv–xvii.

57. Regier DS, Hart TC. Genetics: The future is now with interprofessional collaboration. Dent Clin Am 2016;60(4):943–9.

58. Southerland JH, Webster-Cyriaque J, Bednarsh H. Interprofessional collaborative Practice models in Chronic Disease management. Dent Clin North Am 2016;60(4):789–809.

59. Shaefer J, Barreveld AM, Arnstein P, et al. Interprofessional education for the dentist in managing acute and chronic pain. Dent Clin Am 2016;60(4):825–42.
60. Glassman P, Harrington M, Namakian M, et al. Interprofessional collaboration in improving oral health for special populations. Dent Clin Am 2016;60(4):843–55.
61. Farmer-Dixon Thompson M, Young D, et al. Interprofessional collaborative practice: an oral health paradigm for women. Dent Clin Am 2016;60(4):857–77.
62. Russell SL, More F. Addressing health disparities via coordination of care and interprofessional education: Lesbian, gay, bisexual, and transgender health and oral health care. Dent Clin Am 2016;60(4):891–906.
63. Kaufman LB, Henshaw MM, Brown BP, et al. Oral health and interprofessional collaborative practice: Examples of the team approach to geriatric care. Dent Clin Am 2016;60(4):879–990.
64. Joskow RW. Integrating oral health and primary care: Federal initiatives to drive systems change. Dent Clin Am 2016;60(4):951–68.
65. Busfield J. Assessing the overuse of medicines. Soc Sci Med 2015;131:199–206.
66. Cope AL, Chestnutt IG, Wood F, et al. Dental consultations in UK general practice and antibiotic prescribing rates: a retrospective cohort study. Br J Gen Pract 2016;66(646):e329–36.
67. US Centers for Disease Control and Prevention. Get smart: know when antibiotics work. Available at: http://www.cdc.gov/getsmart/community/. Accessed April 7, 2016.

Genetics

The Future Is Now with Interprofessional Collaboration

Debra S. Regier, MD, PhD[a], Thomas C. Hart, DDS, PhD[b],*

KEYWORDS

- Interprofessional relations • Genetics • Dentistry • Patient care • Health
- Oral health • Medical genetics • Genetic counseling

KEY POINTS

- Application of genetic knowledge to clinical practice is an essential part of interprofessional collaborative practice.
- Interprofessional teams are required to optimize the implementation of genetic technology and information to the total health needs of patients.
- Interprofessional communication improves optimal care for all patients because of the common language among health care providers.
- Opportunities for genetic education as part of an interprofessional team approach are essential for not only oral health care providers but all health care providers.

INTRODUCTION

Given the growing complexity of health care, there is an increasing need for a collaborative approach among all health care providers in providing effective patient care.[1,2] Interprofessional communication and collaboration are especially essential in the combined use of genetic analyses/counseling and how specific genotypes/phenotypes manifest poor oral health outcomes. However, dental clinicians often do not have appropriate training to interact with genetics teams in terms of proper consulting strategies, and often genetic counselors are not fully aware of oral manifestations of genetic diseases. As such, there is a growing need for more effective strategies of communication and collaboration between the two disciplines. In addition, patients or their representatives face the challenge of communicating between the two clinical

[a] Genetics and Metabolism, Children's National Health System, 111 Michigan Avenue, NW Washington, DC 20010, USA; [b] Volpe Research Center, 100 Bureau Drive, Stop 8546, Building 224, Room A-153, NIST, Gaithersburg, MD 20899, USA
* Corresponding author.
E-mail address: Thomas.hart@NIST.gov

Dent Clin N Am 60 (2016) 943–949
http://dx.doi.org/10.1016/j.cden.2016.03.005
0011-8532/16/$ – see front matter © 2016 Elsevier Inc. All rights reserved.

advocates. A lack of an integrated health care record, and separate billing and reimbursement programs, compound the difficulties of getting appropriate clinical care.

Dental education in the United States has traditionally developed along the independent health educational paradigm.[3] The training of students within independent and isolated educational systems contributes to poor communication and inadequate collaboration among clinicians in distinct health disciplines. This situation can result in poor, and in some cases inadequate, patient care in areas that span traditional care areas of health disciplines. This is evident in the emerging field of clinical genetics. Dentists often do not receive training in human genetics and are not prepared to interpret new developments[4] that may support previous observations.[5] The advent of sequencing the human genome has resulted in genetic testing, including some offered direct to consumers and direct to consumers through clinicians, which has created challenges to health care professionals in general[6] because many developments have surpassed clinical training. Challenges include whether genetic testing is available for certain conditions as well as whether the genetic tests offered are valid and useful.[7] In many cases, determination of the clinical validity and utility of genetic testing requires experts from different disciplines. The need for dentists to collaborate interprofessionally is clearly shown in genetics.[8] This article describes an innovative model for integrating genetic counseling and how it applies to the oral and overall health of patients within an interprofessional collaborative practice setting by using a case approach.

AN INTERPROFESSIONAL CASE STUDY OF GENETICS IN HEALTH CARE
Dental Student

A third year dental student is seeing a new patient in her community clinic. Her 14-year-old patient, Sarah, was brought to the clinic by her mother who is concerned that Sarah still has some of her baby teeth, whereas her younger sister has her permanent teeth. The dental student takes a panoramic radiograph and informs Sarah and her mother that Sarah has oligodontia (congenital absence of some of the teeth), because she is missing several molar teeth as well as all eight premolar teeth. The student discusses:

1. The need to wait to do dental implants until Sarah's jaw is more fully formed.
2. Other restorative options to ensure that she has minimal issues with esthetics and function within her oral cavity.

Sarah's mother comments that other relatives also have missing teeth, and says that she is worried that Sarah will die like her grandfather and his mother of colon cancer, because everyone in the family without all their teeth seem to die of cancer. Not knowing how to respond, the dental student reassures her that her teeth can be treated, and advises her not to worry about things that happen to older family members.

That night, the student has a nagging feeling that she gave her patient the wrong information. She therefore uses Google to check for more information. She searches on "oligodontia AND colon cancer." The first three listings are for genetic changes associated with the combination of oligodontia and colon cancer. The next day, she discusses the case with her preceptor and realizes that she needs help to give the best information to this patient. They discuss her next step and it is decided that they should find a clinical geneticist. The preceptor does not know of one, so the student decides to try to find one. She goes back to Google and enters "How to find a geneticist" and an entry from the National Library of Medicine and the American College of Medical Genetics and

Genomics are the first two links. She chooses the top site on the list and goes to the National Library of Medicine site. Opening this web page shows a link to the National Society of Genetic Counselors. Once on the NSGC.com Web site, she enters the city name and finds a genetic counselor's phone number. She decides to call and talk to the genetic counselor. Another resource she saw was The National Institutes of Health Genetics Home Reference at https://ghr.nlm.nih.gov/, which added to her understanding of the people involved with genetic testing and health care.

Genetic Counselor

The genetic counselor who takes the dental student's call is slightly surprised, but extremely pleased by the student's approach to further identify resources for her patient's total health and well-being. They discuss the patient's concerns and the genetic counselor, who, like many, works at the local children's hospital, recognizes that this patient would be best served by being evaluated by a genetic counselor trained in cancer and a medical geneticist (a physician who is trained to identify mild dysmorphisms which can be helpful in identifying an inherited syndrome). Together, they decide to refer the young patient to the medical geneticist and cancer genetic counselor at the children's hospital, because other locations with a cancer genetic counselor do not have a genetic physician to evaluate her noncancer concerns. So far, this approach seems to be forming a foundation for an interprofessional collaborative (IPC) approach to the care of her dental patient.

Cancer Genetic Counselor

On the day of the young girl's appointment, the genetic counselor begins the visit by discussing her concerns and reviewing her family history with the patient and her mother. A full 4-generation pedigree is created (**Fig. 1**). Based on the history, it seems that the oligodontia is autosomal dominant, consistent with a single genetic change leading to the cause. Furthermore, most of the family members with oligodontia did have a cancer diagnosis in their lifetime. However, within the pedigree there was a female relative with normal dentition and breast cancer in her 60s and a male relative with normal dentition with colon cancer in his 70s. The patient's mother is 35 years old, missing her maxillary lateral incisors and third molar teeth, and has no history of screening for colon cancer. Of the ten family members with oligodontia, six had colon polyps diagnosed on their first colonoscopy at age 50 years, and two had colon cancer diagnosed at age 50 years on their first colonoscopy.

Because the patient is 14 years old, her mother asks when Sarah should have her first colonoscopy. The counselor informs her that Sarah should begin screening at 40 years, because this time period precedes the diagnosing of her other family members. In addition, the genetic counselor suggests specific genetic testing for markers of disease and their risk of phenotypic expression.

Medical Geneticist

The next member of this IPC team is the medical geneticist, who performs a dysmorphology examination looking for mild physical findings that could focus the differential diagnosis for colon cancer and oligodontia in this family. Oligodontia has been associated with brain malformation disorders, disorders of the respiratory system, cranial facial syndromes, dermal syndromes, ophthalmic syndromes, skeletal disorders, and genitourinary syndromes. Examples such as ectodermal dysplasia, orofaciodigital syndrome 1, and Mulvihill-Smith syndrome can be found at the Genetic and Rare Diseases Information Center, starting with the center's Web site (https://rarediseases.info.nih.gov/gard/). Based on the normal examination, developmental history, and

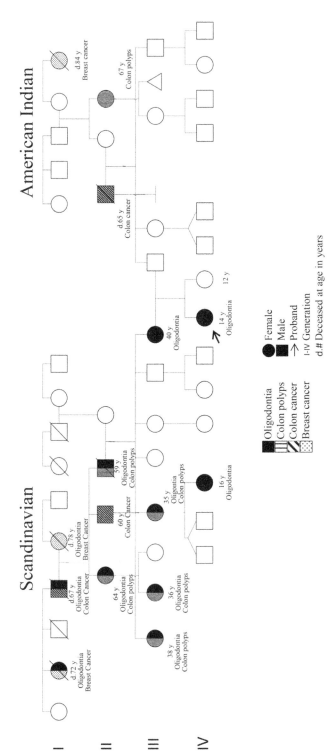

Fig. 1. Sarah's 4-generation pedigree. d, deceased; I-IV indicates generation number where I, generation #1; II, generation #2; III, generation #3, IV, generation #4.

medical history, except for the dental findings, the geneticist and genetic counselor recommend sequencing of the axis inhibition protein, a protein that is encoded by the axin-related protein (AXIN2) gene. Activating mutations in the AXIN2 gene lead to overactivation of the proto-oncogene protein Wnt (WNT) signaling pathway and can lead to severe tooth agenesis and abnormal B-catenin regulation, leading to increased risk of colon polyp formation and subsequent colon cancer.[9] However, because other genes have been associated with colon cancer (as reviewed by Bonds and colleagues[10]) and can affect colon cancer risk, it is deemed necessary to look for genetic changes in AXIN2 to determine her cancer risk and identify her need for cancer screening.

Colorectal Surgeon

Based on her family's history of colon cancer at early ages, the patient's mother is referred to a colorectal surgeon for routine colonoscopy screening. Based on her clinical findings, he will follow her yearly for evaluation with colonoscopy every 1 to 5 years.[11] He agreed with the genetic councelor's recommendation to begin screening for the 14-year-old 10 years before the youngest age a family member was identified with polyps.

Dietician

The colorectal surgeon refers the patient to a dietician to optimize her overall colon health. She recommends a high-fiber diet and they discuss how she can implement these diet changes for herself and how to communicate this information to her extended family. Because of the oligodontia, identifying high-fiber foods that she can also tolerate with her current dentition and after cosmetic repair is also extensively discussed.

Dental Hygienist

While awaiting the AXIN2 testing results, the patient returns for her 6-month dental cleaning with her dental hygienist. After Sarah informs her of the pending tests, the hygienist calls the dental student to ask whether there are other considerations or worries for this patient. They discuss the need to maintain the primary teeth until implants can be placed. If the baby teeth are lost, Sarah may need a removable partial denture to maintain the premolar space, enhance esthetics, and allow better chewing.

Patient Conclusion

The patient was found to have a single base pair change in one of her AXIN2 genes. This mutation changes an amino acid codon to introduce a stop codon, leading to low production of AXIN2, dysregulation of B-catenin, and activation of the WNT signaling pathway.[9,12] Her mother had the same genetic change. Based on this genetic finding, the mother was advised to begin colonoscopy and Sarah was advised to begin colonoscopy at age 40 years. A noncancerous polyp was identified at her mother's first screening. If the polyp had not been identified by the screening guidelines, then the polyp's cells would likely have changed and become cancerous over time suggesting the screening guidelines helped.[11]

The dental student applied an astute knowledge-seeking approach using an IPC model to improve not only her patient's current and future dental health, but also her overall health-related quality of life. This approach exemplifies a well-thought-out IPC model that enables health care providers to deliver patient-centered care using a common thread of communication and treatment hierarchy design.[8] The model presented applies the latest in science, technology, and genetics in order to meld with oral health care for total health. This model is the future of good clinical practice among not only dental practitioners but all health providers because it is essential that they have access to and identify referrals appropriately based on the specific disease of interest. Further insight can be obtained from Johnson and colleagues[13] and Depaula and Slavkin.[14]

Current Educational Practices

How can interprofessional education and IPC practice (IPCP) be made a reality? Although each health care program and profession will find its own answer to this question, some common threads are now in place. The new accreditation standards for predoctoral dental programs state that "Graduates must be competent in communicating and collaborating with other members of the health care team to facilitate the provision of health care," and make clear that interprofessional education is expected to play an important part in dental curricula.[15] As the entering students use their technical knowledge to answer important clinical questions, the interaction with genetic colleagues will expand to allow better patient care.

Role of Interprofessional Relationships in the Care of Genetic Patients: Current and Future Directions

Genomic discovery has significantly changed the understanding of genetic architecture, and has led to new understanding of the complexity of gene-gene and gene-environment interactions. This change has clinical implications for diagnosis and treatment strategies, particularly for common, multifactorial conditions.[16] Surveying US dental schools on their inclusion of genetics education revealed that most schools do not teach a human genetics course.[4] Thus, the combination of low baseline genetic literacy and little understanding of the interprofessional resources available can lead to poor patient care. It has been shown that poor interprofessional collaboration can negatively affect delivery of health services and patient care.[1,2,17]

In 2003, Guttmacher and colleagues[18] foretold the practical applications from the whole-genome project. As genetic technology, the application of genetic knowledge will be an essential part of an IPCP approach in patient-centered care. With modern clinical technologies becoming available to patients, it has become crucial that interprofessional teams form to optimize the implementation of this information on patient care. Misuse of genetic information has led to misrepresentation of clinical risks, mismanagement of patients, overdiagnosis, and underdiagnosis. Thus, patients with genetic variations are at especially high risk of being mismanaged without the support of an interprofessional team that understands their unique needs and can optimize their oral and general health outcomes.

REFERENCES

1. Reeves S, Zwarenstein M, Goldman J, et al. Interprofessional education: effects on professional practice and healthcare outcomes. Cochrane Database Syst Rev 2008;(1):CD002213.
2. Reeves S, Perrier L, Goldman J, et al. Interprofessional education: effects on professional practice and healthcare outcomes (update). Cochrane Database Syst Rev 2013;(3):CD002213.
3. Alfano MC. Connecting dental education to other health professions. J Dent Educ 2012;76(1):46–50.
4. Dudlicek LL, Gettig EA, Etzel KR, et al. Status of genetics education in U.S. dental schools. J Dent Educ 2004;68(8):809–18.
5. Bailit HL. Dental variation among populations. An anthropologic view. Dent Clin North Am 1975;19(1):125–39.

6. Beery TA. Genetic and genomic testing in clinical practice: what you need to know. Rehabil Nurs 2014;39(2):70–5.
7. Richards S, Aziz N, Bale S, et al. ACMG Laboratory Quality Assurance Committee. Standards and guidelines for the interpretation of sequence variants: a joint consensus recommendation of the American College of Medical Genetics and Genomics and the Association for Molecular Pathology. Genet Med 2015;17(5): 405–24.
8. Greiner AC, Knebel E. Health professions education: a bridge to quality. An Institute of Medicine report. Washington, DC: National Academies Press; 2003.
9. Lammi L, Arte S, Somer M, et al. Mutations in AXIN2 cause familial tooth agenesis and predispose to colorectal cancer. Am J Hum Genet 2004;74:1043–50.
10. Bonds J, Pollan-White S, Xiang L, et al. Is there a link between ovarian cancer and tooth agenesis? Eur J Med Genet 2014;57(5):235–9.
11. Garborg K. Colorectal cancer screening. Surg Clin North Am 2015;95(5):979–89.
12. Alves-Ferreira M, Pinho T, Sousa A, et al. Identification of genetic risk factors for maxillary lateral incisor agenesis. J Dent Res 2014;93(5):452–8.
13. Johnson L, Genco RJ, Damsky C, et al. Genetics and its implications for clinical dental practice and education: report of panel 3 of the Macy study. J Dent Educ 2008;72:86–94.
14. DePaola DP, Slavkin HC. Reforming dental health professions education: a white paper. J Dent Educ 2004;68(11):1139–50.
15. Buchanan J. Interprofessional education: why dentistry and why now? Washington, DC: ADEA; 2013. Available at: http://www.adea.org/Blog.aspx?id=21386&blogid=20741. Accessed March 01, 2016.
16. Feero WG, Guttmacher AE, Collins FS. Genomic medicine—an updated primer. N Engl J Med 2010;362(21):2001–11.
17. Zwarenstein M, Goldman J, Reeves S. Interprofessional collaboration: effects of practice-based interventions on professional practice and healthcare outcomes. Cochrane Database Syst Rev 2009;(3):CD000072.
18. Guttmacher AE, Collins FS. Welcome to the genomic era. N Engl J Med 2003; 349(10):996–8.

Integrating Oral Health and Primary Care

Federal Initiatives to Drive Systems Change

CAPT Renée W. Joskow, DDS, MPH, FAGD, FACD

KEYWORDS

- Interprofessional relations • Primary health care • Oral health
- Patient-centered care • United States Health Resources and Services Administration
- Dental education • Medical education • Health literacy

KEY POINTS

- United States federal programs, initiatives, and partnerships have taken action to initiate and institutionalize interprofessional practice.
- Federal activities recognize oral health providers as integral to the provider team.
- Landmark documents and reports, legislation and statutory authority, and the influence of federal program priorities contribute towards a national movement to increase access to care to bridge the chasms between the medical health care system, dental delivery system, and oral health.

INTRODUCTION

Oral health, as a critical component of health, is embedded in the World Health Organization's 1948 broadened definition, "Health is a state of complete physical, mental, and social well-being and not merely the absence of disease or infirmity."[1] Even so, nearly 70 years have passed and oral health, dental education, and dental care delivery remain disconnected and separate from the larger medical system of care. This disconnect and view of the mouth as separate from the body is perpetuated by segmented models of care and delivery and payment systems that have not substantially integrated oral health in overall health. A 1972 Institute of Medicine (IOM) report echoed that "linkages are inadequate between existing models of health delivery and the educational institutions charged with developing the manpower for these

Disclosure Statement: The views expressed in this article are solely the opinions of the author and do not necessarily reflect the official policies of the US Department of Health and Human Services or the Health Resources and Services Administration, nor does mention of the department or agency names imply endorsement by the US government.
US Public Health Service, Health Resources and Services Administration, 5600 Fishers Lane, Rockville, MD 20857, USA
E-mail address: RJoskow@hrsa.gov

Dent Clin N Am 60 (2016) 951–968
http://dx.doi.org/10.1016/j.cden.2016.05.010
0011-8532/16/$ – see front matter Published by Elsevier Inc.

dental.theclinics.com

systems."[2] The report presents the basic argument for interprofessional teams (and integration) in the ambulatory care environment in which the emphasis is on the patient and outcomes of care rather than "on professions, their techniques, or the process of care."[2] With significant disparities in oral health among segments of the population and multifactorial challenges in accessing care, it is in the primary care environment, in particular, that there is an urgent need for the deployment of effective health care teams. Through differing administrations, budget cycles, and economic cycles, the federal government has taken the lead on key issues, such as health promotion and access to care, that affect the nation.

Periodic efforts to move oral health and dental care delivery into the mainstream of health care, and to reunite the mouth with the body in efforts to achieve overall health, have met with mixed results. In *Oral health in America: a report of the Surgeon General*, then Secretary of the Department of Health and Human Services (DHHS), Donna Shalala, stated that oral health is integral to general health because "you cannot be healthy without oral health."[3] She was reflecting the nation's struggle to achieve a systems-level change to implement true integration of oral health and primary care in a consistent and sustainable manner.

This article describes federal programs, initiatives, and partnerships that have the demonstrated potential to initiate and institutionalize interprofessional practice, which includes agreement that oral health providers are integral to the provider team. A discussion of landmark documents and reports, the role of legislation and statutory authority, and the influence of federal program priorities towards a national movement to increase access to care and bridge the chasms separating the medical health care system, the dental delivery system, and oral health is presented.

In 2000, in the first Surgeon General's report on oral health,[3] David Satcher wrote, "There are opportunities for all health professions, individuals, and communities to work together to improve health."[3] Furthermore, this report explicitly states that a principal component of a national oral health plan (NOHP) is an effective health infrastructure that meets the oral health needs of all Americans and integrates oral health effectively into overall health.[3] The DHHS recently took a monumental step forward by promoting an NOHP and publishing the *Oral Health Strategic Framework, 2014–2017*[4] (*Framework*) that "builds upon and outlines a strategic alignment of HHS operating and staff divisions' resources, programs, and leadership commitments to improve oral health with activities of other federal partners."[4]

The recent realignment of federal priorities and programs that recognize the importance and value of integrating oral health and primary care has ignited renewed interest in innovative approaches to continued progress in improving the nation's oral health.

HISTORICAL PERSPECTIVE AND THE ROLE OF FEDERAL PROGRAMS

Throughout history there have been notable occasions when federal policies and programs have made a substantial impact on the health care system in an effort to improve the health of the nation. One example is the 1965 passage of Medicaid and Medicare that today represents the nation's main public health insurance programs for the low-income populations and Americans aged 65 years and older, respectively.[5] The sweeping transformation of the health care system created by these programs continues today.

In the same year, Coggeshall[6] submitted a report to the Association of American Medical Colleges. Although the health care system then was quite different from today, there was awareness and foresight that "the expanding role of government in the health field has been manifesting itself in a growing number of ways and with increasing resources and emphasis in recent years. This can be expected to continue to expand."[7] The Coggeshall Report[6] provided a series of recommendations to the Association of American Medical Colleges that included the need to "maintain productive relationships with government." Nearly 50 years lapsed before efforts to further transform health care delivery resulted in the passage and implementation of the Affordable Care Act (ACA) in 2010.

Partnering with Foundations or Nonprofits

Federal government programs have finite budgets for discretionary programs. Funds availability depends on the specific agency and congressional authorizations and appropriations for that fiscal year (FY). The amount of federal funding is directed by statute or legislation and must be used for specified purposes. Although grants to institutions and states are sometimes used for pilot or demonstration projects, in some circumstances the available federal funding level is insufficient to create permanent widespread change across workforce development education and practice delivery systems. Over the past decade, more and more public-private partnerships between government and nongovernment entities have emerged, such as foundations and nonprofit organizations, in efforts to leverage resources more efficiently and effectively to drive the transformation of health professions education and practice toward a more integrated approach with the goal of improving health outcomes.

An interprofessional education and integrated practice paradigm is not new, although previous efforts did not gain enough momentum to create a fully integrated national network with national visibility, influence, and acceptance. In the late 1980s, Pew Charitable Trusts and the Rockefeller Foundation funded 6 universities as part of their *Health of the Public* national program.[8] One institution, Columbia University, focused on incorporating public health education in the dental, medical, and nursing school curricula by establishing an interdisciplinary clinical curriculum workgroup and a summer *Institute in Clinical Public Health* for entering dental, medical, and bachelor-degree nursing students.

Since then, spurred by the release of the 2000 Surgeon General's Report,[3] increased attention and progress has been made towards incorporating oral health into overall health. Studies have continued to be published that associate oral diseases and conditions with chronic illnesses. A growing number of dental, medical, nursing, and physician assistant education programs, and licensing and credentialing examinations, have begun to emphasize the oral-systemic connection. A summary of the 3-day workshop on the *US Oral Health Workforce in the Coming Decade*[9] was published in 2009. Several relevant conclusions are displayed in **Box 1**.

In February 2011, the Health Resources and Services Administration (HRSA) convened a conference with the Josiah Macy Jr Foundation, the Robert Wood Johnson Foundation, the American Board of Internal Medicine Foundation, and the Interprofessional Education Collaborative (IPEC), to engage a diverse group of leaders in the development of competencies for interprofessional education (IPE) and practice, including dentistry. The final conference report with the IPEC competencies was released May 10, 2011.[10]

Collaborations across a spectrum of funding entities have emerged to promote oral health integration in primary care and reconnect oral health and overall health. In 2012, the DentaQuest Foundation, the Washington Dental Service Foundation, the Highmark Foundation, and the Robert Wood Johnson Foundation provided funding to convene a group of grant makers, researchers, and practitioners to discuss issues

> **Box 1**
> **Selected conclusions from the US Oral Health Workforce in the coming decade workshop summary**
>
> - Interdisciplinary training of all students is required to bridge the gap between medicine and dentistry.
> - The scopes of practice of all health care professionals need to be maximized to improve access to oral health services in rural areas.
> - Integration with the nondental workforce allows for evolution toward true oral health, with dental professionals being an integral part of maintaining the systemic health of their patients.
> - More models are needed for the interdisciplinary education and training of health professions students.
> - Policies need to come into alignment with practice, such as the development and implementation of clinical practice guidelines.
>
> *From* IOM (Institute of Medicine). The U.S. oral health workforce in the coming decade: workshop summary. Washington, DC: The National Academies Press; 2009; with permission.

related to integrating oral health and primary care. This group published an issue brief titled, *Returning the Mouth to the Body: Integrating Oral Health & Primary Care*.[11] The brief makes a strong practical clinical case for integration. It proposes that "by sharing information, providing basic diagnostic services, and consulting each other in a systematic and sustained manner, dental and medical professionals in integrated practice arrangements would have a far better chance of identifying disease precursors and underlying conditions in keeping with a patient-centered model of care. Integration can also raise patients' awareness of the importance of oral health, potentially aiding them in taking advantage of dental services sooner rather than later."[11]

In 2015, the February-March newsletter from the Commonwealth Fund on *Integrating Oral Health into Primary Care*[12] acknowledged that integration is starting to occur through "new approaches to training for both dental and primary care providers, promotion of team-based care, and development of medical, rather than surgical, treatments for oral health problems."[12] The newsletter[12] cites 2 IOM reports from 2011 funded by DHHS and HRSA.[13,14]

The Institute of Medicine

The IOM is a component of the Academies of Sciences, Engineering, and Medicine that was recently renamed the Health and Medicine Division to emphasize a wider range of health matters while building on the rich history of the IOM's previous work.[15] For decades, the federal government has provided substantial support for IOM workshops, conferences, and reports on a variety of topics. The result of the IOM's efforts has fundamentally shifted the landscape to facilitate system-wide change. A similar effect has been seen with federal reports, programs, and initiatives that promote an integrated approach to the delivery of health care and training of health professionals.

A few of the most relevant IOM reports regarding interprofessional practice and oral health integration in primary care are presented here. These IOM efforts were supported at least in part by federal government entities. Specific and relevant federal reports, programs and initiative will be described later.

- In 1972, the IOM held a conference with leaders from allied health, dentistry, medicine, nursing, and pharmacy on the *Interrelationships of Educational*

Programs for Health Professionals to inform national discussions about interprofessional education. The conference resulted in the report "Educating for the Health Team."[2]

- The 2001 IOM report, *Crossing the Quality Chasm: A New Health System for the 21st Century*, recommended that an interdisciplinary summit be held to "reform health professions education to enhance patient care quality and safety."[16] In response and with support from 2 federal agencies in the DHHS (HRSA and AHRQ) and 2 nonprofit organizations (ABIM Foundation and the California Healthcare Foundation) a summit was held to enhance health care quality in the United States.
- The resulting 2003 report, *Health Professions Education: A Bridge to Quality,*[17] underscores the importance of recognizing each profession's essential contribution to not only the educational system and training of health professionals but also the practice environment and interfacing systems in which care is provided. The report focuses on "integrating a core set of competencies—patient-centered care, interdisciplinary teams, evidence-based practice, quality improvement and informatics—into health professions education."[17] Education and practice-based competencies and the federal policies and investments that spur the development of the health workforce must meet the needs of patients, communities and society overall, and the requirements of a changing or evolving health system. Recognizing the role, influence, and capability of the federal government to drive health professions systems change, this 2003 IOM report included 10 recommendations of which 5 were specifically directed to federal entities (**Table 1**).

LANDMARK PUBLICATIONS AND REPORTS

Landmark documents have established the foundation for understanding of the relationship between oral and systemic health, the prevalence of dental diseases in the population, barriers to access to care, the adequacy of the dental workforce, and health disparities of certain subpopulations in the United States. Federal agencies have provided funding to develop these documents, establish national priorities, take strategic actions, and implement policies to accelerate the translation of ideas into practice. For example, the aforementioned Surgeon General's report on oral health,[3] addressed the importance of building a science and evidence base to improve oral health, building the infrastructure to address oral health, removing barriers to oral health services, and developing public-private partnerships to address disparities in oral health. Oral health is essential to overall general health and well-being; however, the Healthy People 2020[18] national oral health objectives illustrate that many challenges identified 16 years ago have not been adequately addressed.

Federal Initiatives

Over the past 6 years, there have been significant federal investments and efforts to move the needle on improving oral health access to care and integrating oral health and primary care. In 2010, leadership from DHHS and HRSA announced the Oral Health Initiative 2010[19] (OHI2010), which renewed the DHHS commitment to work with national and state partners and continue building on the recommendations set forth in the 2000 Surgeon General's Report on Oral Health[3] and A National Call to Action to Promote Oral Health.[20] The key message of the OHI2010[19] is that oral health is integral to overall health. This initiative[19] used a systems-approach to create and finance programs to

Table 1 Selected Institute of Medicine recommendations to federal agencies	
Recommendation 1	DHHS and leading foundations should support an interdisciplinary effort focused on developing a common language, with the ultimate aim of achieving consensus across the health professions on a core set of competencies that includes patient-centered care, interdisciplinary teams, evidence-based practice, quality improvement, and informatics.
Recommendation 2	DHHS should provide a forum and support for a series of meetings involving the spectrum of oversight organizations across and within the disciplines. Participants in these meetings would be charged with developing strategies for incorporating a core set of competencies into oversight activities, based on definitions shared across the professions. These meetings would actively solicit the input of health professions associations and the education community.
Recommendation 7	Through Medicare demonstration projects, the Centers for Medicare and Medicaid Services should take the lead in funding experiments that will enable and create incentives for health professionals to integrate interdisciplinary approaches into educational or practice settings, with the goal of providing a training ground for students and clinicians that incorporates the 5 core competencies.
Recommendation 8	Agency for Healthcare Research and Quality and private foundations should support ongoing research projects addressing the 5 core competencies and their association with individual and population health, as well as research related to the link between the competencies and evidence-based education. Such projects should involve researchers across 2 or more disciplines.
Recommendation 9	AHRQ should work with a representative group of health care leaders to develop measures reflecting the core set of competencies, set national goals for improvement, and issue a report to the public evaluating progress toward these goals. AHRQ should issue the first report, focused on clinical educational institutions, in 2005 and produce annual reports thereafter.

From Greiner AC, Knebel E, editors. Health professions education: a bridge to quality. Washington, DC: Institute of Medicine of the National Academies of Science, National Academies; 2003. Available at: http://www.nap.edu/catalog/10681.html. Accessed April 8, 2016; with permission.

- Emphasize oral health promotion and disease prevention
- Increase access to care
- Enhance oral health workforce
- Eliminate oral health disparities.

The OHI2010[19] featured 9 activities to maximize the impact of federal programs on the oral health of the nation. One of the highlighted activities was the development of 2 landmark IOM reports that have been widely studied, cited extensively, and have served as the impetus for actions federal agencies have taken and those planned. With the strategic priority to advance oral health for underserved populations, HRSA commissioned the IOM to assess current oral health and the oral health care system and make recommendations to DHHS to improve the oral health of the nation, especially for vulnerable and underserved Americans. In April and July of 2011, 2 significant oral health reports were published: *Advancing Oral Health in America*[13] and *Improving Access to Oral Health Care for Vulnerable and Underserved Populations*.[14]

These IOM reports are cornerstones in the conversation about access to care and have created new benchmarks for oral health in America, almost 2 decades after the release of the Surgeon General's report on oral health.[3]

The first of these 2011 reports assesses the current oral health care delivery system and explores ways to promote use of preventive oral health interventions and improve oral health literacy.[13] The second report focuses on issues of access to oral health care for underserved and vulnerable populations.[14] Each report contains recommendations for action, including the development of core competencies for health care professionals in oral health care. Specific recommendations related to interprofessional collaboration and integrating oral health and primary care practice are shown in **Boxes 2** and **3**.

HRSA, in response to these IOM recommendations, developed the Integration of Oral Health and Primary Care Practice (IOHPCP)[21] initiative to expand the oral health clinical competency of primary care clinicians and to integrate oral health and primary care practice. The initiative was founded on 3 inter-related components:

- Develop oral health domains and associated core clinical competencies
- Use a systems approach to identify and prioritize the elements that affect the adoption of oral health competencies by primary care clinicians
- Characterize foundational elements for successful implementation strategies that translate into primary care practice.

As part of the IOHPCP initiative, HRSA invited a diverse cross-section of individuals from the public and private sectors to participate alongside HRSA staff in facilitated discussions. The initial meeting focused on an essential set of Interprofessional Oral Health Core Clinical Competencies (IPOHCCC or IPOHC[3]) (**Table 2**) for nondental primary care providers. The second meeting used a systems approach and process that revealed complexities and interdependent relationships that are critical to successful integration in the practice setting. The systems analysis uncovered 12 cross-cutting systems (**Fig. 1**) at the environment-organization level that are involved in the implementation of clinical oral health competencies for primary care providers. During the third meeting, presentations followed by facilitated discussions about strategies and approaches for implementing IPOHC[3] were framed around the importance of 3 essential systems, with communication as an overarching requirement (**Fig. 2**).

HRSA synthesized recommendations (**Box 4**) to support core competency adoption by primary care clinicians and to promote the integration of oral health and primary

---

Box 2
Advancing oral health in America recommendation to increase the oral health workforce

- Recommendation 4: DHHS should invest in workforce innovations to improve oral health that focuses on:
  - Core competency development, education, and training, to allow for the use of all health care professionals in oral health care
  - Interprofessional, team-based approaches to the prevention and treatment of oral diseases
  - Best use of new and existing oral health care professionals
  - Increasing the diversity and improving the cultural competence of the workforce providing oral health care.

From IOM (Institute of Medicine). Advancing oral health in America. Washington, DC: The National Academies Press; 2011; with permission.

Box 3
Improving access to oral health care for vulnerable and underserved populations recommendations on oral health competencies for health professionals

- Recommendation 1a: The HRSA should convene key stakeholders from both the private and public sectors to develop a core set of competencies for health care professionals
- Recommendation 1b: Following the development of a core set of oral health competencies for nondental health care professionals
  ○ Accrediting bodies for undergraduate and graduate-level nondental health care professional education programs should integrate these core competencies into their requirements for accreditation
  ○ All certification and maintenance of certification for health care professionals should include demonstration of competence in oral health care as a criterion.

From IOM (Institute of Medicine), NRC (National Research Council). Improving access to oral health care for vulnerable and underserved populations. Washington, DC: The National Academies Press; 2011; with permission.

---

care practice. The IOHPCP report and its recommendations serve as guiding principles and provide a framework for the design of a competency-based, interprofessional practice model to integrate oral health and primary care.[21]

HRSA's commitment to improving access to quality dental care by integrating oral health has not been limited to the release of the IOHPCP report.[21] HRSA also funded a pilot project to demonstrate the validity of the IPOHC[3] and potential implementation strategies for primary care practice at 3 health centers. The results are available as *A User's Guide for Implementation of Interprofessional Oral Health Core Clinical Competencies.*[22] Dental and medical education and training program priorities and funding opportunities reflect recognition of the importance of oral health and primary care

---

Table 2
Interprofessional oral health core clinical domains

Domains	
Risk Assessment	Identifies factors that impact oral health and overall health.
Oral Health Evaluation	Integrates subjective and objective findings based on completion of a focused oral health history, risk assessment, and performance of clinical oral screening.
Preventive Intervention	Recognizes options and strategies to address oral health needs identified by a comprehensive risk assessment and health evaluation.
Communication and Education	Targets individuals and groups regarding the relationship between oral and systemic health, risk factors for oral health disorders, effect of nutrition on oral health, and preventive measures appropriate to mitigate risk on both individual and population levels.
Interprofessional Collaborative Practice	Shares responsibility and collaboration among health care professionals in the care of patients and populations with, or at risk of, oral disorders to assure optimal health outcomes.

Data from U.S. Department of Health and Human Services. Integration of oral health and primary care practice. Rockville (MD): U.S. Department of Health and Human Services, Health Resources and Services Administration; 2014. Available at: http://www.hrsa.gov/publichealth/clinical/oralhealth/primarycare/integrationoforalhealth.pdf. Accessed March 29, 2016; with permission.

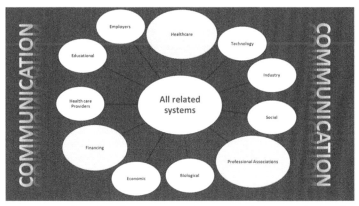

Fig. 1. Systems approach analysis for 12 cross-cutting systems in interprofessional oral health core competencies. (*Data from* U.S. Department of Health and Human Services. Integration of oral health and primary care practice. Rockville (MD): U.S. Department of Health and Human Services, Health Resources and Services Administration; 2014. Available at: http://www.hrsa.gov/publichealth/clinical/oralhealth/primarycare/integrationoforalhealth.pdf. Accessed March 29, 2016; with permission.)

integration. In FY 2015, HRSA grants for predoctoral dental and primary care medical training programs included a focus on enhancing training to support integration of oral health within the broader health care delivery system and models of training for integrated oral health[23] and medicine or primary care.[24]

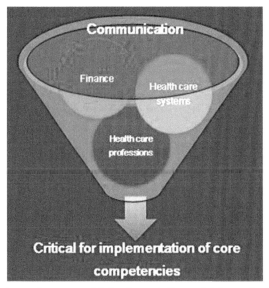

Fig. 2. Critical systems for successful implementation of interprofessional oral health competencies. (*Data from* U.S. Department of Health and Human Services. Integration of oral health and primary care practice. Rockville (MD): U.S. Department of Health and Human Services, Health Resources and Services Administration; 2014. Available at: http://www.hrsa.gov/publichealth/clinical/oralhealth/primarycare/integrationoforalhealth.pdf. Accessed March 29, 2016; with permission.)

Box 4
HRSA integration of oral health and primary care report recommendations

1. Apply oral health core clinical competencies within primary care practices to increase oral health care access for safety net populations in the United States.
   a. Clinicians should incorporate the oral health core clinical competencies in patient care.
   b. Health care professional education and training, as well as continuing education curricula, should incorporate the oral health core clinical competencies.
   c. Accreditation and certification bodies should integrate the oral health core clinical competencies into primary care practitioner standards.

2. Develop infrastructure that is interoperable, accessible across clinical settings, and enhances adoption of the oral health core clinical competencies. The defined, essential elements of the oral health core clinical competencies should be used to inform decision-making and measure health outcomes. Health care systems should
   a. Establish technological infrastructure to support and facilitate referrals, knowledge exchange, and a follow up with clinicians to improve health outcomes.
   b. Identify and support executive level champions to enhance communications and prioritize incorporation of the oral health core clinical competencies into primary care practice.
   c. Engage and educate consumers about oral health in primary care as an expected standard of interprofessional practice.
   d. Evaluate effectiveness of the application of the oral health core clinical competencies by assessing patient satisfaction and health outcomes.
   e. Use common language, interoperable electronic health records, and interprofessional collaboration in patient-centered medical and health homes to facilitate high quality accessible oral health care.

3. Modify payment policies to efficiently address costs of implementing oral health competencies and provide incentives to health care systems and practitioners.
   a. Include or enhance public and private health care payment for oral health care throughout the lifespan.
   b. Use safety net settings to pilot payment methodologies that lower dental care costs.
   c. Build partnerships and coalitions that educate policy makers and the public about the benefit of integrating oral health care and primary care.

4. Execute programs to develop and evaluate implementation strategies of the oral health core clinical competencies into primary care practice.
   a. Implement pilot projects to identify innovative and promising practices that inform and support the broader implementation of the oral health core clinical competencies.
   b. Develop demonstration projects to validate and replicate the oral health core clinical competencies implementation.
   c. Evaluate implementation of the oral health core clinical competencies by clinicians and the systems in which they practice.
   d. Assess the cost-effectiveness and efficiency of implementing the oral health core clinical competencies in primary care practice.

From U.S. Department of Health and Human Services. Integration of oral health and primary care practice. Rockville (MD): U.S. Department of Health and Human Services, Health Resources and Services Administration; 2014. Available at: http://www.hrsa.gov/publichealth/clinical/oralhealth/primarycare/integrationoforalhealth.pdf. Accessed December 23, 2015; with permission.

PUBLIC-PRIVATE PARTNERSHIPS AND BUILDING ON A FOUNDATION

Additional examples of areas of investment and collaboration aimed at maximizing opportunities to improve oral health for the persons with and without access to dental care are include in this section. The IOHPCP initiative has served as a national call to action and has contributed to the increased interest and focus on integrating oral health and primary care by federal and nonfederal entities alike. Many integration efforts across health professions are underway and it seems that a tipping point for gaining momentum has been reached. Cross-cutting efforts by entities such as non-profits, foundations, insurers, and federal programs have been leveraging resources and building on programmatic successes and increased collaboration. Recently, a Qualis Health White Paper, *Oral health: an essential component of primary care*,[25] describes the "complementary roles of primary care and dentistry in addressing oral disease, and describes the benefits of providing preventive oral health care in the primary care setting."[25] The paper outlines an *"Oral health delivery framework"* that "delineates the activities for which a primary care team can take accountability to protect and promote oral health."[25] The influence and impact of the federal government's efforts to drive change is exemplified in the Qualis effort because their framework[25] was built on the HRSA IOHPCP initiative and report.[21]

In addition, the thirteenth annual report[26] to the Secretary of the DHHS and the Congress of the United States from the Advisory Committee on Interdisciplinary, Community-Based Linkages emphasized, "Interprofessional education and collaborative practice can play an important role in improving patient care quality, satisfaction, safety, and efficiency. Health professions training, continuing education, continuing professional development, faculty development, and community-based training need to change to provide healthcare professionals, educators, and students with the collaborative care tools needed to improve the health of populations."[26]

Educational Resources for Clinicians, Academics, and Researchers

- HRSA contracted with the American Academy of Pediatrics to develop a Web-based oral health module for pediatricians. The information is also available as an electronic document that may be used as the basis to educate primary care providers working with children. The content can be used to increase knowledge and integration of oral health preventive interventions into systems of care.[27]
- HRSA funded the Association of American Medical Colleges to build oral health training capacity in medical education (MedEdPortal) with the aim to advance physician understanding of the oral-systemic impact on overall health and to prepare clinicians to provide comprehensive coordinated care.[28]
- HRSA convened an expert workgroup to promote integrated health care and interprofessional collaboration and published *Oral health care during pregnancy: a national consensus statement–summary of an expert workgroup meeting*[29] to shape the practices of both medical and dental professionals serving pregnant women. In addition, a valuable user-friendly resource document was developed for dental professionals, medical or prenatal care providers, and patients regarding dental care and pharmacologic considerations during pregnancy.[30] Clinicians will find this a useful tool in caring for pregnant women in the dental setting. (See related information, Farmer-Dixon C, Thompson M, Young D, et al: Interprofessional Collaborative Practice (IPC): An Oral Health Paradigm for Women, in this issue.)
- HRSA established a National Center for Interprofessional Practice and Education at the University of Minnesota. The interprofessional coordinating center provides an infrastructure for leadership, expertise, and support to enhance the coordination and capacity-building of interprofessional education and collaborative practice among health professions.[31]
- HRSA conducted interviews, convened expert panel meetings, and commissioned a report on women's health curricula across health professions to identify actionable strategies and develop a dissemination plan to increase the

awareness of women's health education needs.[32] The report includes details and resources leading to increased integration of women's health content and inter-professional collaboration.[32] Additional information and an in-depth discussion (see Farmer-Dixon C, Thompson M, Young D, et al: Interprofessional Collaborative Practice (IPC): An Oral Health Paradigm for Women, in this issue.)

FEDERAL PROGRAMS THAT PROMOTE ORAL HEALTH INTEGRATION AND INTERPROFESSIONAL COLLABORATION

The previously mentioned DHHS *Framework*[4] articulates the vision of DHHS and other federal partners to increase the public's understanding that oral health is integral to overall health. By leveraging public and private sector partnerships to achieve better oral health and overall health for all populations across the lifespan, *Framework*[4] provides the roadmap for engaging and resolving ongoing disparities in oral health.

Organized around 5 overarching goals: (1) integrate oral health and primary health care, (2) prevent disease and promote oral health, (3) increase access to oral health care and eliminate disparities, (4) increase the dissemination of oral health information and improve health literacy, and (5) advance oral health in public policy and research, *Framework*[4] illustrates the commitment across multiple federal entities to "serve as the catalyst for moving a national oral health agenda forward."[4] These goals provide the foundation for development, execution, and evaluation of implementation strategies and actions that federal agencies and partners alike may use to address the nation's oral health and workforce needs.

In addition to DHHS and federal partners' recognition of the importance of oral health integration and interprofessional collaboration, a HRSA strategic priority is the integration of oral health and primary care. As a follow up to the *OHI2010*,[19] the agency has continued to lead efforts to increase access to quality care for vulnerable and underserved populations by investing in activities that promote oral health integration and improve access for early detection and preventive interventions by expanding the oral health clinical competency of primary care clinicians. HRSA has undertaken multiple activities designed to accelerate the integration of oral health and primary care at the level of training and education and the practice interface.

Training and Education Grant Programs

Beginning in the early 1980s, recognition of aging trends in the US population coupled with research indicating insufficient training of health care professionals in geriatrics led to the development of the Veterans Affairs (VA) Geriatric Dental Fellowships the and DHHS HRSA Geriatric Education Centers (GEC) grant program. The VA fellow-ships were analogous to the Geriatric Medical Fellowships and represented a partner-ship between a VA Medical Center and a university. The HRSA "Geriatrics Education Centers funded health professions schools [including dentistry] to provide interprofes-sional/interdisciplinary education and training to health professions students, faculty, and practitioners in the diagnosis, treatment, and prevention of disease, disability, and other health problems of older adults."[33] The VA geriatric fellowship program continued for about 10 years while the HRSA programs persisted. The GEC and other similar HRSA programs have evolved over the decades with renewed efforts to integrate geriatrics with primary care with an emphasis on increasing the knowledge and skills of the primary care workforce to care for older adults as the focus of the new Geriatrics Workforce Enhancement Program (GWEP).[34] The GWEP, established in 2015, resulted from the consolidation 4 geriatric education programs, including the GEC; Geriatric Training for Physicians, Dentists, and Behavioral/Mental Health

Providers; Comprehensive Geriatric Education Program; and Geriatric Academic Career Award.[34] For further insight into IPE and interprofessional collaborative practice [IPCP] with geriatrics (see Kaufman LB, Henshaw MM, Brown BP, et al: Oral Health and Interprofessional Collaborative Practice: Examples of the TEAM Approach to Geriatric Care, in this issue.)

With the enactment of the ACA in October 2010, HRSA oral health training programs were expanded and continue to provide funding to universities and institutions for pre-doctoral and postdoctoral training, faculty development, faculty loan repayment, and grants to states to support oral health workforce activities to improve oral health by increasing the number of and improving the quality of well-trained primary oral health care providers working in underserved areas. In 2015, the grant programs were updated to reflect the growing importance of interprofessional education and collaboration in support of IPCP. For example, the *Pre-doctoral Training in General, Pediatric, and Public Health Dentistry and Dental Hygiene* grant program includes a focus on "Enhancing training to support integration of oral health within the broader health care delivery system to improve access to oral health care for vulnerable, underserved, or rural communities."[23]

Additional leverage to promote interprofessional training and practice was implemented in the 2015 postdoctoral grant program. Institutions receiving HRSA grants are required to develop or enhance integrated health care delivery systems that serve as training sites for postdoctoral dental trainees, including partnerships with primary care delivery organizations and other community-based organizations. HRSA oral health program support spans the continuum from training and education to practice. Ten states received funding for activities in a new focus area, "Integrating oral and primary care medical delivery systems for underserved communities" under the *Grants to Support Oral Health Workforce Activities* program.[35] In addition to grant programs administered with funds directed for oral health, many other health professional grant programs have encouraged interprofessional education and practice, thereby magnifying the oral health footprint supported by HRSA funds. Examples include

- HRSA GWEP[34] (see previous discussion of the history of this program and geriatric training supported by the VA).
- HRSA funding to Area Health Education Centers nationwide to enhance "access to high quality, culturally competent health care through academic-community partnerships to ultimately improve the distribution, diversity, and supply of the primary care health professions workforce who serve in rural and underserved health care delivery sites."[36]

AHEC programs and centers along with state and local partners

- Promote interprofessional education and collaborative teams to improve quality of care
- Recruit and train students from minority and disadvantaged backgrounds into health careers
- Place health professions students in community-based clinical practice settings, with a focus on primary care
- Facilitate continuing education resources and programs for health professionals, particularly in rural and underserved areas.

HRSA also funds Advanced Nursing Education Grants[37,38] that "support projects that develop and test innovative academic-practice partnership models for clinical training." Several grants have been made for training-based collaborations between schools of dentistry and nursing. Examples include

- Enhanced oral-systemic IPE and IPCP through collaboration between the University at Buffalo Schools of Nursing and Dental Medicine to develop innovative IPE experiences and new IPCP teams that include dental and advanced practice registered nurse (APRN) students and faculty.[37]
- Teaching Oral-Systemic Health is an interprofessional initiative of New York University (NYU) College of Nursing, to engage APRN students, together with medical students from NYU School of Medicine and dental students from NYU College of Dentistry in simulation learning with standardized patients and virtual patient cases.[38] Note: this HRSA funded program is discussed in detail (see Gordon S, Donoff RB: Problems and Solutions for Interprofessional Education in North American Dental Schools, in this issue.)
- The Academic Unit-Primary Care Training and Enhancement grant program focuses on academic units that integrate oral health and primary care models, such as increasing oral health core clinical competencies for primary care trainees, training in integrated or virtually integrated oral health and primary care practices, and new interprofessional education models for integrated oral health and primary care; in particular, on models that support the training of providers in advanced roles. The academic unit must understand the challenges, limitations, and levels of a fully integrated model and understand and disseminate how training programs can promote and achieve successful integration.[25]

Clinical Practice Investments

Agencies such as HRSA, the Federal Bureau of Prisons, Office of Minority Health, and the Indian Health Service foster activities that promote interprofessional collaboration. Examples of federal activities that have implications for clinical care are presented in the DHHS *Framework*[4] under the Goal 1 strategy, "Create programs and support innovation using a systems change approach that facilitates a unified patient-centered health home."[4] Furthermore, a Qualis paper on the patient-centered medical home (PCMH) states that, "embracing comprehensive care, the PCMH model provides the perfect environment for strengthening access to oral health care, improving provider and patient understanding of oral health, and providing the needed oral health care screening, preventive and restorative services that are essential to optimal health status."[39] The PCMH or health home provides a conceptual platform in which IPCP can be actualized to maximize health outcomes for individuals and populations.

Over the past several years, HRSA Health Center Program has made substantial investments in new service delivery sites, expansion of existing health centers, and school-based health centers. In FY 2014, nearly 300 HRSA Health Center grantees expanded oral health services. An additional FY2016 commitment of $156 million was made specifically for oral health expansion of 420 existing health centers to increase access to oral health care services and improve oral health outcomes for Health Center Program patients. Health centers are required to provide "all required primary, preventive, enabling health services and additional health services as appropriate and necessary, either directly or through established written arrangements and referrals"[40] and, therefore, provide the opportunity to integrate oral health and primary care practice and capitalize on interprofessional collaboration.

Federal program initiatives and investments may serve to facilitate systems change and demonstrate value and the opportunity for quality improvement with improved health outcomes attainable through a truly integrated model of care. The HRSA Health Center Program promotes formalized PCMH recognition, which "includes an emphasis on care coordination, patient self-management, and ongoing quality improvement in all areas including oral health." As of June 2015, 61% of health centers had achieved National Committee for Quality Assurance PCMH recognition,[41] "the most widely-used way to transform primary care practices into medical homes"[42] and 96% of health centers use electronic health records, including the electronic dental records.[41]

The IOHPCP Report's Recommendation 2 (see **Box 4**) accentuates the importance of interoperable and accessible health care systems infrastructure that "use common language, interoperable electronic health records, and interprofessional collaboration in patient-centered medical and health homes to facilitate high quality accessible oral health care."[21] Furthermore, oral health integration in a PCMH environment has the imperative for funders to "support integration/interface of health center electronic dental and medical records systems [with the understanding that] bi-directional sharing of dental and medical records will allow the care teams in both services to better address the needs of their patient population(s) and enable fully coordinated care."[39]

The important take-away message is that dental and other health professional students and recent graduates increasingly have training and practice experience working collaboratively across health disciplines. Through community-based clinical experiences, targeted training programs such as those previously discussed, and increasing exposure to interprofessional faculty, graduates of health professional programs will be more comfortable working in mixed or diverse practice environments, will have the familiarity and knowledge of the roles of other clinicians, and be able to work together to assure overall health of the patients they serve. In addition, the increase in availability of patient-centered interprofessional practice settings that use integrated electronic health records provides the opportunity to facilitate the provision of quality competent care and improved health outcomes through prevention, early detection and treatment, and increased patient education to maintain health.

SUMMARY

For more than 50 years, experts have weighed in on the benefits of integrated collaborative care and the challenges of translating interprofessional training and education into sustainable, disseminated clinical practice models. Numerous workshops, conferences, and published reports have examined the issues and recognized the important role of the federal government in supporting health professional's training and educational programs; as well as health care delivery for vulnerable population groups, especially those who are underserved, geographically isolated, poor or disadvantaged, and those with special needs.

The United States federal government has taken the lead on key issues that affect the nation, such as health promotion and access to care. It serves as an essential partner working collaboratively with states and local governments, academic institutions, professional organizations, health care providers, and nonfederal entities in efforts to improve the quality of health care and overall health across the lifespan. The historical and present day perspective presented in this article shows that the federal government's programs, initiatives, and public-private partnerships play a critical role to influence, incentivize, initiate, and institutionalize interprofessional practice in which oral health providers are an integral part of the patient-centered provider team. The federal government has provided support for innovation, infrastructure expansion, clinical services delivery, and policy development to drive systems change. As a result, great progress has been made in establishing and promoting integrated training experiences for interprofessional health professional students, residents, and practicing clinicians to integrate oral health and primary care while endorsing a patient-centered interprofessional approach dedicated to improving health outcomes.

REFERENCES

1. Preamble to the Constitution of the World Health Organization as adopted by the International Health Conference. New York, June 19-22, 1946. Signed on 22 July 1946 by the representatives of 61 States (Official Records of the World Health Organization, no. 2, p. 100) and entered into force on 7 April 1948.
2. IOM. Educating for the Health team: Report of the Conference on the Interrelationships of Educational Programs for Health Professionals. Washington, DC: National Academy of Sciences; 1972. Available at: http://files.eric.ed.gov/fulltext/ED110819.pdf. Accessed March 19, 2016.
3. U.S. Department of Health and Human Services. Oral health in America: a report of the Surgeon General. Rockville (MD): U.S. Department of Health and Human Services, National Institute of Dental and Craniofacial Research, National Institutes of Health; 2000.
4. U.S. Department of Health and Human Services Oral Health Coordinating Committee. U.S. Department of Health and Human Services Oral Health Strategic Framework, 2014-2017. Public Health Rep 2016;131(2):242–57.
5. CMS' program history, Medicare & Medicaid. Available at: https://www.cms.gov/About-CMS/Agency-Information/History/index.html?redirect=/History/. Accessed March 31, 2016.
6. Coggeshall LT. Planning for medical progress through education: a report submitted to the Executive Council of the Association of American Medical Colleges. Evanston (IL): Association of American Medical Colleges; 1965.
7. The Coggeshall Report. J Med Educ 1965;7:700–2.
8. Schroeder SA. Health of the public: an academic challenge. J Gen Intern Med 1990;5(Suppl 5):S3–10.
9. IOM (Institute of Medicine). The U.S. oral health workforce in the coming decade: workshop summary. Washington, DC: The National Academies Press; 2009.
10. Interprofessional Education Collaborative Expert Panel. Core competencies for interprofessional collaborative practice: Report of an expert panel. Washington, DC: Interprofessional Education Collaborative; 2011. Available at: https://ipecollaborative.org/uploads/IPEC-Core-Competencies.pdf.
11. Grant Makers in Health. Returning the Mouth to the Body: Integrating Oral Health & Primary Care. Washington, DC; 2012. Issue Brief No. 40. Available at: www.gih.org/files/FileDownloads/Returning_the_Mouth_to_the_Body_no40_September_2012.pdf. Accessed March 29, 2016.
12. The Commonwealth Fund. Quality matters archive. In focus: integrating oral health into primary care. 2015. Available at: http://www.commonwealthfund.org/publications/newsletters/quality-matters/2015/february-march/in-focus. Accessed March 29, 2016.
13. IOM (Institute of Medicine). Advancing oral health in America. Washington, DC: The National Academies Press; 2011.
14. IOM (Institute of Medicine), NRC (National Research Council). Improving access to oral health care for vulnerable and underserved populations. Washington, DC: The National Academies Press; 2011.
15. The National Academies of Sciences, Engineering, and Medicine: Health and Medicine Division. Available at: http://www.nationalacademies.org/hmd/. Accessed March 29, 2016.

16. IOM (Institute of Medicine). Crossing the quality chasm: a new health system for the 21st century. Washington, DC: The National Academies Press; 2001. Available at: http://nap.edu/10027. Accessed April 8, 2016.

17. Greiner AC, Knebel E, editors. Health professions education: a bridge to quality. Washington, DC: Institute of Medicine of the National Academies of Science, National Academies; 2003. Available at: http://www.nap.edu/catalog/10681.html. Accessed April 8, 2016.

18. Healthy People 2020 Topics and Objectives: Oral Health. Available at: http://www.healthypeople.gov/2020/topics-objectives/topic/oral-health/objectives Accessed March 29, 2016.

19. US Department of Health and Human Services. HHS Oral Health Initiative. 2010. Available at: http://www.hrsa.gov/publichealth/clinical/oralhealth/hhsinitiative.pdf Accessed March 19, 2016.

20. U.S. Department of Health and Human Services. A National call to action to promote oral health. Rockville (MD): U.S. Department of Health and Human Services, Public Health Service, Centers for Disease Control and Prevention, National Institutes of Health, National Institute of Dental and Craniofacial Research; 2003. NIH Publication No. 03–5303.

21. U.S. Department of Health and Human Services. Integration of oral health and primary care practice. Rockville (MD): U.S. Department of Health and Human Services, Health Resources and Services Administration; 2014. Available at: http://www.hrsa.gov/publichealth/clinical/oralhealth/primarycare/integrationoforalhealth.pdf. Accessed March 29, 2016.

22. National Network for Oral Health Access. A User's Guide for Implementation of Interprofessional Oral Health Core Clinical Competencies: Results of a Pilot Project. 2015. Available at: http://www.nnoha.org/nnoha-content/uploads/2015/01/IPOHCCC-Users-Guide-Final_01-23-2015.pdf. Accessed March 29, 2016.

23. HRSA Bureau of Health Workforce. Predoctoral Training in General Dentistry, Pediatric Dentistry and Dental Public Health and Dental Hygiene. Available at: http://apply07.grants.gov/apply/opportunities/instructions/oppHRSA-15-050-cfda93.059-cidHRSA-15-050-instructions.pdf. Accessed March 29, 2016.

24. HRSA Bureau of Health Workforce. Medicine Grant Programs. Academic Units for Primary Care Training and Enhancement. Available at: http://bhw.hrsa.gov/grants/medicine/aupcte.html. Accessed March 29, 2016.

25. Hummel J, Phillips KE, Holt B, et al. Oral health: an essential component of primary care. Seattle (WA): Qualis Health; 2015. Available at: http://www.safetynetmedicalhome.org/sites/default/files/White-Paper-Oral-Health-Primary-Care.pdf. Accessed March 19, 2016.

26. Transforming Interprofessional Health Education and Practice: Moving Learners from the Campus to the Community to Improve Population Health. Thirteenth Annual Report to the Secretary of the United States Department of Health and Human Services and the Congress of the United States. Advisory Committee on Interdisciplinary, Community-Based Linkages (ACICBL), October 2014.Available at: http://www.hrsa.gov/advisorycommittees/bhpradvisory/acicbl/reports/thirteenthreport.pdf. Accessed December 28, 2015.

27. U.S. Department of Health and Human Services, Health Resources and Services Administration. Oral health in primary care. Rockville (MD): U.S. Department of Health and Human Services; 2012.

28. AAMC MedEdPORTAL. Building an Oral Health in Medicine Model Curriculum. Available at: https://www.mededportal.org/about/initiatives/oralhealth/oralhealth/. Accessed January 20, 2016.

29. Oral Health Care During Pregnancy Expert Workgroup. Oral health care during pregnancy: a national consensus statement–summary of an expert workgroup meeting. Washington, DC: National Maternal and Child Oral Health Resource Center; 2012. Available at: http://mchoralhealth.org/PDFs/Oralhealthpregnancy consensusmeetingsummary.pdf. Accessed March 30, 2016.

30. Oral Health Care During Pregnancy Expert Workgroup. Oral health care during pregnancy: a National Consensus Statement. Washington, DC: National Maternal and Child Oral Health Resource Center; 2012. Available at: http://mchoralhealth. org/PDFs/OralHealthPregnancyConsensus.pdf. Accessed March 30, 2016.

31. National Center for Interprofessional Practice and Education. Available at: https:// nexusipe.org/. Accessed January 12, 2016.

32. U.S. Department of Health and Human Services, Health Resources and Services Administration, Office of Women's Health. Women's health curricula: final report on expert panel recommendations for interprofessional collaborations across the Health Professions. Rockville (MD): U.S. Department of Health and Human Services; 2013.

33. Geriatric Education Centers. Available at: http://bhw.hrsa.gov/grants/ geriatricsalliedhealth/gec.html. Accessed March 17, 2016.

34. Geriatrics Workforce Enhancement Program. Available at: http://bhw.hrsa.gov/ grants/geriatricsalliedhealth/gwep.html. Accessed March 17, 2016.

35. HRSA Bureau of Health Workforce. Grants to States to Support Oral Health Workforce Activities. Available at: http://apply07.grants.gov/apply/opportunities/ instructions/oppHRSA-15-052-cfda93.236-cidHRSA-15-052-instructions.pdf. Accessed June 25, 2016.

36. Area Health Education Centers. Available at: http://bhw.hrsa.gov/grants/ areahealtheducationcenters/. Accessed April 8, 2016.

37. Active Grants for HRSA Program(s): Advanced Nursing Education Grants. Available at: https://ersrs.hrsa.gov/ReportServer?/HGDW_Reports/FindGrants/ GRANT_FIND&ACTIVITY=D09&rs:Format=HTML4.0%20https://ersrs.hrsa.gov/ ReportServer/Pages/ReportViewer.aspx?/HGDW_Reports/FindGrants/GRANT_ FIND&ACTIVITY=D09&rs:Format=HTML4.0. Accessed February 1, 2016. Grant # D09HP25931.

38. Active Grants for HRSA Program(s): Advanced Nursing Education Grants. Available at: https://ersrs.hrsa.gov/ReportServer?/HGDW_Reports/FindGrants/ GRANT_FIND&ACTIVITY=D09&rs:Format=HTML4.0%20https://ersrs.hrsa.gov/ ReportServer/Pages/ReportViewer.aspx?/HGDW_Reports/FindGrants/GRANT_ FIND&ACTIVITY=D09&rs:Format=HTML4.0. Accessed February 1, 2016. Grant # D09HP25019.

39. Brownlee B. Oral Health Integration in the Patient-Centered Medical Home (PCMH) environment: case studies from Community Health Centers. Seattle (WA): Qualis Health; 2012.

40. HRSA Health Center Program Requirements. Available at: http://bphc.hrsa.gov/ programrequirements/index.html#services1. Accessed March 15, 2016.

41. Health Center Program Fact Sheet – America's Primary Care Safety Net Working to Address Oral Health. Available at: http://bphc.hrsa.gov/qualityimprovement/ clinicalquality/oralhealth/factsheet2014.pdf. Accessed March 15, 2016.

42. Patient-Centered Medical Home Recognition. Available at: http://www.ncqa.org/ programs/recognition/practices/patient-centered-medical-home-pcmh. Accessed April 8, 2016.

Index

Note: Page numbers of articles titles are in **boldface** type.

Dent Clin N Am 60 (2016) 969–974
http://dx.doi.org/10.1016/S0011-8532(16)30091-X
0011-8532/16/$ – see front matter

dental.theclinics.com

UNITED STATES POSTAL SERVICE®

Statement of Ownership, Management, and Circulation (All Periodicals Publications Except Requester Publications)

1. Publication Title	DENTAL CLINICS OF NORTH AMERICA
2. Publication Number	566 - 480
3. Filing Date	9/18/2016
4. Issue Frequency	JAN, APR, JUL, OCT
5. Number of Issues Published Annually	4
6. Annual Subscription Price	$269.00

7. Complete Mailing Address of Known Office of Publication (Not printer) (Street, city, county, state, and ZIP+4®)

ELSEVIER INC.
360 PARK AVENUE SOUTH
NEW YORK, NY 10010-1710

Contact Person
STEPHEN R. BUSHING

Telephone (Include area code)
215-239-3688

8. Complete Mailing Address of Headquarters or General Business Office of Publisher (Not printer)

ELSEVIER INC.
360 PARK AVENUE SOUTH
NEW YORK, NY 10010-1710

9. Full Names and Complete Mailing Addresses of Publisher, Editor, and Managing Editor (Do not leave blank)

Publisher (Name and complete mailing address)

ADRIANNE BRIGIDO, ELSEVIER INC.
1600 JOHN F KENNEDY BLVD. SUITE 1800
PHILADELPHIA, PA 19103-2899

Editor (Name and complete mailing address)

JOHN VASSALLO ELSEVIER INC.
1600 JOHN F KENNEDY BLVD. SUITE 1800
PHILADELPHIA, PA 19103-2899

Managing Editor (Name and complete mailing address)

PATRICK MANLEY, ELSEVIER INC.
1600 JOHN F KENNEDY BLVD. SUITE 1800
PHILADELPHIA, PA 19103-2899

10. Owner (Do not leave blank. If the publication is owned by a corporation, give the name and address of the corporation immediately followed by the names and addresses of all stockholders owning or holding 1 percent or more of the total amount of stock. If not owned by a corporation, give the names and addresses of the individual owners. If owned by a partnership or other unincorporated firm, give its name and address as well as those of each individual owner. If the publication is published by a nonprofit organization, give its name and address.)

Full Name	Complete Mailing Address
WHOLLY OWNED SUBSIDIARY OF REED/ELSEVIER, ES HOLDINGS	1600 JOHN F KENNEDY BLVD. SUITE 1800 PHILADELPHIA, PA 19103-2899

11. Known Bondholders, Mortgagees, and Other Security Holders Owning or Holding 1 Percent or More of Total Amount of Bonds, Mortgages, or Other Securities. If none, check box. ▶ ☐ None

Full Name	Complete Mailing Address
N/A	

12. Tax Status (For completion by nonprofit organizations authorized to mail at nonprofit rates) (Check one)
The purpose, function, and nonprofit status of this organization and the exempt status for federal income tax purposes:
☐ Has Not Changed During Preceding 12 Months
☐ Has Changed During Preceding 12 Months (Publisher must submit explanation of change with this statement)

13. Publication Title	14. Issue Date for Circulation Data Below
DENTAL CLINICS OF NORTH AMERICA	JULY 2016

15. Extent and Nature of Circulation		Average No. Copies Each Issue During Preceding 12 Months	No. Copies of Single Issue Published Nearest to Filing Date
a. Total Number of Copies (Net press run)		603	750
b. Paid Circulation (By Mail and Outside the Mail)	(1) Mailed Outside-County Paid Subscriptions Stated on PS Form 3541 (Include paid distribution above nominal rate, advertiser's proof copies, and exchange copies)	187	236
	(2) Mailed In-County Paid Subscriptions Stated on PS Form 3541 (Include paid distribution above nominal rate, advertiser's proof copies, and exchange copies)	0	0
	(3) Paid Distribution Outside the Mails Including Sales Through Dealers and Carriers, Street Vendors, Counter Sales, and Other Paid Distribution Outside USPS®	145	201
	(4) Paid Distribution by Other Classes of Mail Through the USPS (e.g., First-Class Mail®)	0	0
c. Total Paid Distribution (Sum of 15b (1), (2), (3), and (4))		332	437
d. Free or Nominal Rate Distribution (By Mail and Outside the Mail)	(1) Free or Nominal Rate Outside-County Copies included on PS Form 3541	43	43
	(2) Free or Nominal Rate In-County Copies Included on PS Form 3541	0	0
	(3) Free or Nominal Rate Copies Mailed at Other Classes Through the USPS (e.g., First-Class Mail)	0	0
	(4) Free or Nominal Rate Distribution Outside the Mail (Carriers or other means)	0	0
e. Total Free or Nominal Rate Distribution (Sum of 15d (1), (2), (3) and (4))		43	43
f. Total Distribution (Sum of 15c and 15e)		375	480
g. Copies not Distributed (See Instructions to Publishers #4 (page #3))		228	270
h. Total (Sum of 15f and g)		603	750
i. Percent Paid (15c divided by 15f times 100)		89%	91%

* If you are claiming electronic copies, go to line 16 on page 3. If you are not claiming electronic copies, skip to line 17 on page 3.

16. Electronic Copy Circulation	Average No. Copies Each Issue During Preceding 12 Months	No. Copies of Single Issue Published Nearest to Filing Date
a. Paid Electronic Copies	0	0
b. Total Paid Print Copies (Line 15c) + Paid Electronic Copies (Line 16a)	332	437
c. Total Print Distribution (Line 15f) + Paid Electronic Copies (Line 16a)	375	480
d. Percent Paid (Both Print & Electronic Copies) (16b divided by 16c × 100)	89%	91%

☒ I certify that 50% of all my distributed copies (electronic and print) are paid above a nominal price.

17. Publication of Statement of Ownership

☒ If the publication is a general publication, publication of this statement is required. Will be printed ☐ Publication not required.

in the OCTOBER 2016 issue of this publication

18. Signature and Title of Editor, Publisher, Business Manager or Owner

STEPHEN R. BUSHING - INVENTORY DISTRIBUTION CONTROL MANAGER

Date 9/18/2016

I certify that all information furnished on this form is true and complete. I understand that anyone who furnishes false or misleading information on this form or who omits material or information requested on the form may be subject to criminal sanctions (including fines and imprisonment) and/or civil sanctions (including civil penalties).

Moving?

Make sure your subscription moves with you!

To notify us of your new address, find your **Clinics Account Number** (located on your mailing label above your name), and contact customer service at:

Email: journalscustomerservice-usa@elsevier.com

800-654-2452 (subscribers in the U.S. & Canada)
314-447-8871 (subscribers outside of the U.S. & Canada)

Fax number: 314-447-8029

Elsevier Health Sciences Division
Subscription Customer Service
3251 Riverport Lane
Maryland Heights, MO 63043

*To ensure uninterrupted delivery of your subscription, please notify us at least 4 weeks in advance of move.

Printed and bound by CPI Group (UK) Ltd, Croydon, CR0 4YY

07/10/2024

01040501-0002